Ovulation Induction:
Basic Science and Clinical Advances

OVULATION INDUCTION: BASIC SCIENCE AND CLINICAL ADVANCES

Proceedings of the Symposium on Ovulation Induction: Basic Science and Clinical Advances, 20–22 January 1994, Palm Beach, Florida, USA

Editors:

Marco Filicori

and

Carlo Flamigni

Reproductive Medicine Unit, University of Bologna, Bologna, Italy

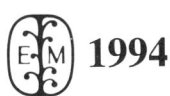 **1994**

Excerpta Medica, Amsterdam – London – New York – Tokyo

©1994 Elsevier Science B.V. All rights reserved.

No part of this publication may be reproduced, stored in a retrieval system or transmitted in any form or by any means, electronic, mechanical, photocopying, recording or otherwise without the prior written permission of the publisher, Elsevier Science B.V., Permissions Department, P.O. Box 521, 1000 AM Amsterdam, The Netherlands.
No responsibility is assumed by the Publisher for any injury and/or damage to persons or property as a matter of products liability, negligence or otherwise, or from use or operation of any methods, products, instructions or ideas contained in the material herein. Because of rapid advances in the medical sciences, the Publisher recommends that independent verification of diagnoses and drug dosages should be made.
Special regulations for readers in the USA — This publication has been registered with the Copyright Clearance Center Inc. (CCC), 27 Congress Street, Salem, MA 01970, USA. Information can be obtained from the CCC about conditions under which photocopies of parts of this publication may be made in the USA. All other copyright questions, including photocopying outside the USA should be referred to the copyright owner, Elsevier Science B.V., unless otherwise specified.

International Congress Series No. 1046
ISBN 0 444 81696 8

This book is printed on acid-free paper.

Published by:
Elsevier Science B.V.
P.O. Box 211
1000 AE Amsterdam
The Netherlands

Library of Congress Cataloging in Publication Data:

```
Symposium on Ovulation Induction: Basic Science and Clinical Advances
  (1994 : Palm Beach, Fla.)
    Ovulation induction : basic science and clinical advances :
  proceedings of the Symposium on Ovulation Induction: Basic Science
  and Clinical Advances, 20-22 January 1994, Palm Beach, Florida, USA
  / editors, Marco Filicori and Carlo Flamigni.
        p.   cm. -- (International congress series ; no. 1046)
    Includes indexes.
    ISBN 0-444-81696-8
    1. Ovulation--Induction--Congresses.  2. Ovulation--Regulation-
  -Congresses.   I. Filicori, M.  II. Flamigni, C.  III. Title.
  IV. Series.
    [DNLM: 1. Ovulation Induction--congresses.  2. Gonadotropins-
  -congresses.    W3 EX89 no. 1046 1994 / WP 540 S989 1994]
  RG133.7.S96   1994
  618.1'78--dc20
  DNLM/DLC
  for Library of Congress                                    94-18241
                                                                 CIP
```

In order to ensure rapid publication this volume was prepared using a method of electronic text processing known as Optical Character Recognition (OCR). Scientific accuracy and consistency of style were handled by the author. Time did not allow for the usual extensive editing process of the Publisher.

Printed in the Netherlands

Preface

This volume contains the proceedings of the Conference "Ovulation Induction: Basic Science and Clinical Advances" which was held in Palm Beach, Florida, January 20–22, 1994. This scientific area has undergone profound changes in recent years thanks to a greater understanding of the physiology and pathophysiology of ovulation and the availability of new and more selective therapeutic tools such as purified FSH, GnRH agonists and pulsatile GnRH. The imminent introduction in clinical practice of recombinant gonadotropins and GnRH antagonists will further advance our knowledge and therapeutic options. This conference certainly came at a timely moment, and several issues that were debated and that are included in these proceedings will have a profound impact on the clinical conduct of ovulation induction for many years to come.

"Ovulation Induction: Basic Science and Clinical Advances" was attended by over 400 scientists from 30 countries. Invited speakers gave an invaluable contribution to the success of the meeting with their high-level scientific presentations; timely manuscript submission permitted the publication of this volume within a few months after the conference ended. We wish to thank the other members of the Scientific Committee: Drs Adashi, Crowley, Jacobs, Meldrum and Schoemaker, for providing their advice in the preparation of the Scientific Program; and Mr Filler and Ms Zeissler of Communications Media for Education, Inc. for efficiently running the Organizing Secretariat.

Finally, this onerous endeavor would not have been possible without the unconditional support provided by Ferring Arzneimittel GmbH; our special thanks go to Mr Chris Thomas, Managing Director, and to Dr Farid Saad, Marketing Manager of Ferring in Kiel.

Bologna, 1 March 1994

Marco Filicori
Carlo Flamigni

Contents

Preface   v

Hypothalamic-pituitary control of ovulation

Some modulations of GnRH pulse generator activity in the rhesus monkey
   E. Knobil   3
Pituitary translation of the pulsatile GnRH message
   J.C. Marshall, A.C. Dalkin, D.J. Haisenleder, J.R. Kerrigan, S.E. Kirk and M. Yasin   11
Ovulation and LH-regulated genes
   J.S. Richards   21
Follicular development: the role of LH
   D.A. Magoffin, T.J. Gelety and P.C. Magarelli   25
Gonadotropic control of folliculogenesis: the threshold theory
   A.J. Zeleznik   37

Nongonadotropic regulation of ovarian function

Nongonadotropic regulation of ovarian function: roles of follicular sex steroids
   S.G. Hillier   47
The effect of exogenous recombinant human activin A on pituitary and ovarian hormone secretion and ovarian folliculogenesis in female rats and monkeys
   T.K. Woodruff, T.A. Molskness, K.D. Dahl, J.P. Mather and R.L. Stouffer   57
Nongonadotropic regulation of ovarian function: insulin
   J.F. Cara   65
Nongonadotropic regulation of ovarian function: growth hormone and IGFs
   G.F. Erickson   73
Nongonadotropic regulation of ovarian function: interleukin-1
   E.Y. Adashi   85

Pathophysiology of anovulation

LH-dependent polycystic ovary syndrome
   S.L. Berga   91

Role of obesity and insulin in the development of anovulation
  J.E. Nestler 103
Hypergonadotropic amenorrhea
  R.W. Rebar and M.I. Cedars 115

Ovulation induction with gonadotropins

Purified FSH: characteristics and applications
  C. Flamigni, S. Venturoli, L. Dal Prato and E. Porcu 125
Induction of ovulation with gonadotrophins: hMG versus purified FSH
  D.T. Baird and C.M. Howles 135
Low-dose gonadotropin regimens for induction of ovulation
  S. Franks, D.W. Polson, M. Sagle, D. Hamilton-Fairley and
  D.M. White 145
Step-down follicle-stimulating hormone regimens in polycystic ovary syndrome
  B.C.J.M. Fauser 153
Use of FSH threshold administration in polycystic ovarian disease
  J. Schoemaker, M.M. van Weissenbruch and M. van der Meer ... 163
Endometrial receptivity in controlled ovarian hyperstimulation (COH): the hormonal factor
  D. de Ziegler and R. Fanchin 167

Recombinant gonadotropins: basic aspects

Structure-function studies of gonadotropins using site-directed mutagenesis and gene transfer: design of a long-acting gonadotropin agonist
  I. Boime, F. Fares, M. Furuhashi, P.D. LaPolt, K. Nishimori,
  T. Shikone, T. Sugahara and A.J.W. Hsueh 177
Control of gonadotropin-binding specificity
  R.K. Campbell 185
New recombinant hCG analogs with potent FSH activity in vivo
  Y. Wang, Y. Han, R.V. Myers, G.J. Macdonald and W.R. Moyle ... 191

Recombinant gonadotropins: clinical aspects

Pharmacokinetics of natural/recombinant FSH (follitropin) and some analogs
  M.R. Sairam and K. Sebok 199
Biological action of recombinant human FSH (Puregon®) during induction of multiple follicular growth
  B. Mannaerts, R. de Leeuw and P. Devroey 209

Potential clinical applications of recombinant FSH
  H.J.T. Coelingh Bennink, P. Bouchard, P. Devroey, B.C.J.M. Fauser,
  J. Harlin and Z. Shoham 219
Ovulation induction with recombinant human follicle-stimulating hormone
and luteinizing hormone
  E. Loumaye, H.C. Porchet, V. Beltrami, D. Giroud, J.-Y. Le Cotonnec,
  L. O'Dea, A. Piazzi, C.M. Howles and A. Galazka 227

Ovulation induction with pulsatile GnRH

Use of GnRH and its analogs in the treatment of ovulatory disorders:
an overview
  M. Filicori 239
Appropriate regimens of pulsatile gonadotropin-releasing hormone (GnRH)
administration
  G.B. Wilshire and N. Santoro 245
Pulsatile GnRH in hypogonadotropic hypogonadism
  K.A. Martin, J. Hall, J. Adams and W.F. Crowley Jr 255
Pulsatile GnRH in multifollicular and polycystic ovary patients
  H.S. Jacobs 267

Add-on regimens

Long-term GnRH agonist suppression and gonadotropins
  D.R. Meldrum 277
Flare-up protocols in assisted reproductive technologies (ART):
a re-evaluation
  R. Frydman and R. Fanchin 283
The role of GnRH during the periovulatory period: a basis for the use of
GnRH antagonists in ovulation induction
  P. Bouchard, B. Charbonnel, A. Caraty, H.M. Fraser, S. Dubourdieu,
  I. Leroy, F. Olivennes and R. Frydman 291
Potential for embryo damage by GnRH analogs
  T.M. Siler-Khodr, I.S. Kang, T.J. Kuehl and G.S. Khodr 297
Gonadotropins and growth hormone regimens for ovarian stimulation
  R. Homburg and H. Østergaard 307

Ovarian hyperstimulation

Pathophysiology and clinical management of ovarian hyperstimulation
  D. Navot, P.A. Bergh and R. Palermo 319
Prevention of ovarian hyperstimulation
  J. Blankstein 331

Pregnancy reduction in iatrogenic multifetal pregnancies
    M. Dommergues, Y. Dumez and M.I. Evans 339

Pregnancy complications

Infertility and spontaneous abortion — the role of luteinizing hormone
    A. Zosmer and S.-L. Tan 347
Predictors of miscarriage in menotropin ovulation induction for anovulatory polycystic ovarian syndrome
    M. Wingfield, S. Clarke, X. Li, P.I. McCloud, H.G. Burger, G. Kovacs, N. McClure and D.L. Healy 353
Management and obstetrical outcome of multiple pregnancies
    J. Salat-Baroux and J.M. Antoine 361

General discussion

Ovulation induction regimens: is a consensus possible?
    M. Filicori and C. Flamigni 371

Index of authors 389

Keyword index 391

Hypothalamic-pituitary control of ovulation

Some modulations of GnRH pulse generator activity in the rhesus monkey

E. Knobil

Laboratory for Neuroendocrinology, The University of Texas Medical School, P.O. Box 20708, Houston, TX 77225, USA

Since the discovery of the gonadotropin-releasing hormone (GnRH) pulse generator nearly a quarter of a century ago [1] a vast body of literature has been amassed describing a host of inputs that impact on this fundamental neuronal system and on its neuroendocrine sequelae. The purpose of this brief discussion is to describe some unexpected interactions between the GnRH pulse generator and the internal and external environments.

Many strategies have been used to monitor GnRH pulse generator activity, including the detection of luteinizing hormone (LH) pulses in peripheral blood [2], the measurement of pulsatile GnRH in pituitary portal blood [3-5], in cerebrospinal fluid [6] and in hypothalamic extracellular fluid sampled by microperfusion [7,8]. Efforts in our own laboratory have centered on monitoring the electrophysiological manifestations of GnRH pulse generator activity in the rhesus monkey. Using the classic neuroendocrine techniques of radiofrequency lesions [9] and surgical disconnection [10], the GnRH pulse generator has been localized to the arcuate nucleus area of mediobasal hypothalamus in this species. Knowing its location and the unambiguous marker of its activity, LH pulses in the peripheral circulation, bilateral arrays of recording electrodes were chronically implanted in the mediobasal hypothalamus in an attempt to detect the neural correlates of pulsatile LH secretion. An invariable association between abrupt increases in frequency of hypothalamic multiunit electrical activity (MUA volleys) and the initiation of LH pulses was observed under a variety of experimental circumstances [11-17], with the conclusion that these volleys of increased electrical activity represent GnRH pulse generator activity as reliably as the various LH pulse detection methods. More recently, we have been able to adduce evidence in support of the view that the rhythmic increases in MUA activity indeed represent synchronous increases in unit activity [18].

The electrophysiological approach to the study of the GnRH pulse generator proffered the possibility of monitoring its activity in freely behaving animals, using radiotelemetry [16]. This gave us the opportunity to re-examine the precise pattern of GnRH pulse generator activity throughout the normal menstrual cycle, particularly around the time of the preovulatory LH surge. As previously shown in women [19] pulse generator frequency increased during the first few days of the follicular phase, reaching a plateau of approximately 1 volley/h that was maintained until the advent of the phenomenon described below. Unexpectedly, a marked slowing of pulse generator frequency was observed just before the initiation of the LH surge, coincidentally with the preovulatory rise in serum estradiol, with a virtual arrest of activity throughout the mid-cycle LH peak. Resumption of activity then followed at the lower frequency characteristic of the luteal phase in many species [20], before reaccelerating towards the follicular phase frequency as luteolysis progressed [16]. It would appear that the marked deceleration in pulse generator frequency at mid-cycle is a consequence of the preovulatory rise in serum estradiol because the induction of LH surges by estradiol administration in the early follicular phase of the cycle is associated with identical changes in pulse generator frequency [16]. These preovulatory events in the monkey recall reports in the rat showing that pulsatile LH secretion ceases at the beginning of the LH surge [21], and the more recent findings in sheep that estradiol-induced LH surges are preceded by a marked slowing in GnRH pulses measured in pituitary portal blood [5,22], followed by a virtual absence of pulsatile GnRH secretion during the LH surge [23]. Similar observations have been made in the goat [24] and in the rat [25] using electrophysiological monitoring of the pulse generator. These findings, however, contrast with those in women of continued high frequency LH pulsatility during the LH surge [19,26,27]. But the physiological significance of these frequency changes throughout the normal menstrual cycle remains unclear, because the pulsatile administration of exogenous GnRH at an unvarying frequency and amplitude to monkeys bereft of endogenous GnRH secretion can re-establish normal ovulatory menstrual cycles [28].

The unexpected and dramatic inhibitory effects of estradiol on GnRH pulse generator activity in the physiological setting of the monkey menstrual cycle were adumbrated by earlier studies in ovariectomized animals, wherein it was found that re-establishment of follicular phase estradiol levels by either infusion of the steroid, or implantation of estradiol containing Silastic capsules, first reduced pulse generator frequency and then abolished pulsatile LH secretion altogether [14]. We attributed these findings to a pharmacologic curiosity occasioned by the absence of the ovary, because, in the intact monkey, follicular phase levels of estradiol are obviously not incompatible with follicular development and ovulation in response to circhoral pulsatile gonadotropin stimulation, and concluded that the presence of the ovary normally protects the GnRH pulse generator from the inhibitory effect of physiological levels of estradiol. We still believe that this interpretation is correct, but that it has to be modified by the recognition that at the high physiologic concentrations characteristic of the time just preceding the initiation of the LH surge, estradiol is, in fact, inhibitory, first reducing the frequency of the GnRH pulse generator and then arresting it altogether, albeit but for a brief time. The nature of the putative "ovarian protection factor", however, remains unknown.

Another aspect of the electrophysiological investigations of the GnRH pulse generator has been the unveiling of a dramatic difference between the hypothalamic signal recorded from intact and ovariectomized monkeys (Fig. 1) that is also attributable to an action of estrogens [29]. The increase in hypothalamic MUA lasts only 1–3 min in the intact monkey, while in the ovariectomized female the duration

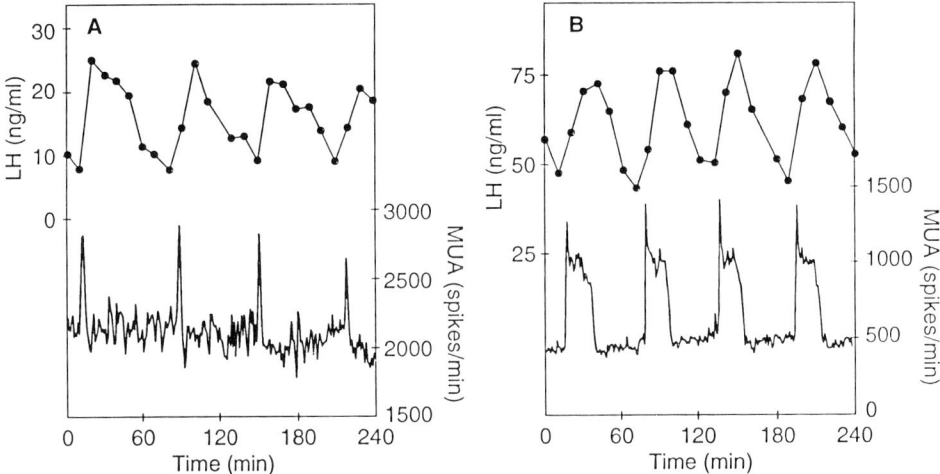

Fig. 1. Multiunit electrical activity (MUA) recorded from the mediobasal hypothalamus in an ovary-intact animal on day 5 of the follicular phase of the menstrual cycle (A), and in a long-term (8 month) ovariectomized monkey (B) [29].

of the MUA volley is increased to 20 min or longer. In the castrate, the MUA volley consists of a brief initial "overshoot", which is equivalent in duration to the entire volley of the intact animal, followed by a plateau phase that ends in a rapid decline to baseline. Estradiol given to ovariectomized monkeys causes, within 3–5 h, a reduction in the duration of the MUA volleys to that characteristic of intact animals [14,29]. In contrast to this acute effect of estradiol, the prolongation of the MUA volley duration following ovariectomy is a surprisingly protracted phenomenon, with 4–6 weeks required to achieve the extended period of firing seen in long-term ovariectomized monkeys [29]. The mechanisms underlying the striking discrepancy in the time required to shorten MUA volley duration by estradiol administration on the one hand and for its prolongation following ovariectomy on the other remain obscure, despite an abundance of possible explanations. The physiological significance of the differences in MUA volley duration between normal and ovariectomized monkeys is also unclear, because the magnitude of the resulting LH pulse is the same, whether the GnRH pulse generator MUA volleys last 2 or 20 min, suggesting that the brief initial "overshoot" phase of the MUA volley triggers the release of the entire bolus of GnRH responsible for each LH pulse and that the subsequent electrical activity has no additional effect on LH secretion [30]. It has been suggested, however, that the marked prolongation in hypothalamic electrical activity following ovariectomy may be related to the hot flushes of postmenopausal women, but, unfortunately, such a phenomenon has not yet been described in monkeys. It should be mentioned parenthetically that the inhibitory effect of estradiol on pulse generator frequency, but not that on duration, can be prevented by naloxone administration [31].

The electrophysiological approach to GnRH pulse generator activity uncovered yet another unanticipated role of the ovary in the hypothalamic control of gonadotropin secretion. When the pulsatile nature of LH secretion was first discovered, it was noted that LH pulses could only be clearly discerned in ovariectomized rhesus monkeys restrained in primate chairs. In identically treated intact animals, the time courses of LH appeared to be nonpulsatile [32]. This was ascribed at the time to the insensitivity of the radioimmunoassay employed, with the conclusion that the high amplitude LH pulses in the open feedback loop situation could easily be measured, but that the supposedly smaller pulses secreted when the negative feedback loop was closed, could not. Some years later, when the electrophysiological monitoring technique became available, we noted that not only did intact, chaired animals not have LH pulses, MUA volleys were also absent. The problem was not the insensitivity of the radioimmunoassay; LH pulses were not discernable because they were not there. Yet, these animals had normal, ovulatory menstrual cycles indicating a normally functioning pulse generator, except on the day of the experiment. We belatedly concluded that the stress of removing the monkeys from their home cage, transporting them to the laboratory and restraining them in the primate chairs "turned off" their pulse generators. The very same procedures, however, had no effect on ovariectomized animals suggesting that the presence of the ovary somehow sensitized the GnRH

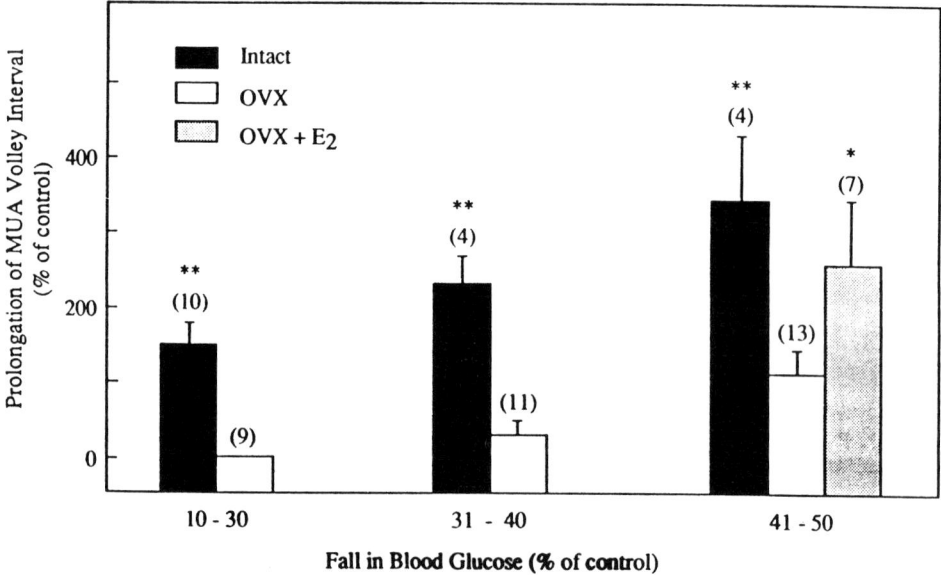

Fig. 2. GnRH pulse generator activity in intact, ovariectomized (OVX) and Estradiol (E_2)-treated OVX monkeys in response to reductions in blood glucose concentrations of increasing magnitude. Inhibition of pulse generator activity, expressed on the ordinate as a prolongation of the interval between MUA volleys, is presented as percent of pretreatment control (mean ± SEM). Hypoglycemia (10–40% reduction in blood sugar) did not significantly prolong the interval between MUA volleys in OVX animals, whereas the same reduction in blood sugar markedly inhibited pulse generator activity in intact animals (**$p < 0.01$). E_2 administration to OVX monkeys significantly (*$p < 0.05$) increased the inhibitory response compared to that seen in intact monkeys. Numbers in parentheses indicate the number of experiments performed in 4–7 monkeys [17].

pulse generator to the inhibitory effects of "stress". This notion was confirmed in the course of a formal study, wherein the responses to the stress of insulin hypoglycemia in ovariectomized and intact rhesus monkeys were compared [17]. It was found that, indeed, normal female monkeys were considerably more sensitive to the inhibitory effects of insulin hypoglycemia than ovariectomized animals. Furthermore, estradiol administration restored the sensitivity of the ovariectomized monkeys to this rather severe stress (Fig. 2). Again, the mechanisms of action of the steroid in this regard remain unknown and represent a challenging subject for future investigation.

The continuous monitoring of hypothalamic MUA volleys revealed a significant nocturnal slowing of pulse generator frequency during the follicular phase of the cycle, as reported previously in women [19,27,33]. Because it was noticed that the nocturnal slowing of pulse generator frequency occurred immediately after the lights were turned off at 7 pm, and that the frequency increased immediately when the lights were turned on again at 7 am, the normal lighting schedule, the effect of light per se on pulse generator frequency was investigated. When "lights off" was delayed until 10 pm or "lights on" advanced to 1 am or 4 am, identical, albeit somewhat attenuated, changes in pulse generator frequency were observed, suggesting the possibility that the diurnal fluctuation in GnRH pulse generator frequency under normal lighting conditions may be attributable to a direct effect of light on pulse generator activity. That this was not simply an effect of arousal was demonstrated by awakening the animals with loud noises in total darkness at 1 am and 4 am, without an effect on pulse generator frequency (Fig. 3). Nevertheless, when monkeys were

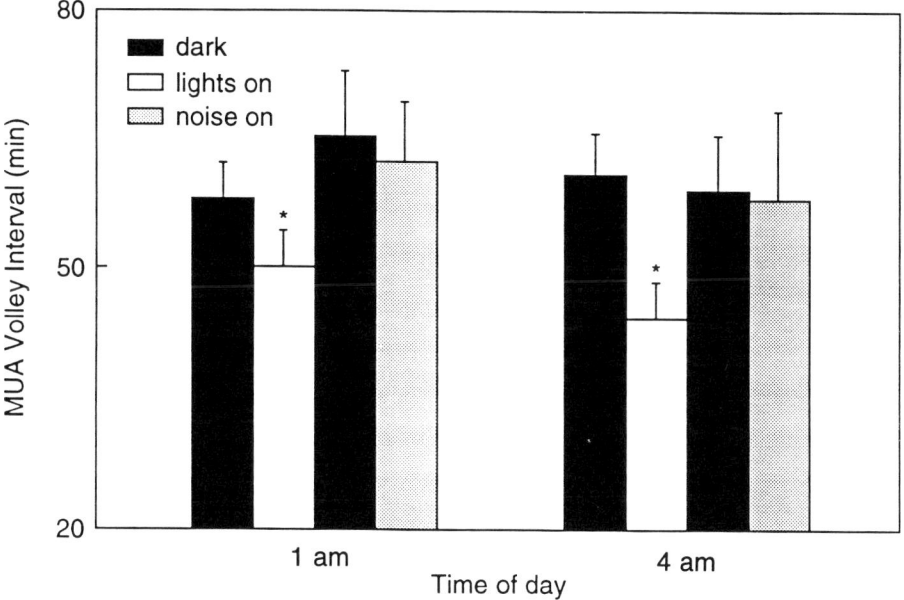

Fig. 3. Effect of light or noise on hypothalamic MUA volley frequency. Each bar represents the mean and SE of the first three MUA volley intervals before and after lights on or noise on, in four or five monkeys. Arousal by noise in total darkness at 1 am and 4 am did not affect pulse generator frequency, whereas turning the lights on at these times increased pulse generator frequency ($\star$, $p < 0.05$) [34].

exposed to both constant light and constant darkness for periods of 2—3 days, the diurnal rhythm in pulse generator frequency was found to persist. Thus, it would appear that an acute effect of light is superimposed on the diurnal rhythm of pulse generator frequency, perhaps mediated by the retino-hypothalamic tract [34].

The foregoing studies underline the utility of the electrophysiological approach to the GnRH pulse generator by providing an unambiguous, on-line, marker of its activity in freely behaving animals and proffers the possibility of physiological studies in relation to exercise, stress, caloric restriction, puberty and lactation.

Acknowledgements

This work was supported by grants HD 8610 and HD 17438 from the National Institutes of Health, and by a grant from the Clayton and Ellwood Foundations.

References

1. Knobil E. Endocrinology 1992;131:1005—1006.
2. Crowley Jr WF, Filicori M, Spratt DI, Santoro NF. Recent Prog Horm Res 1985;41:473—531.
3. Carmel PW, Araki S, Ferin M. Endocrinology 1976;99:243—248.
4. Clarke IJ, Cummins JT. Endocrinology 1982;111:1737—1739.
5. Caraty A, Locatelli A, Martin GB. J Endocrinol 1989;123:375—382.
6. Van Vugt DA, Diefenbach WD, Alston E, Ferin M. Endocrinology 1985;117:1550—1558.
7. Levine JE, Norman RL, Gliessman PM, Oyama TT, Bangsberg DR, Spies HG. Endocrinology 1985; 117:711—721.
8. Gearing M, Terasawa E. Brain Res Bull 1988;21:117—121.
9. Plant TM, Krey LC, Moossy J, McCormack JT, Hess DL, Knobil E. Endocrinology 1978;102:52—62.
10. Krey KC, Butler WR, Knobil E. Endocrinology 1975;1073—1087.
11. Wilson RC, Kesner JS, Kaufman J-M, Uemura T, Akema T, Knobil E. Neuroendocrinology 1984; 39:256—260.
12. Kaufman J-M, Kesner JS, Wilson RC, Knobil E. Endocrinology 1985;116:1327—1333.
13. Kesner JS, Kaufman J-M, Wilson RC, Kuroda G, Knobil E. Neuroendocrinology 1986;43:686—688.
14. Kesner JS, Wilson RC, Kaufman J-M, Hotchkiss J, Chen Y, Yamamoto H, Pardo RR, Knobil E. Proc Natl Acad Sci USA 1987;84:8745—8749.
15. Williams CL, Nishihara M, Thalabard J-C, Grosser PM, Hotchkiss J, Knobil E. Neuroendocrinology 1990;52:133—137.
16. O'Byrne KT, Thalabard J-C, Grosser PM, Wilson RC, Williams CL, Chen M-D, Ladendorf D, Hotchkiss J, Knobil E. Endocrinology 1991;129:1207—1214.
17. Chen M-D, O'Byrne KT, Chiappini SE, Hotchkiss J, Knobil E. Neuroendocrinology, 1992;56:666—673.
18. Cardenas H, Ördög T, O'Byrne KT, Knobil E. Proc Natl Acad Sci USA 1993;90:9630—9634.
19. Filicori M, Santoro N, Merriam GR, Crowley Jr WF. J Clin Endocrinol Metab 1986;62:1136—1144.
20. Hotchkiss J, Knobil E. In: Knobil E, Neill JD (eds) The Physiology of Reproduction 2. New York: Raven Press, 1994;711—749.
21. Fox SR, Smith MS. Endocrinology 1985;116:1485—1492.
22. Moenter SM, Caraty A, Karsch FJ. Endocrinology 1990;127:1375—1384.
23. Moenter SM, Brand RC, Karsch FJ. Endocrinology 1992;130:2978—2984.
24. Tanaka T, Mori Y, Hoshino K. Neuroendocrinology 1992;56:641—645.

25. Nishihara M, Sano A, Kimura F. Cessation of the electrical activity of gonadotropin-releasing hormone pulse generator during the steroid-induced surge of luteinizing hormone in the rat. Neuroendocrinology (in press).
26. Reame N, Saunder SE, Kelch RP, Marshall JC. J Clin Endocrinol Metab 1984;59:328–337.
27. Rossmanith WG, Liu CH, Laughlin GA, Mortola JF, Suh BY, Yen SSC. Clin Endocrinol (Oxford) 1990;32:647–660.
28. Knobil E, Plant TM, Wildt L, Belchetz PE, Marshall G. Science 1980;207:1371–1373.
29. O'Byrne KT, Chen M-D, Nishihara M, Williams CL, Thalabard J-C, Hotchkiss J, Knobil E. Neuroendocrinology 1993;57:588–592.
30. Williams CL, Thalabard J-C, O'Byrne KT, Grosser PM, Nishihara M, Hotchkiss J, Knobil E. Proc Natl Acad Sci USA 1990;87:8580–8582.
31. Grosser PM, O'Byrne KT, Williams CL, Thalabard J-C, Hotchkiss J, Knobil E. Neuroendocrinology 1993;57:115–119.
32. Dierschke DJ, Bhattacharya AN, Atkinson LE, Knobil E. Endocrinology 1970;87:850–853.
33. Soules MR, Steiner RA, Cohen NY, Bremner WJ, Clifton DK. J Clin Endocrinol Metab 1985;61:43–49.
34. O'Byrne KT, Thalabard J-C, Chiappini SE, Chen M-D, Hotchkiss J, Knobil E. Endocrinology 1993;133:1520–1524.

Pituitary translation of the pulsatile GnRH message

John C. Marshall[1], Alan C. Dalkin[1], Daniel J. Haisenleder[1], James R. Kerrigan[2], Susan E. Kirk[1] and Murat Yasin[1]

Division of Endocrinology, Departments of [1]Internal Medicine and [2]Pediatrics, University of Virginia Health Sciences Center, Charlottesville, VA 22908, USA

Abstract. Gonadotropin-releasing hormone (GnRH) regulates gonadotropin subunit gene expression and a pulsatile GnRH signal is required for β subunit transcription. The pattern of GnRH pulses can differentially regulate β subunit mRNA expression — fast frequencies favor α and slow frequencies β mRNA. mRNA stability may be an important regulatory factor. Testosterone increases follicle-stimulating hormone (FSH) β mRNA stability, as does activin, while inhibin and follistatin reduce mRNA stability. Thus alterations in the pulse GnRH signal appear to regulate gene transcription, which together with variation in mRNA half life, allows differential expression of the β subunit mRNAs. In GnRH-deficient female rats pulsatile GnRH increases α and FSH β, but not LH β mRNA expression. Further, LH β mRNA was unchanged by GnRH pulses and replacement of gonadal steroids, and addition of other hypothalamic peptides, such as GAP, NPY or galanin to the GnRH pulses did not increase LH β mRNA. These latter data suggest that the rapid increase in LH β mRNA on proestrus may require the presence of other factors besides GnRH.

Introduction

The pituitary gonadotropic hormones, LH and follicle-stimulating hormone (FSH) consist of a common α and different β subunits which are encoded by three genes [1]. LH and FSH are present in the gonadotrope cells and both synthesis and secretion appear to be regulated by gonadotropin-releasing hormone (GnRH). GnRH is secreted by the hypothalamus in a series of pulses [2–4]. In different physiologic situations the amplitude and frequency of GnRH pulses vary and are associated with differential secretion of LH and FSH [5–10]. The pattern of GnRH secretion can be modified by gonadal steroids, and gonadotrope responses to GnRH are modified by both gonadal steroids and gonadal peptides such as inhibin, activin and follistatin [11–16]. Activin increases FSH β mRNA concentrations and FSH secretion and while inhibin and follistatin reduce mRNA concentration and serum FSH levels. Thus, regulation of LH and FSH synthesis and secretion results from changes in the pattern of the GnRH pulse stimulus, together with the direct actions of the gonadal steroids and peptides on the gonadotrope cells.

This review examines regulation of gonadotropin subunit gene expression and LH and FSH secretion, using male and female rat models.

Regulation of gonadotropin subunit mRNAs in rats

Effects of gonadectomy and gonadal hormone replacement

LH and FSH secretion and concentrations of all three subunit mRNAs increase, following gonadectomy. However, the patterns of subunit mRNA responses differ between the sexes and appear to involve different mechanisms [17–21]. In male rats, serum gonadotropins increase rapidly (within 24 h) and α and LH β mRNA concentrations also rise in the first 24 h after castration. Alpha mRNA achieves 3- to 4-fold elevations after 10 days, while LH β mRNA continues to rise to a plateau (5-fold) after 14 days. FSH β mRNA shows a slower and smaller increase, rising 2-fold after 7 days. In female rats, ovariectomy is followed by a rapid increase in serum FSH and a slower rise, over several days, in serum LH. The increase in LH is paralleled by a gradual increase in both α and LH β mRNA concentrations, which initially rise over 2–4 days and plateau 2–3 weeks later (α, 5-fold; LH β mRNA, 15-fold). In contrast, serum FSH increases within 12 h of ovariectomy and FSH β mRNA increases even more rapidly, within 2 h. This rapid increase in FSH β mRNA can be reproduced in intact female rats by immunoneutralization of inhibin, suggesting that the initial increase in FSH β mRNA reflects the loss of ovarian inhibin [22]. The later elevations of all three subunit mRNAs can be abolished by a GnRH antagonist suggesting that they reflect the gradual increase in GnRH secretion over several days [21].

In male rats, replacement of testosterone at the time of castration prevents the increases in all three subunit mRNAs [23,24]. In other studies, higher doses of testosterone do not fully suppress FSH β mRNA in long-term castrates, and testosterone appears to exert a direct action on mRNA stability [25,26]. Both testosterone and a GnRH antagonist prevent the increase in α, LH β and FSH β mRNAs. The parallel effects of testosterone and a GnRH antagonist suggest that testosterone acts by preventing the increase in GnRH secretion following castration. In contrast to females, immunoneutralization of inhibin has little or no effect in adult male rats [22].

In ovariectomized females, estradiol only partially suppresses subunit mRNAs and differential effects are seen, with α mRNA actually increasing during the first 2–3 days [21]. When both estradiol and progesterone are given at ovariectomy, the increase in α and LH β mRNAs is prevented, but FSH β mRNA is only partially reduced. Similar effects were seen after administration of a GnRH antagonist, suggesting that estradiol and progesterone together prevent the increase in GnRH secretion after ovariectomy. For FSH β mRNA the acute increase, reflecting the loss of ovarian inhibin, is maintained in the presence of a GnRH antagonist. The subsequent further increase 2–4 days after ovariectomy does not occur, indicating dependence on increasing GnRH stimulation of the gonadotrope.

The above data indicate that gonadal steroids and peptides regulate expression of all three subunit mRNAs. However, the mechanisms vary, and combinations of estradiol and progesterone in females, or testosterone in males suppress GnRH secretion. Testosterone can also stabilize FSH β mRNA in males [26], an effect that progesterone may exert in females [27]. In vitro studies have shown that inhibin and follistatin can decrease FSH β mRNA by direct actions on the gonadotrope [28]. These appear to involve a reduction of FSH mRNA stability, rather than a change in transcription rate. Conversely, activin increases FSH β mRNA by enhancing stability [28]. The inhibin subunits (components of both inhibin and activin) and follistatin have been shown to be present in pituitary gonadotropes. This finding suggests that the peptides have a paracrine and/or autocrine role in regulating gonadotropin synthesis and secretion [29–31], in addition to the endocrine effects of peptides of gonadal origin.

Gonadotropin subunit mRNA expression during the estrous cycle

Evidence for regulation of all three subunit mRNAs is seen during the 4-day estrous cycle in rats [32–34]. On metestrus a selective increase in FSH β mRNA (2-fold) occurs, while α and LH β mRNAs are stable. Both α and LH β transiently increase on diestrus when FSH β mRNA is unchanged. On the afternoon of proestrus, LH β mRNA increases 3-fold prior to the evening LH surge. FSH β mRNA also increases (4-fold) later during the proestrus gonadotropin surge, while α mRNA is unchanged. The proestrus increase in LH and FSH β mRNAs appears to reflect increased transcription [35].

Previous studies have shown that both the amplitude and frequency of GnRH pulsatile secretion are altered during the estrous cycle [36,37]. Low amplitude slow frequency pulses on metestrus increase in both amplitude and frequency by proestrus. The exact mechanisms involved in regulating mRNA expression in females remain uncertain, but probably involve changes in the pattern of GnRH stimulation, in addition to the direct effects of ovarian steroids and peptides on the gonadotrope. Plasma inhibin levels during the estrous cycle generally show an inverse relationship to FSH β mRNA concentrations [34].

The above physiologic studies have provided clear evidence for regulation of subunit mRNA expression, which, like gonadotropin secretion, appear to be differentially regulated. This differential regulation is effected by complex interplay between GnRH secretory pulse patterns, which are modified by gonadal steroids, and the direct effects of steroids and peptides on mRNA stability. In the subsequent sections, we will examine the role played by pulsatile GnRH secretion in regulating subunit mRNA expression.

GnRH pulses and differential regulation of gonadotropin subunit gene expression

GnRH-deficient rat models

To investigate the role of altered GnRH stimulation we have utilized GnRH-deficient rat models. GnRH-deficient rats, in which the gonadotrope can be stimulated by exogenous GnRH, can be produced by lesions of the hypothalamus, pharmacologic blockade of GnRH secretion, or inhibition of GnRH secretion by gonadal steroids. In male rats, a practical GnRH-deficient model is found when castrated male rats are replaced with a constant level of testosterone from a subcutaneous silastic implant [38]. In females, a similar approach would involve the use of both estrogen and progesterone, as estradiol alone does not fully suppress GnRH secretion. In order to study the potential modifying effects of ovarian steroids on gene expression, we have developed a GnRH-deficient rat model using pharmacologic blockade of GnRH secretion. The latter allows administration of exogenous GnRH pulses, given at known amplitudes and frequencies, in either the absence or presence of ovarian steroids and peptides.

Studies in GnRH-deficient female rats

We recently characterized a GnRH-deficient model produced by administering the α-adrenergic antagonist phenoxybenzamine (PBZ) to ovariectomized (OVX) rats [27]. Earlier studies have shown that PBZ could block the LH surge on proestrus, while responsiveness of LH secretion to exogenous GnRH was preserved. A regimen of PBZ given intraperitoneally (15 mg/kg at OVX, 10 mg/kg 24 h, and 5 mg/kg 48 h post-OVX) prevents the increase in LH and FSH secretion and the rise in α and LH β mRNAs for 72 h post-OVX. This regimen partially reduced the increase in FSH β mRNA, the partial rise (50% over intact females) reflecting the loss of ovarian inhibin.

We administered exogenous GnRH pulses by i.v. cannulae to this animal model. The results have shown that GnRH pulses given at 30 min intervals (to mimic the frequency of GnRH secretion during the LH surge) produced small increases in α mRNA concentrations over 12–24 h and larger (5-fold) increases in FSH β mRNA. Interestingly, LH β mRNA was not increased, despite administration of a wide range of GnRH pulses with amplitudes between 5–250 ng/pulse (25 ng/pulse produces a peak plasma GnRH level of 200 pg/ml). These regimens increased LH and FSH secretion to values similar to those seen during the proestrus gonadotropin surge. In intact animals, the gonadotropin surge on proestrus was accompanied by rapid (over 4–8 h) 3-fold increase in LH β mRNA and this was not reproduced by administration of GnRH pulses [27].

We also examined whether the rapid proestrus expression of LH β mRNA requires the presence of estradiol and/or progesterone. Using the female PBZ-treated model with replacement of estradiol and progesterone to mimic proestrus plasma concentrations, we administered GnRH pulses for 12 h. These regimens produced similar increases of α and FSH β mRNA, 2- and 3-fold, respectively, in either the presence or absence of estradiol. LH β mRNA, however, was not increased. Of interest was that the addition of progesterone to estradiol produced an additional increase in FSH β mRNA [27], perhaps suggesting stabilization of the FSH β mRNA, similar to that exerted by testosterone in males.

These data were of interest in that they suggested that GnRH pulses, together with ovarian steroids, were not adequate to reproduce the rapid increase in LH β mRNA seen on proestrus. An alternative explanation was that PBZ, in addition to blocking GnRH secretion, also inhibited LH β mRNA responsiveness to GnRH pulses. We studied this latter possibility utilizing a GnRH-deficient male rat model, produced by using a similar PBZ treatment regimen. In male rats, GnRH pulses increased LH β mRNA 2-fold, in addition to increasing both α and FSH β concentrations.

The above experiment indicated that α-adrenergic blockade by PBZ did not inhibit LH β gene expression in response to GnRH pulses. Thus, the absence of response in our GnRH-deficient female rat model suggested that PBZ may have other actions besides inhibition of GnRH release from the hypothalamus. Other hypothalamic compounds whose secretion is known to increase on proestrus include GnRH-associated peptide (GAP, a product of the GnRH gene) [39], neuropeptide-Y (NP-Y) [40], and galanin (GAL) [41]. Both NP-Y and galanin are known to increase GnRH secretion or enhance LH responses to GnRH. Thus, we administered GnRH pulses to GnRH-deficient female rats in the presence of GAP, NP-Y or galanin, given in concentrations aimed to mimic those present in portal blood during the proestrus surge. These studies revealed similar responses to those seen using GnRH pulses alone. Alpha and FSH β mRNAs were increased, but LH β mRNA concentrations remained unchanged after either 12 or 24 h of GnRH plus peptide pulses [42].

These experiments indicated that α-adrenergic blockade produces a practical GnRH-deficient female rat model and have shown that GnRH pulses are required to increase α and FSH β gene expression. However, our data suggest that other factors in addition to GnRH are required to produce the rapid 3-fold increase in LH β mRNA concentrations which occur during proestrus afternoon in a 4-day estrous cycle.

Studies in GnRH-deficient male rats

The experimental approach of using α-adrenergic blockade to produce a GnRH-deficient model is also applicable to male rats. However, a more practical approach is to suppress endogenous GnRH secretion, utilizing constant replacement of testosterone [43]. We have used the latter model to study the role of different patterns of pulsatile GnRH secretion in the regulation of gonadotropin subunit mRNA expression.

Prior studies have clearly indicated the requirement for a pulsatile GnRH stimulus to maintain LH and FSH secretion. GnRH pulses are also required to stimulate LH and FSH β gene transcription, though α gene expression can be elevated by a continuous GnRH stimulus [44]. The pattern of GnRH pulse secretion is known to change in different physiologic circumstances. Both the amplitude and frequency of GnRH pulses are increased after gonadectomy. Thus, we have used the testosterone-replaced castrate rat as the GnRH-deficient model, and delivered exogenous GnRH pulses at various amplitudes and frequencies to examine the role of GnRH pulse patterns. At castration, male rats were given subcutaneous implants containing testosterone to produce a constant serum testosterone concentration of 2.5–3 ng/ml.

Effects of altered GnRH pulse amplitude
In castrate male rats, LH and (by inference) GnRH pulses occur every 30 min. Thus, we administered GnRH pulses at 30 min intervals for 24–48 h to the castrate testosterone-replaced rat model. The dose of GnRH per pulse ranged from 10–250 ng/pulse, and pulse doses of 25 ng/pulse produced physiologic concentrations of GnRH (approximately 200 pg/ml). Measurement of steady-state subunit mRNA concentrations revealed that a wide range of GnRH pulse amplitudes (10–250 ng/pulse) increased both α and FSH β mRNA to a similar degree (2- to 3-fold). In contrast, LH β mRNA concentrations showed a biphasic response, with maximum values being observed after 25 ng GnRH pulses; higher doses produced a smaller LH β mRNA response. Thus, altered amplitude of the pulsatile GnRH signal can regulate expression of the LH β subunit mRNA [45–48].

Effects of altered GnRH pulse frequency
We examined the effects of GnRH pulse frequency by giving exogenous pulses at the optimal amplitude (25 ng/pulse). Pulses were given at intervals between 8 min and 480 min for 24–48 h. GnRH pulses given at 8 min intervals increased both α and LH β mRNAs, with maximum responses (similar to values in castrate males) being seen after 30 min pulses. Slower pulse frequencies, every 120 min or longer, did not increase α or LH β mRNAs. For FSH β, faster frequencies (8 min) did not increase mRNA concentrations, while pulse intervals of every 30 min or longer maintained a 3-fold increase in FSH β mRNA concentration. Thus, GnRH pulses given at a fast physiologic frequency of every 30 min increase all three subunit mRNAs, while slower pulse stimuli (every 120 min intervals or longer) only elevate FSH β mRNA [45,49].

These data indicate that pulse frequency can differentially regulate subunit mRNA expression and this effect is exerted in part by altered gene transcription rates. Alpha and LH β gene transcription were increased by fast frequency (every 8 or 30 min) GnRH pulses, but was not altered by slower pulse frequencies. Slow pulse frequencies, however, selectively increased FSH β gene transcription [50]. Continuous GnRH stimulation did not increase LH β or FSH β mRNA transcription rates. Thus, a pulsatile GnRH stimulus appears essential for β subunit expression and the differential effects of frequency involve altered β subunit transcription rates.

Our recent studies have suggested that other mechanisms play a role in GnRH-stimulated β subunit mRNA expression. We have used a quantitative reverse transcriptase-polymerase chain reaction assay to measure follistatin mRNA in RNA extracted from rat pituitaries [51]. Follistatin mRNA was increased 4-fold in castrate male rats. Administration of a GnRH antagonist abolished the increase, suggesting that the rise in follistatin mRNA was dependent upon GnRH. This was confirmed by administering GnRH pulses to GnRH-deficient male rats. Of interest was that GnRH pulses given at different frequencies altered follistatin mRNA expression. Maximal follistatin mRNA levels (3-fold increase) were produced by fast frequency (every 8 and 30 min) pulses, while slower frequencies did not increase follistatin mRNA. These changes were the exact opposite of FSH β mRNA concentrations after stimulation by GnRH pulses. The data suggest that the absence of an increase in FSH β mRNA after fast frequency GnRH pulses may be due to follistatin reducing FSH β mRNA stability. Conversely, the increase in FSH β mRNA after the slow frequency GnRH pulses may reflect increased mRNA synthesis without a reduction in mRNA half-life.

Summary

The data reviewed above have established the importance of the GnRH pulsatile signal in increasing expression of the gonadotropin subunit genes by increasing transcription of β subunit mRNAs. In addition, altered patterns of GnRH amplitude and frequency can exert differential expression of subunit mRNAs; fast frequencies favor α and LH β, slower frequencies increasing only FSH β mRNA. The mechanisms of the differential effect in part involve transcription, but other factors may play a role. Gonadal steroids modify the pattern of GnRH pulsatile secretion, but also appear able to exert direct effects on the stability of subunit mRNAs in the gonadotrope. Testosterone can increase FSH β mRNA concentrations in the absence of GnRH stimulation of gene transcription. It is unclear whether these steroid effects are direct or are mediated through altered gonadotrope concentrations of activin and follistatin. Further studies should elucidate the exact mechanisms involved. This should allow clarification of complex systems which are operative to allow a single gonadotropin-releasing hormone to exert differential expression of the three subunit genes and secretion of the two gonadotropin hormones. In addition, the rapid increase in LH β mRNA seen in females on proestrus afternoon has not yet been reproduced by GnRH pulses, suggesting that other factors may be required for LH β mRNA expression over the course of a few hours.

Acknowledgements

This work was supported by USPS grants (HD11489 and HD23736) to John C. Marshall, and by a clinical investigator award (HD00926) to James R. Kerrigan.

References

1. Chin WW. In: Habener JF (ed) Genes Encoding Hormones and Regulatory Peptides. Clifton, NJ: Human Press, 1987;137–149.
2. Clarke IJ, Cummins JT. Endocrinology 1982;111:1737–1739.
3. Belchetz PE, Plant TM, Nakai Y. Keogh EG, Knobil E. Science 1978;202:631–633.
4. Marshall JC, Kelch RP. N Engl J Med 1986;315:1459–1468.
5. Yen SSC, Tsai CC, Naftolin F, Vanderberg G, Ajabor, L. J Clin Endocrinol Metab 1972;34:671–675.
6. Hale PM, Khoury S, Foster CM, Beitins IZ, Hopwood NJ, Marshall JC, Kelch RP. J Clin Endocrinol Metab 1988;66:785–791.
7. Wu FCW, Butler GE, Kelnar CJH, Sellar RE. J Clin Endocrinol Metab 1990;70:629–637.

8. Backstrom CT, McNeilly AS, Leask RM, Baird DT. Clin Endocrinol (Oxford) 1982;17:29–49.
9. Reame N, Sauder SE, Kelch RP, Marshall JC. J Clin Endocrinol Metab 1984;59:328–338.
10. Crowley WF, Filicori M, Spratt DI, Santoro NF. Recent Prog Horm Res 1985;41:473–531.
11. Gay VL, Bogdanove EM. Endocrinology 1969;84:1132–1137.
12. Schanbacher BD, Ford JJ. Endocrinology 1977;100:342–347.
13. Kennedy J, Chapel S. Endocrinology 1985;116:747–748.
14. Strobl FJ, Levine JE. Endocrinology 1988;123:622–630.
15. Carroll RS, Corrigan AZ, Gharib SD, Vale W, Chin WW. Mol Endocrinol 1989;3:1969–1976.
16. Rivier C, Rivier J, Vale W. Science 1986;234:205–208.
17. Mercer JE, Clements JE, Funder JW, Clarke IJ. Neuroendocrinology 1988;47:563–566.
18. Wierman ME, Gharib SD, LaRovere JM, Badger TM, Chin WW. Mol Endocrinol 1989;2:492–498.
19. Papavasiliou SS, Zmeili S, Herbon L, Duncan-Weldon J, Marshall JC. Landefeld TD. Endocrinology 1986;119:691–698.
20. Charlton HM, Jones AJ, Ward BJ, Detta A, Clayton RN. Neuroendocrinology 1987;45:376–380.
21. Dalkin AC, Haisenleder DJ, Ortolano GA, Suhr A, Marshall JC. Endocrinology 1990;127:798–806.
22. Dalkin AC, Knight DC, Shupnik MA, Haisenleder DJ, Aloi J, Kirk S, Yasin M, Marshall JC. Endocrinology 1993;132:1292–1296.
23. Haisenleder DJ, Katt JA, Ortolano GA, El-Gewely MR, Duncan JA, Dee C, Marshall JC. Mol Endocrinol 1988;2:338–343.
24. Gharib SD, Bower SM, Need LR, Chin WW. J Clin Invest 1986;77:582–589.
25. Paul SJ, Ortolano GA, Haisenleder DJ, Stewart JM, Shupnik MA, Marshall JC. Mol Endocrinol 1990;4:1943–1955.
26. Gharib SD, Leung PCK, Carroll RS, Chin WW. Mol Endocrinol 1990;4:1620–1626.
27. Kerrigan JR, Dalkin AC, Haisenleder DJ, Yasin M, Marshall JC. Endocrinology 1993;133:2071–2079.
28. Carroll RS, Corrigan AZ, Gharib SD, Vale WW, Chin WW. Mol Endocrinol 1989;3:1969–1976.
29. Shimasaki S, Koga M, Buscaglia ML, Simmons DM, Bicsak TA, Ling N. Mol Endocrinol 1989;3:651–659.
30. Kogawa K, Nakamura T, Sugino K, Takio K, Titani K, Sugino H. Endocrinology 1989;128:1434–1437.
31. Roberts V, Meunier H, Vaughan J et al. Endocrinology 1991;124:552–555.
32. Zmeili SM, Papavasiliou SS, Thorner MO, Evans WS, Marshall JC, Landefeld TD. Endocrinology 1986;119:1867–1870.
33. Ortolano GA, Haisenleder DJ, Dalkin AC, Iliff-Sizemore SA, Landefeld TD, Marshall JC. Endocrinology 1988;123:2149–2151.
34. Haisenleder DJ, Ortolano GA, Jolly D et al. Life Sci 1990;47:1769–1773.
35. Shupnik MA, Gharib SD, Chin WW. Mol Endocrinol 1989;3:474–480.
36. Levine JE, Ramirez VD. Endocrinology 1982;111:1439–1448.
37. Fox SE, Smith MMS. Endocrinology 1985;116:1485–1492.
38. Steiner, RA, Bremner WJ, Clifton DK. Endocrinology 1982;111:2055–2061.
39. Clarke IJ, Cummins JT, Karsch FJ, Seeburg PH, Nikolics K. Biochem Biophys Res Comm 1987;143:665–671.
40. Sutton SW, Toyama TT, Otto S, Plotsky PM. Endocrinology 1988;123:1208–1210.
41. Lopez, FJ, Merchanthaler I, Ching M, Wisniewski MG, Negro-Vilar A. Proc Natl Acad Sci USA 1991;88:4508–4512.
42. Kerrigan W Jr, Haisenleder DJ, Marshall JC. Proc 35th Meeting Endocrine Soc, Las Vegas, 1993;929(abstract):283.
43. Papavasiliou SS, Zmeili S, Khoury S, Landefeld TD, Chin WW, Marshall JC. Proc Natl Acad Sci USA 1986;83:4026–4029.
44. Shupnik MA. Mol Endocrinol 1990;4:1444–1450.
45. Haisenleder DJ, Katt JA, Ortolano GA et al. Mol Endocrinol 1988;2:338–343.

46. Iliff-Sizemore SA, Ortolano GA, Haisenleder DJ, Dalkin AC, Krueger KA, Marshall JC. Endocrinology 1990;127:2876—2883.
47. Marshall JC, Dalkin AC, Haisenleder DJ, Paul SJ, Ortolano GA, Kelch RP. Recent Prog Horm Res 1991;47:155—189.
48. Haisenleder DJ, Ortolano GA, Yasin M, Dalkin AC, Marshall JC. Endocrinology 1993;132:1297—1304.
49. Dalkin, AC, Haisenleder DJ, Ortolano GA, Ellis T, Marshall JC. Endocrinology 1989;125:917—924.
50. Haisenleder DJ, Dalkin AC, Ortolano GA, Marshall JC, Shupnik MA. Endocrinology 1991;128:509—517.
51. Kirk SE, Dalkin AC, Marshall JC. Proc 3rd Int Pituitary Congress, Los Angeles, 1993;19(abstract).

Ovulation and LH-regulated genes

JoAnne S. Richards
Department of Cell Biology, Baylor College of Medicine, One Baylor Plaza, Houston, TX 77030, USA

Introduction

Ovulation of the ovarian Graafian follicle is a unique biological process triggered in mammals by the surge of LH. This event is preceded by the growth, development and selection of the preovulatory follicle [1] and is associated with specific changes in the differentiation of the theca cells and granulosa cells [2,3]. Of particular significance is the increased synthesis of theca-derived androgens and their conversion to estradiol by the aromatase enzyme system in granulosa cells of the preovulatory follicle. The increase in estradiol is obligatory to initiate the LH surge from the pituitary. In the ovary, androgens, as well as estradiol, exert autocrine and intracrine effects by mediating certain biochemical changes in granulosa cells via ligand specific receptors. Although the precise biochemical and molecular changes which occur in response to these steroids are not yet known, the steroids do act to increase the responsiveness of granulosa cells to gonadotropins. This effect is mediated, in part, by the induction of receptors for LH, as well as by increased production of cAMP in response to both follicle-stimulating hormone (FSH) and LH. The increase in cAMP appears to be independent of changes in FSH receptor number suggesting that changes in components of the intracellular signaling pathway (type of G protein?) may occur.

One of the major questions regarding the LH surge is why it is biologically necessary for such a bolus of hormone to be released in order to trigger ovulation and luteinization? One possibility is that the surge of hormone released must be sufficient (in amount and duration) to ensure that ovulation will be successful and coordinated with other biological events, including behavior. This contrasts with the regulation of basal concentrations of hormone which are finely tuned to allow only a select number of follicles to develop to the preovulatory stage. Another possibility is that surge concentrations of hormone will stimulate different intracellular signaling events than basal concentrations of hormone. Both of these possibilities are likely to be important. Two examples will be discussed to provide evidence that the LH surge induces a specific set of genes which are associated with ovulation and luteinization.

Prostaglandin synthase

Ovulation has been likened to an inflammatory response [4]. The LH surge increases prostaglandin production and induces the expression of the enzyme prostaglandin endoperoxide synthase (PGS) in granulosa cells prior to ovulation [5,6]. Until recently, it has generally been assumed that there was only one gene encoding the PGS enzyme. However, recent evidence has now refuted this idea [7–17]. The enzyme induced in granulosa cells of rat preovulatory follicles exhibits immunological characteristics which are distinct from ovine PGS [7]. The purified granulosa cell protein has N-terminal amino acid sequences which differ from ovine PGS [9]. Lastly, two immediate-early genes which exhibit PGS-like homology have been shown to encode a specific isoform of PGS, identical to that induced in rat ovarian granulosa cells [13,15]. The isoform of PGS induced by the LH surge in granulosa cells is now referred to as PGS-2, whereas the other isoform of PGS which is expressed constitutively in many tissues (kidney, uterus, endothelial cells) is called PGS-1 [9]. These two enzymes are encoded by distinct genes [11–17], are differentially regulated in a variety of tissues [7–9] and exhibit distinct biochemical characteristics [7,9,16].

Induction of PGS-2 mRNA (4.4 kb transcript) and protein by LH in granulosa cells is rapid and transient [5,6,10] and can be mimicked by agonists such as GnRH [8,18]. Whereas LH (and FSH) bind serpentine receptors coupled to the adenylyl cyclase/cAMP/A-kinase pathway [19,20], GnRH binds a serpentine receptor coupled to the phospholipase C/IP3-DAG-Ca^{2+}/C-kinase pathway [21]. These observations indicate that the PGS-2 gene can be regulated by multiple signals [8,18]. These observations also indicate that the LH surge may activate more than one intracellular signaling pathway. Evidence to support the latter hypothesis has recently been provided by a number of studies. The cloned LH receptor when expressed in non-endocrine L cells can stimulate cAMP production at low concentrations of LH and IP3 production at higher concentrations [22]. Low doses of LH which are unable to induce PGS-2 can act synergistically with a C-kinase activator, the phorbol ester, PMA, to induce this enzyme [18]. Furthermore, induction of PGS-2 by LH can be blocked by the tyrosine kinase inhibitors, genistein [8] and AG18 [18].

One of the transcription factors regulating LH-induced expression of the PGS-2 gene is the CAAT enhancer binding protein (C/EBP) [11,12]. A C/EBPβ consensus sequence is present in the 5' flanking region of the gene. Mutation of this sequence reduces functional activity of chimeric promoter-reporter constructs [12]. Nuclear extracts of granulosa cells from preovulatory follicles contain C/EBPα, one isoform of the C/EBP family. This isoform binds to the consensus sequence in the PGS-2 gene [12]. In addition, the LH surge induces expression of C/EBPβ mRNA within 30 min [12]. C/EBPβ protein is present by 2 h and remains high at 10 h. These observations indicate that C/EBPα and C/EBPβ may both be important for regulating transcriptional events associated with ovulation, one of which is the induction of the PGS-2 gene.

Progesterone receptor

The progesterone receptor (PR) is also induced in granulosa cells of rat preovulatory follicles by the LH surge in a rapid and transient manner [23]. The effect of LH in vivo [23] can be mimicked in differentiated (preovulatory) granulosa cells in vitro by LH, FSH, GnRH and epidermal growth factor (EGF) [24,25]. Multiple transcripts have been observed by Northern blotting [25]. Both the A and B forms of the receptor have been observed by immunoblotting procedures and are synthesized in an agonist- and time-dependent manner [25]. Indirect immunofluorescent analyses verified that the induced PR protein was localized to nuclei [25]. A functional role of progesterone in ovulation has been proposed based on numerous observations [4]. In addition, progesterone has been implicated to play a role in luteinization. When preovulatory follicles were incubated with surge concentrations (500 ng/ml) LH for 7 h, the granulosa cells obtained from these follicles spontaneously luteinize in culture in the absence of hormones [26,27]. These cells maintain a stable luteal cell phenotype for 10−14 days, produce high levels of progesterone, express high levels of P450$_{SCC}$ mRNA and exhibit luteal cell morphology [18,26,27]. However, if the follicles are incubated in the presence of LH and progesterone antagonists (RU486 or ZK98299) they fail to luteinize [25]. These observations indicate that the induction of PR and the action of progesterone are involved in early events leading to luteinization.

The progesterone receptor, like PGS-2, appears to be regulated by multiple cellular signaling pathways. However, the transcription factors involved have yet to be identified.

Summary

The LH surge is a unique event and plays a specific role in the reproductive physiology of the female mammal. Based on recent studies, the LH surge appears to regulate the expression of specific genes by activating multiple cellular signaling pathways, including A-kinases, C-kinases and tyrosine kinases [18,22,28,29]. The identity of the specific factors involved in ovulation and luteinization will no doubt be the continued focus of research in the coming years. In addition, the proteolytic cascade which permits release of the fertilizable oocyte also remains to be clearly defined.

References

1. Richards JS. Physiol Rev 1980;60:51−89.
2. Richards JS, Kurten RC, Fitzpatrick SL, Oonk RB, Wong WYL. In: Hunzicker-Dunn M, Schwartz NB (eds) Regulation and Actions of Follicle Stimulating Hormone. New York: Springer-Verlag, 1990;145−155.
3. Richards JS. Recent Prog Horm Res 1979;35:343−373.

4. Espey LL. Biol Reprod 1980;22:73–106.
5. Hedin L, Gaddy-Kurten D, Kurten R, DeWitt DL, Smith WL, Richards JS. Endocrinology 1987; 121:722–731.
6. Wong WYL, DeWitt DL, Smith WL, Richards JS. Mol Endocrinol 1989;3:1714–1723.
7. Wong WYL, Richards JS. Mol Endocrinol 1991;5:1269–1279.
8. Wong WYL, Richards JS. Endocrinology 1992;130:3512–3521.
9. Sirois J, Richards JS. J Biol Chem 1992;267:6382–6388.
10. Sirois J, Simmons DL, Richards JS. J Biol Chem 1992;267:11586–11592.
11. Sirois J, Levy LO, Simmons DL, Richards JS. J Biol Chem 1993;268:12199–12206.
12. Sirois J, Richards JS. J Biol Chem 1993;268:21931–21938.
13. Xie W, Chipman JG, Robertson DL,, Erickson RL, Simmons DL. Proc Natl Acad Sci USA 1992; 88:2692–2696.
14. Xie W, Merrill JR, Bradshaw WS, Simmons DS. Arch Biochem Biophys 1993;300:247–252.
15. Kubuju DA, Fletcher BS, Varnum BC, Lim RW, Hershman HR. J Biol Chem 1991;266:12866–12872.
16. Kubuju DA, Reddy ST, Fletcher BS, Hershman HR. J Biol Chem 1993;268:5425–5430.
17. Fletcher BS, Kubuju DA, Perrin DM, Hershman HR. J Biol Chem 1992;267:4338–4344.
18. Morris JK, Richards JS. Endocrinology 1993;133:770–779.
19. McFarland KC, Sprengel R, Phillips HS, Kohler M, Rosenblitt N, Nikolics K, Segaloff DL, Seeburg PH. Science 1989;245:494–499.
20. Sprengel R, Braun T, Nikolics N, Segaloff DL, Seeburg PH. Mol Endocrinol 1990;4:525–530.
21. Tsutsumi M, Zhou W, Millar RP, Mellon PL, Roberts JL, Flanagan CA, Dong K, Gillo B, Sealfon SC. Mol Endocrinol 1992;6:1163–1169.
22. Gudermann T, Birnbaumer M, Birnbaumer L. J Biol Chem 1992;267:4479–4488.
23. Park O-K, Mayo KE. Mol Endocrinol 1991;5:967–978.
24. Iwai M, Yasuda K, Fukuoka M, Iwai T, Takakura K, Taii S, Nakanishi S, Mori T. Endocrinology 1991;129:1621–1627.
25. Natraj U, Richards JS. Endocrinology 1993;133:761–769.
26. Oonk RB, Krasnow JS, Beattie WG, Richards JS. J Biol Chem 1989;264:21934-21942.
27. Oonk RB, Parker KL, Gibson JL, Richards JS. J Biol Chem 1990;65:22392-22401.
28. Gomberg-Malool S, Ziv R, Posner I, Levitski A, Orly J. Endocrinology 1993;133:362–370.
29. Richards JS. In: Adashi EY, Leung PCK (eds) The Ovary. New York: Raven Press, 1993;93–111.

Follicular development: the role of LH

Denis A. Magoffin, Timothy J. Gelety and Paul C. Magarelli
Department of Obstetrics and Gynecology, Cedars-Sinai Research Institute, Cedars-Sinai Medical Center/UCLA School of Medicine, 8700 Beverly Boulevard, DRB 2066, Los Angeles, CA 90048, USA

Abstract. In primordial and small preantral follicles there are no LH receptors, consequently the follicle cells cannot respond to LH. Follicle-stimulating hormone (FSH) appears to be the important gonadotropin early in follicle development that initiates the expression of LH receptors and steroidogenic enzymes in the theca interna by an indirect paracrine mechanism. When the theca interna (TC) express LH receptors, LH appears to be essential for the large increases in steroidogenic capacity that occur as the follicle grows to ovulatory size. Thus, the first important role of LH is to stimulate androgen biosynthesis by TC. The androgen is essential for biosynthesis of the estrogen that is necessary to trigger the ovulatory surge of LH and stimulate the female reproductive tract. The granulosa cells (GC) only express LH receptors late in follicle development. LH does not play a direct role in regulating GC throughout most of follicle development and does not appear to be important for follicle cell proliferation and follicle growth. LH appears to play a role in selection of the dominant follicle through its tonic stimulation of thecal androgen production. The stimulatory effects of LH are augmented and limited by intraovarian modulators to ensure selection of the dominant follicle and atresia of the cohort follicles. Paracrine mechanisms increase the sensitivity of the dominant follicle to gonadotropic stimulation. In cohort follicles the unaromatized androgen promotes atresia. Finally, the preovulatory surge of LH triggers luteinization of both the theca and granulosa compartments of the follicle and initiates the formation of the corpus luteum and breakdown of the follicle wall. Although FSH appears to be the major hormone regulating follicle growth, there is also strong evidence that low but not excessive levels of LH are also required for normal follicle development.

Ovarian follicle development begins when a primordial follicle is recruited into the population of growing follicles. The oocyte grows to full size, the granulosa cells (GC) proliferate into a multilayered band of endocrine cells surrounding a fluid-filled antrum, and several layers of steroidogenic cells differentiate into the theca interna. These events occur with varying degrees of dependence on gonadotropin stimulation and culminate with a preovulatory follicle capable of ovulating a fertilizable oocyte. This chapter will explore the role of LH as a regulator of ovarian follicle development.

LH is known to produce its effects on ovarian cells through binding to a specific cell surface receptor [1,2]. Cells which do not contain LH receptors are incapable of directly responding to LH. Granulosa cells in developing follicles do not contain LH receptors until relatively late in follicle development [3–6]. Consequently, it is highly unlikely that LH plays a significant role in recruiting primordial follicles into the population of growing follicles or the earliest stages of follicle development. In contrast, the endocrine cells in the theca interna (TC) contain LH receptors and can respond to LH throughout follicle development [3,4]. These facts are fundamental to the two-cell, two-gonadotropin concept of follicle estrogen biosynthesis [7,8]. LH stimulates the TC to secrete androgens that are metabolized to estrogens in the GC by the aromatase enzyme under the control of FSH. Because the TC are the only cells that contain LH receptors throughout most of follicle development we will concentrate on the role of LH with respect to the TC in developing follicles.

LH regulation of the theca interna in developing follicles

There are numerous studies demonstrating the stimulatory effects of LH on the TC in vivo and in vitro leading to the concept that LH is the principal hormone regulating thecal differentiation and function [9,10]. Not only does LH stimulate thecal steroidogenesis, but there is a marked hypertrophy and hyperplasia of the theca interna in response to LH treatment [11–13]. The proliferative effects of LH are not understood well, but the role of LH in stimulating thecal differentiation and steroid hormone production is becoming increasingly clear.

The trophic actions of LH on TC are mediated through activation of the cAMP/PKA signaling pathway. Studies in isolated rat theca-interstitial cells (TIC) have shown that activation of either type I or type II PKA leads to expression of steroidogenic enzyme genes [14]. LH stimulates the expression of cholesterol side chain cleavage cytochrome P450 ($P450_{SCC}$), 3β-hydroxysteroid dehydrogenase (3β-HSD), 17α-hydroxylase/C_{17-20} lyase cytochrome P450 ($P450_{17\alpha}$) mRNAs, and translation of the mRNAs into functional proteins [15–17]. Although there is evidence that LH also stimulates inositol phosphate formation in granulosa [18,19] and luteal cells [20,21], LH has not been shown to activate the inositol phosphate signaling pathway in TC. There is evidence demonstrating that activation of PKC with angiotensin II sensitizes TIC to LH [22] and that depletion of PKC with phorbol esters inhibits the ability of LH to stimulate steroidogenesis [23], but the role, if any, of PKC in mediating the effects of LH in TC is unknown. LH stimulates marked increases in progesterone and androgen production in differentiated TIC [9,10]. Similar stimulatory effects on androgen production have been demonstrated in rats, mice, sheep, swine, cows, horses, nonhuman primates and women, indicating that the trophic effects of LH on TC are universal in mammals. Thus, it is apparent that LH stimulation alone is sufficient to stimulate differentiation of TC into active androgen-producing cells.

Stimulation of androgen production by the TC is one of the most prominent effects of LH on the follicle. It is these androgens that are the essential substrates for follicle estrogen biosynthesis. Although it is well known that estrogen has important effects on the endometrium, oviduct and the breast, and is required to trigger the midcycle surge of LH that stimulates ovulation, follicle development in women has little or no requirement for estrogen. This concept is supported by two lines of evidence. First, small follicles have the capacity to synthesize androgens in response to LH, but it is not until the antral stage of development prior to selection of the dominant follicle that aromatase is expressed and the follicle begins to produce significant amounts of estrogen [24]. Follicle development proceeds through the preantral and early antral stages, even though the follicle is incapable of producing estrogens. Second, FSH was capable of stimulating follicle development in a woman with 17α-hydroxylase deficiency. This woman was able to ovulate fertile oocytes, even though her follicular fluid levels of estrogen were more that 1,000-fold lower than normal [25]. The lack of a requirement for estrogen in the developing follicles of women is further supported by the observation that estrogen receptors were not detected in primate ovaries [26]. Thus, it appears that human follicles are not dependent on estrogen to support their development.

Detrimental effects of LH

Although LH has a clearly positive effect on differentiation of the thecal compartment, its effects on follicle development in general are not exclusively trophic [27]. Given the lack of requirement for estrogens in developing follicles, it follows that there is not a requirement for large amounts of androgens in developing follicles either. In fact, the deleterious effects of LH on follicle development may be largely mediated by androgens. Increased production of androgens causes follicles to undergo atresia [28] and inhibits aromatase activity [29]. This concept is supported by the observations that decreasing circulating levels of LH by passive immunization to LH reduces atresia [30], and immunization to androstenedione increases the ovulation rate [31]. These concepts may be clinically relevant in hyperandrogenic states such as polycystic ovarian disease (PCO) where follicle development is arrested in the presence of high levels of androgens.

In PCO, as in euandrogenic women, elevated levels of LH correlate with decreased fertility and appear to be detrimental to developing follicles [32]. In women treated with clomiphene citrate, increased levels of LH during follicle development were associated with a decreased incidence of pregnancy [33,34], suggesting that even small elevations in LH levels interfere with the optimal development of preovulatory follicles and the production of viable oocytes. It has been suggested that elevated levels of LH may prematurely allow resumption of meiotic maturation [35]. This hypothesis is based on the observation that the midcycle surge of LH decreases the activity of oocyte maturation inhibitor (OMI), a peptide that maintains the meiotic arrest of oocytes in developing follicles [36]. Elevated LH levels during the follicular phase of the cycle could prematurely decrease OMI, causing ovulation of postmature oocytes. The resulting embryos might have decreased viability, producing lower implantation rates and increased incidence of miscarriage early in pregnancy.

Taken together it seems clear that even modest increases in LH concentrations during the follicular phase are deleterious to follicle development. These effects are likely mediated at several levels, in particular through increased androgen production and decreased production of OMI. It is also clear that the follicle must produce estrogen in order for the female reproductive system to function properly and for selection of the dominant follicle and ovulation to occur. Without LH stimulation of the TC to produce androgens, estrogen production will be deficient, yet increases in LH interfere with follicle development. How can the follicle produce sufficient androgen substrate while LH concentrations remain low?

The effects of LH on thecal cells are modulated by intraovarian mechanisms

The ovary has developed autocrine and paracrine mechanisms by which the granulosa and thecal compartments can modulate the actions of the gonadotropins. Table 1 lists regulatory molecules that are produced in the ovary and their modulatory effects on LH action in TIC. Some of the modulators augment the stimulatory effects of LH and some inhibit LH stimulation. Without discussing the nuances of the effects of each modulator, there are several important points that were discovered by studying the intraovarian growth and differentiation factors.

The positive modulatory factors such as IGF-I and inhibin provide a mechanism whereby the granulosa cells can increase androgen substrate production by the thecal cells in developing follicles without alterations in circulating concentrations of LH. Although without effect on androgen production alone, physiological concentrations of IGF-I, for example, increase thecal androgen production approximately 3-fold at a given concentration of LH [37,38]. Thus, at low follicular phase, concentrations of LH androgen production by the theca of a dominant follicle could be significantly higher than the basal production observed in cohort follicles. A similar effect would be expected with inhibin [39]. Indeed, such mechanisms may be critical to selection

Table 1. Intraovarian modulators of LH action on theca-interstitial cells

Modulator	Origin	Effect on theca-interstitial cells	References
Activin	GC	Inhibition of androgen synthesis	[40–42]
Angiotensin II	GC/TC/FF	Sensitization to LH	[43–46]
Catecholamines	Nerves	Augmentation of androgen synthesis	[47,48]
Estrogen	GC	Inhibition of androgen synthesis	[49–54]
Inhibin	GC	Augmentation of androgen synthesis	[41,42,55–57]
IGF-I	GC	Augmentation of androgen synthesis Stimulation of steroidogenic enzyme gene expression	[15–17,37,38,58]
IGF-II	GC/TC	Unknown	[59,60]
Interleukin 1	GC/TC Macrophage	Inhibition of androgen synthesis	[61–63]
TGFα	TC	Inhibition of androgen synthesis	[64–66]
TGFβ	TC/GC	Inhibition of androgen synthesis Stimulates $P450_{scc}$ content	[67–72]
TNFα	Macrophage	Inhibition of androgen synthesis Morphological alterations	[73–75]

IGF-I: insulin-like growth factor-I; IGF-II: insulin-like growth factor-II; TGFα: transforming growth factor-α; TGFβ: transforming growth factor-β; TNFα: tumor necrosis factor-α; GC: granulosa cells; TC: theca cells; $P450_{scc}$: cholesterol side-chain cleavage cytochrome P450.

of the dominant follicle [24]. As follicles grow in response to FSH stimulation during the follicular phase of the cycle, the granulosa compartment proliferates and secretes increasing amounts of IGF-I and inhibin. When the largest follicle reaches sufficient size the inhibin causes a subtle decrease in FSH secretion that has the effect of limiting gonadotropic support of the growing follicles. The largest follicle becomes dominant, because it has compensated for the lack of gonadotropic support in part by increasing the effective potency of LH to stimulate thecal androgen production. This is accomplished by a paracrine augmentation of thecal androgen biosynthesis by IGF-I, inhibin, and perhaps other unidentified molecules. Similar mechanisms occur with respect to aromatase expression by the GC [76]. The cohort follicles cannot adequately compensate for the decrease in FSH and undergo atresia. Exogenous treatment with FSH can overcome this process and promote development of a large number of follicles to ovulatory size, a fact that forms the physiologic basis for the superovulation protocols employed to obtain oocytes for in vitro fertilization.

The inhibitory modulators provide a mechanism by which the follicle can limit the amount of androgen produced by the theca. As discussed above, excessive androgen production is deleterious to normal follicle development and ovulation. Molecules such as estrogen [49–54] and TGF-β [67,70] can inhibit LH stimulation of androgen production, without decreasing the ability of the theca to synthesize progesterone. Such a mechanism could limit the amount of androgen produced during the follicular phase of the cycle, but not interfere with the ability of the theca to luteinize and contribute to the formation of a corpus luteum.

The second major concept that has emerged from the study of intraovarian regulators of thecal function is that putative autocrine and paracrine regulators alone can stimulate the expression of genes in TIC that are associated with thecal differentiation. IGF-I has been shown to stimulate the expression of LH receptor [77,78], P450$_{SCC}$ [17] and 3β-HSD [16] mRNA in TIC and to selectively stimulate translation of P450$_{SCC}$ protein [37]. IGF-I is not unique in this regard as TGFα causes a similar stimulation of 3β-HSD mRNA and inhibin stimulates the expression of both P450$_{SCC}$ and 3β-HSD mRNA [79]. It was not long ago that the only recognized stimulator of thecal gene expression was LH. Although LH is a potent regulator of thecal differentiation, we now know that intraovarian peptides can play an important role in stimulating thecal differentiation in the absence of LH. The significance of this concept with regard to follicle development remains unclear, because the follicle is continuously exposed to varying concentrations of LH. Further studies will need to be completed to determine the physiological importance of paracrine and autocrine mechanisms in vivo when superimposed on the low follicular phase levels of LH.

The third important concept discovered from the study of intraovarian peptides is that thecal steroid hormone biosynthesis is dissociated from expression of steroidogenic enzyme genes. This concept was initially demonstrated by the observation that IGF-I alone induced the expression of P450$_{SCC}$ mRNA in TIC, but had no effect on steroid hormone production [37]. Only after stimulation of the TIC with molecules that increase intracellular cAMP or bypass the need for cholesterol transport across the mitochondrial membranes was steroidogenesis increased [37]. The implication of this observation is that it is possible to stimulate gene expression in TIC and even the presence of catalytically active $P450_{SCC}$ enzyme, without increasing the conversion of cholesterol to pregnenolone. Thus, the potential exists for theca cells to begin differentiation in the absence of LH stimulation and later respond to LH by secreting steroid hormones.

The role of paracrine differentiation factors in initiating thecal differentiation

For many years the two-cell, two-gonadotropin concept of follicular estrogen biosynthesis has dominated our thinking about how theca and granulosa cell differentiation is regulated. Until recently, little was known regarding the effects of regulators other than LH on thecal gene expression. Consequently, the available data supported the conclusion that LH is the principal hormone regulating thecal differentiation, because LH is capable of stimulating expression of all of the enzymes necessary for androgen biosynthesis. There is, however, a serious flaw in this line of reasoning. There are no LH receptors present on theca precursor cells [9], therefore LH cannot be the hormone that initiates thecal differentiation. The fact that theca only differentiate adjacent to growing follicles supports this conclusion, since all follicles are exposed to LH.

As summarized in Table 2, primordial follicles begin to grow before there are morphologically identifiable theca cells associated with the follicles, and in the absence of LH receptors. Evidence from ^{3}H-thymidine incorporation studies in rats has suggested that theca precursor (stem?) cells adjacent to small developing follicles begin to replicate DNA and presumably proliferate prior to the functional differentiation of LH-responsive steroidogenic cells and the appearance of morphologically recognizable TC [80]. Recent work in intact rats from our laboratory has revealed that the genes for LH receptors, $P450_{SCC}$, 3β-HSD and $P450_{17\alpha}$ begin to be coordinately expressed immediately prior to the appearance of morphologically differentiated TC. Within 24 h morphologically distinct TC appear adjacent to the basal lamina. These

Table 2. Differentiation of theca interna cells during follicle development

Layers of cells		Steroid production		LH stimulation	Gene expression			
Granulosa	Theca	P^4	A^4		LH R	$P450_{SCC}$	3β-HSD	$P450_{17\alpha}$
Primordial	0	–	–	–	–	–	–	–
1	0	–	–	–	–	–	–	–
3	Partial	–	–	–	+	+	+	+
4	1–2	+	+	+	+	+	+	+
Early antral	2–3	++	++	++	++	++	++	++
Antral	>3	+++	+++	+++	++	+++	+++	+++

P^4: progesterone; A^4: androstenedione; LH R: luteinizing hormone receptor; $P450_{SCC}$: cholesterol side-chain cleavage cytochrome P450; 3β-HSD: 3β-hydroxysteroid dehydrogenase; $P450_{17\alpha}$: 17α-hydroxylase/C_{17-20} lyase cytochrome P450; –: not detectable; +: low; ++: moderate; +++: high.

TC are responsive to LH and are capable of secreting low levels of androstenedione. Taken together, these findings indicate that when primordial follicles begin to grow, a specific population of undifferentiated stromal cells in close proximity to the growing follicles begin to express the unique pattern of gene expression that leads to differentiation of the theca interna. The evidence indicates that TC assume their characteristic morphology concurrently with translation of these specific genes into protein.

The implication of these findings is that the growing follicle secretes one or more substances that stimulate the expression of both LH receptors and steroidogenic enzymes. It is interesting to note that this substance must have the capacity to stimulate steroidogenic enzyme gene expression as well as LH receptor gene expression, because the differentiating TC express steroidogenic enzyme genes before becoming responsive to LH. To test this hypothesis we have recently isolated preantral ovarian follicles from intact rats with 1–4 layers of granulosa cells [81] and examined their capacity to secrete substances in vitro that can stimulate thecal differentiation. Conditioned mediums from the follicle cultures were assayed for androgen-stimulating activity, using isolated TIC cultures as a bioassay. As shown in Fig. 1, conditioned medium from growing follicles with a single layer of granulosa

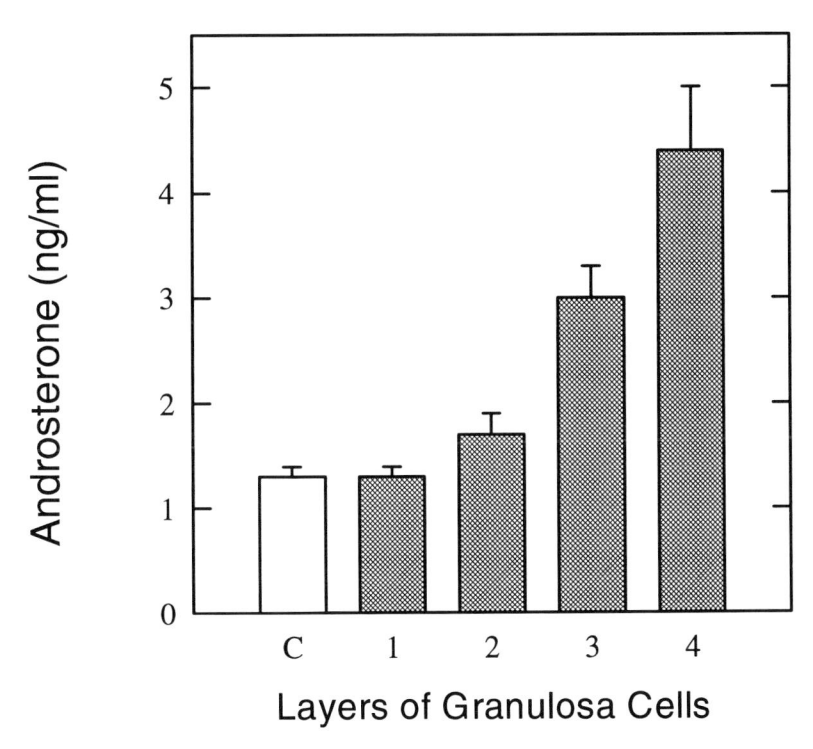

Fig. 1. Stimulation of thecal androgen production by substances secreted from primary follicles. Follicles were isolated from enzymatically dissociated 26-day-old rat ovaries [81], then cultured in serum-free medium for 2 days. The conditioned medium (100 µl) was added to isolated theca-interstitial cell cultures (2×10^4 viable cells) containing 100 µl of fresh medium for 2 days. Androsterone was measured by RIA [82]. Data are mean ± SEM (n = 3).

cells did not stimulate TIC androgen production. Beginning with two layers of granulosa cells the follicles secreted increasing amounts of an androgen-stimulating substance into the medium. It is known from earlier studies that androgen production in this model requires stimulation of steroidogenic enzyme gene expression [14]. This is the first evidence supporting the hypothesis that the follicle secretes bioactive substances that can stimulate thecal differentiation. The secretion of the androgen-stimulating substance was increased by FSH. When the follicles were treated with FSH that was immunopurified to remove the LH contamination there was a marked increase in the amount of bioactivity in the conditioned medium (Fig. 2). Thus, we have shown that small growing follicles secrete one or more substances that are hormonally and developmentally regulated, which appear to stimulate thecal differentiation and androgen production.

Based on these findings it is reasonable to hypothesize that the initial differentiation of the theca interna is not regulated by LH, but is stimulated indirectly by FSH through a paracrine mechanism involving one or more mediators secreted by the growing follicle. This hypothesis is supported by studies in which recombinant FSH was shown to stimulate $P450_{17\alpha}$ gene expression and androgen production in the ovary by a paracrine mechanism [83]. Interestingly, in this study the effects of FSH were abolished in hypophysectomized rats, suggesting that the paracrine signals modulated LH-stimulated thecal differentiation rather than producing their effects de novo. These results are not inconsistent with ours, because large follicles predominate

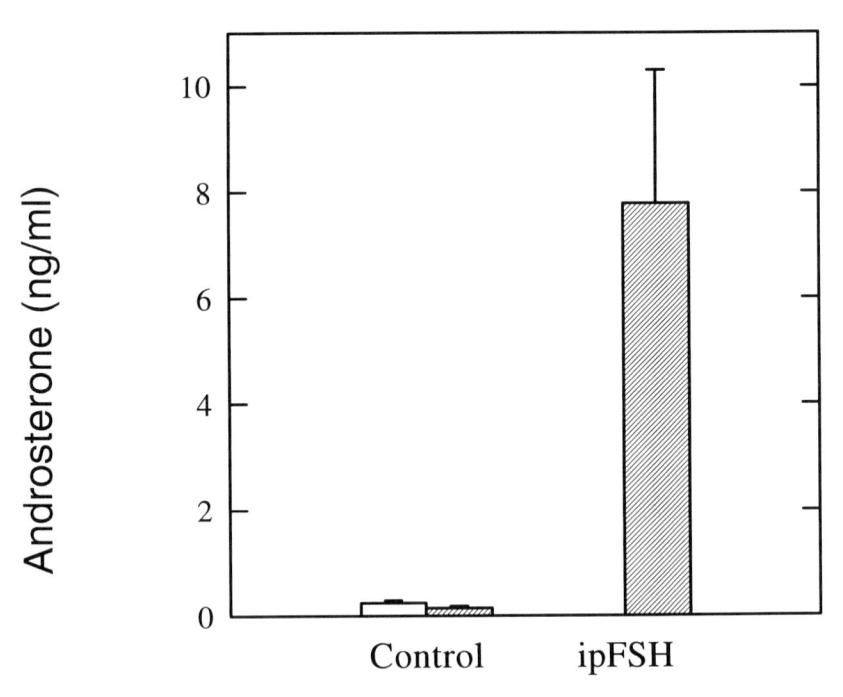

Fig. 2. FSH stimulation of follicular thecal differentiation factors. Preantral follicles with 1–4 layers of granulosa cells were cultured in serum-free medium for 2 days with and without immunopurified FSH (50 ng/ml). The conditioned medium was bioassayed as in Fig. 1. Data represent mean ± SEM (n = 3).

in the in vivo studies, whereas we focused on very small preantral follicles. It is possible that the effects we observed may be limited to specific stages of preantral follicle development. The data suggest that the initial phases of thecal differentiation may be regulated by one paracrine mechanism responsive to FSH and that, as the follicle develops LH responsiveness, additional paracrine mechanisms predominate that are dependent on the low physiologic levels of LH during the follicular phase. These LH-dependent mechanisms appear to be responsible for increasing the androgenic capacity of the TC to the high levels that are present in antral follicles.

Summary

Figure 3 summarizes the current information regarding the role of LH in follicle development. In primordial and small preantral follicles there are no LH receptors, consequently the follicle cells cannot respond to LH. FSH appears to be the important gonadotropin early in follicle development that initiates the expression of LH receptors and steroidogenic enzymes in the theca interna by an indirect paracrine mechanism. When the TC express LH receptors, LH appears to be essential for the large increases in steroidogenic capacity that occur as the follicle grows to ovulatory size. Thus, the first important role of LH is to stimulate androgen biosynthesis by TC.

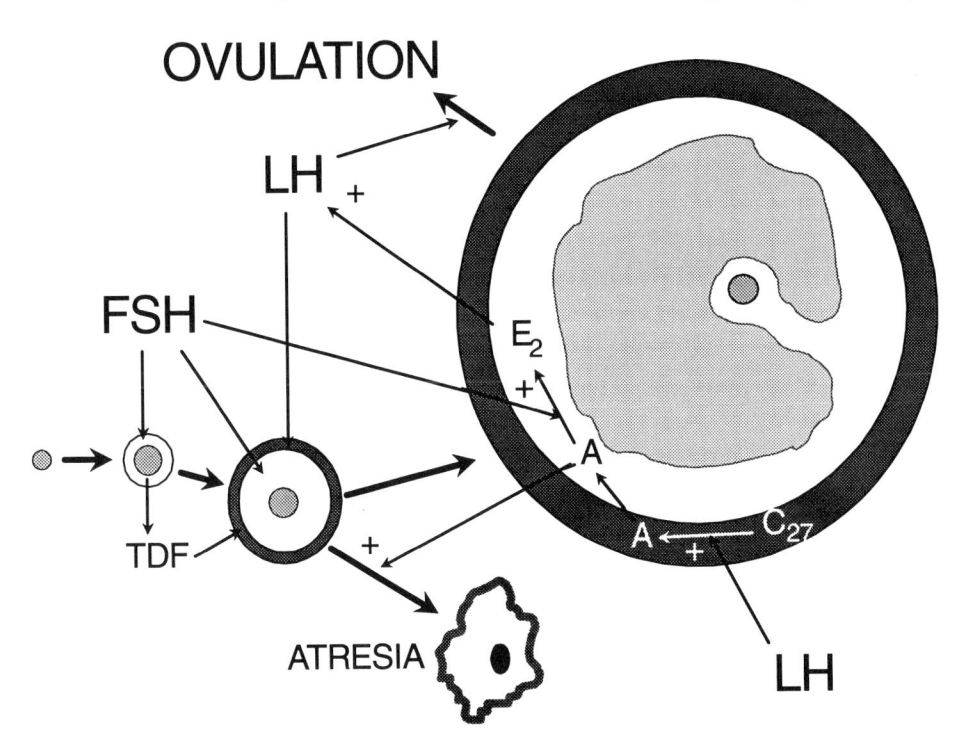

Fig. 3. The role of LH in ovarian follicle development. TDF: theca differentiating factors; E_2: estradiol-17β; A: androstenedione; C_{27}: cholesterol.

The androgen is essential for biosynthesis of the estrogen that is necessary to trigger the ovulatory surge of LH and stimulate the female reproductive tract. The GC only express LH receptors late in follicle development. LH does not play a direct role in regulating GC throughout most of follicle development and does not appear to be important for follicle cell proliferation and follicle growth. LH appears to play a role in selection of the dominant follicle through its tonic stimulation of thecal androgen production. The stimulatory effects of LH are augmented and limited by intraovarian modulators to ensure selection of the dominant follicle and atresia of the cohort follicles. Paracrine mechanisms increase the sensitivity of the dominant follicle to gonadotropic stimulation. In cohort follicles the unaromatized androgen promotes atresia. Finally, the preovulatory surge of LH triggers luteinization of both the theca and granulosa compartments of the follicle, and initiates the formation of the corpus luteum and breakdown of the follicle wall. Although FSH appears to be the major hormone regulating follicle growth, there is also strong evidence that low but not excessive levels of LH are also required for normal follicle development.

References

1. Jia X, Oikawa M, Bot M, Ny T, Boime I, Hsueh AJ. Mol Endocrinol 1991;5:759–768.
2. Frazier AL, Robbins LS, Stork PJ, Sprengel R, Segaloff DL, Cone RD. Mol Endocrinol 1990;4: 1264–1276.
3. Peluso JJ, Steger RW, Hafez ESE. J Reprod Fertil 1976;47:55–58.
4. Siebers JW, Peters F, Zenzes MT, Schmidtke J, Engel W. J Endocrinol 1977;73:491–496.
5. Zeleznik AJ, Midgley AR, Reichert LE. Endocrinology 1974;95:818–825.
6. Erickson GF, Wang C, Hsueh AJW. Nature 1979;279:336–338.
7. Falck B. Acta Physiol Scand 1959;47(suppl):1–101.
8. Bjersing L. Acta Endocrinol Copenh 1967;125(suppl):1–23.
9. Erickson GF, Magoffin DA, Dyer CA, Hofeditz C. Endocr Rev 1985;6:371–399.
10. Magoffin DA. Sem Reprod Endocrinol 1991;9:321–331.
11. Rennels EG. Am J Anat 1951;88:63–107.
12. Selye H, Collip JB. Proc Soc Exp Biol Med 1933;30:647–649.
13. Selye H, Collip JB, Thomson DL. Proc Soc Exp Biol Med 1933;30:780–783.
14. Magoffin DA. Endocrinology 1989;125:1464–1473.
15. Magoffin DA, Weitsman SR. Endocrinology 1993;132:1945–1951.
16. Magoffin DA, Weitsman SR. Biol Reprod 1993;48:1166–1173.
17. Magoffin DA, Weitsman SR. Mol Cell Endocrinol 1993;96:45–51.
18. Davis JS, Weakland LL, West LA, Farese RV. Biochem J 1986;238:597–604.
19. Dimino MJ, Snitzer J, Brown KM. Biol Reprod 1987;37:1129–1134.
20. Allen RB, Su HC, Snitzer J, Dimino MJ. Biol Reprod 1988;38:79–83.
21. Davis JS, Weakland LL, Farese RV, West LA. J Biol Chem 1987;262:8515–8521.
22. Magoffin DA. In: Gibori G (ed) Signaling Mechanisms and Gene Expression in the Ovary. Norwell, MA: Serono Symposia, 1991;417–422.
23. Hofeditz C, Magoffin DA, Erickson GF. Biol Reprod 1988;39:873–881.
24. Hirshfield AN. Int Rev Cytol 1991;124:43–101.
25. Rabinovici J, Blankstein J, Goldman B, Rudak E, Dor Y, Pariente C, Geier A, Lunenfeld B, Mashiach S. J Clin Endocrinol Metab 1989;68:693–697.
26. Hild-Petito S, Stouffer RL, Brenner RM. Endocrinology 1988;123:2896–2905.
27. Stanger JD, Yovich JL. Br J Obstet Gynecol 1985;92:385–393.

28. Louvet JP, Harman SM, Schreiber JR, Ross GT. Endocrinology 1975;97:366−372.
29. Hillier SG, van den Boogard AM, Reichert LE, van Hall EV. J Endocrinol 1980;84:409−419.
30. Terranova PF, Greenwald GS. J Reprod Fertil 1981;61:37−42.
31. Scaramuzzi RJ, Davidson WG, Van Look PFA. Nature 1977;269:817−818.
32. Homburg R, Armar NA, Eshel A, Adams J, Jacobs HS. Br Med J 1988;297:1024−1026.
33. Quigley MM, Berkowitz AS, Gilbert SA, Wolf DP. Fertil Steril 1984;41:809−815.
34. Shorham Z, Borenstein R, Lunenfeld B, Pariente C. Clin Endocrinol 1990;33:271−278.
35. Jacobs HS, Porter R, Eshel A, Craft I. In: Vickery BH, Nestor IJ (eds) LHRH and its Analogues: Contraception and Therapeutic Application, II. Lancaster: MTP Press, 1987;303−319.
36. Tsafriri A, Pomerantz SH. J Clin Endocrinol Metab 1986;15:157−170.
37. Magoffin DA, Kurtz KM, Erickson GF. Mol Endocrinol 1990;4:489−496.
38. Hernandez ER, Resnick CE, Svoboda ME, Van Wyk JJ, Payne DW, Adashi EY. Endocrinology 1988;122:1603−1612.
39. Hillier SG, Miro F. Ann NY Acad Sci 1993;687:29−38.
40. Hillier SG, Yong EL, Illingsworth PJ, Baird DT, Schwall RH, Mason AJ. J Clin Endocrinol Metab 1991;72:1206−1211.
41. Hsueh AJW, Dahl KD, Vaughan J, Tucker E, River J, Bardin CW, Vale W. Proc Natl Acad Sci 1987;84:5082−5086.
42. Schwall RH, Mason AJ, Wilcox JN, Bassett SG, Zeleznik AJ. Mol Endocrinol 1990;4:75−79.
43. Do YS, Sherrod A, Lobo RA, Paulson RJ, Shinagawa T, Chen S, Kjos S, Hsueh WA. Proc Natl Acad Sci USA 1988;85:1957−1961.
44. Speth RC, Husain A. Biol Reprod 1988;38:695−702.
45. Husain A, Bumpus FM, De Silva P, Speth RC. Proc Natl Acad Sci USA 1987;84:2489−2493.
46. Schultze D, Brunswig B, Mukhopadhyay AK. Endocrinology 1989;124:1389−1398.
47. Dyer CA, Erickson GF. Endocrinology 1985;116:1645−1652.
48. Hernandez ER, Jimenez JL, Payne DW, Adashi EY. Endocrinology 1988;122:1592−1602.
49. Magoffin DA, Erickson GF. Endocrinology 1981;108:962−969.
50. Magoffin DA, Erickson GF. Mol Cell Endocrinol 1982;28:81−89.
51. Leung PCK, Goff AK, Kennedy TG, Armstrong DT. Biol Reprod 1978;19:641−647.
52. Leung PCK, Armstrong DT. Endocrinology 1979;104:1411−1417.
53. Tsang BK, Leung PCK, Armstrong DT. Mol Cell Endocrinol 1979;14:131−139.
54. Leung PCK, Armstrong DT. Biol Reprod 1979;21:1035−1042.
55. Engelhardt H, Smith KB, McNeilly AS, Baird DT. Biol Reprod 1993;49:281−294.
56. Hillier SG, Yong EL, Illingworth PJ, Baird DT, Schwall RH, Mason AJ. Mol Cell Endocrinol 1991;75:R1−6.
57. Hillier SG, Wickings EJ, Illingworth PI, Yong EL, Reichert LE, Baird DT, Mcneilly AS. Clin Endocrinol 1991;35:71−78.
58. Cara JF, Rosenfield RL. Endocrinology 1988;123:733−739.
59. Ramasharma K, Li CH. Proc Natl Acad Sci 1987;84:2643−2647.
60. Hernandez ER, Roberts Jr CT, Hurwitz A, LeRoith D, Adashi EY. Endocrinology 1990;127:3249−3251.
61. Hurwitz A, Payne DW, Packman JN, Andreani CL, Resnick CE, Hernandez ER, Adashi EY. Endocrinology 1991;129:1250−1256.
62. Hurwitz A, Ricciarelli E, Botero L, Rohan RM, Hernandez ER, Adashi EY. Endocrinology 1991;129:3427−3429.
63. Hurwitz A, Loukides J, Ricciarelli E, Botero L, Katz E, McAllister JM, Garcia JE, Rohan R, Adashi EY, Hernandez ER. J Clin Invest 1992;89:1746−1754.
65. Skinner MK, Coffey RJ. Endocrinology 1988;123:2632−2638.
66. Kudlow JE, Kobrin MS, Purchio AF, Twardzik DR, Hernandez ER, Asa SL, Adashi EY. Endocrinology 1987;121:1577−1579.
67. Magoffin DA, Gancedo B, Erickson GF. Endocrinology 1989;125:1951−1958.
68. Skinner MK, Keski-Oja J, Osteen KG, Moses HL. Endocrinology 1987;121:786−792.

69. Mulheron GW, Danielpour D, Schomberg DW. Endocrinology 1991;129:368–374.
70. Hernandez ER, Hurwitz A, Payne DW, Dharmarajan AM, Purchio AF, Adashi EY. Endocrinology 1990;127:2804–2811.
71. Mulheron GW, Schomberg DW. Biol Reprod 1992;46:546–550.
72. Kim I, Schomberg DW. Endocrinology 1989;124:1345–1351.
73. Zachow RJ, Tash JS, Terranova PF. Endocrinology 1992;131:2503–2513.
74. Zachow RJ, Tash JS, Terranova PF. Endocrinology 1993;133:2269–2276.
75. Andreani CL, Payne DW, Packman JN, Resnick CE, Hurwitz A, Adashi EY. J Biol Chem 1991;266:6761–6766.
76. Erickson GF, Garzo VG, Magoffin DA. J Clin Endocrinol Metab 1989;69:716–724.
77. Cara JF, Fan J, Azzarello J, Rosenfield RL. J Clin Invest 1990;86:560–565.
78. Magoffin DA, Weitsman SR. Biol Reprod 1993;48(suppl):74.
79. Magoffin DA, Erickson GF. In: Findlay JK (ed) Cellular and Molecular Mechanisms of Female Reproduction. Orlando: Academic Press, 1994;39–65.
80. Hirshfield AN. Biol Reprod 1991;44:1157–1162.
81. Roy SK, Greenwald GS. Biol Reprod 1985;32:203–215.
82. Zamecnik J, Barbe G, Moger WH, Armstrong DT. Steroids 1977;30:679–689.
83. Smyth CD, Miro F, Whitelaw PF, Howles CM, Hillier SG. Endocrinology 1993;133:1532–1538.

Gonadotropic control of folliculogenesis: the threshold theory

Anthony J. Zeleznik

Departments of Cell Biology and Physiology, and Obstetrics, Gynecology and Reproductive Sciences, The University of Pittsburgh School of Medicine, Magee Women's Research Institute, Pittsburgh, PA 15213, USA

Historical overview on the role of gonadotropins on follicular development

A little over 50 years ago, the classic studies of Greep et al. demonstrated the presence of two distinct gonadotropin hormones of the anterior pituitary gland [1]. In this study, the biological effects of purified thylakentrin (follicle-stimulating hormone, FSH) and metakentrin (interstitial cell stimulation hormone, ICSH or luteinizing hormone, LH) were studied in hypophysectomized rats and it was shown that while FSH alone was capable of stimulating antral follicular development, the stimulation of the follicle to produce estrogen and to ovulate required treatment with both FSH and LH. This paper is the seminal study on ovulation induction, not only because it identified the distinct biological activities of FSH and LH, but also because it demonstrated that there must be synergistic actions between FSH and LH in the maturation of the preovulatory follicle, its production of estrogen, its ovulation and the transition of the ruptured follicle into a corpus luteum. Over the subsequent 50 years since the publication of this paper, many, but clearly not all, of the interactions between FSH and LH in the control of folliculogenesis have been elucidated. Thus, the requirement for both FSH and LH in the secretion of estrogen can be accounted for by the "two-cell two-gonadotropin" model for estrogen secretion in which the theca cells, under the stimulation of LH, produce C_{19} androgens which serve as obligatory substrates for the FSH-induced aromatase activity [2,3]. The requirement for both FSH and LH in the process of ovulation and luteinization is now explained by the knowledge that FSH induces cell surface receptor for luteinizing hormone as the follicle matures to the preovulatory stage, which allows only those follicles with LH receptors on the granulosa cells to respond to the midcycle gonadotropin surge [4].

The direct application of Greep's findings to ovulation induction in humans and subhuman primates was made by Gemzell et al., in which it was shown that injection of purified preparations of FSH, LH and/or hCG could provoke follicular development and ovulation [5–7]. However, despite being able to induce ovulation with exogenous gonadotropins, the initial results were often associated with uncontrolled ovarian responses leading to ovarian hyperstimulation. In 1978, Brown [8] published a summary of his experiences at the University of Melbourne regarding the use of human pituitary gonadotropins to produce ovulation in humans and concluded that the ovarian requirement for FSH operates in a very narrow range, such that incremental doses of 10—30% are sufficient to initiate follicular development. In this paper, Brown likened the ovarian requirement to a "threshold" in which, once a critical concentration of FSH is achieved, follicles readily enter the final trajectory of preovulatory development. Over the past 15 years this concept has been studied extensively and refined to provide a physiological account, not only for the initiation of preovulatory follicular development by FSH, but also for the interactions between FSH, LH and intraovarian factors that govern the selective maturation of a single preovulatory follicle in humans and subhuman primates. The purpose of this chapter is to review current concepts regarding the hormonal control of preovulatory follicular development in humans and subhuman primates. More extensive discussions of this topic have been published elsewhere [9,10].

Physiology of the follicular phase of the menstrual cycle

A successful follicular phase requires the complete interplay between the ovary and the hypothalamic-pituitary axis; disturbances of function at either location result in abnormal follicular development and/or anovulation. Accordingly, an examination of the gonadotropic control of follicular development must include a description of both the process of folliculogenesis, as well as the interrelationships between the ovary and the hypothalamic-pituitary axis.

Folliculogenesis in primates

Follicular growth begins with the exit of follicles from the pool of nonproliferating primordial follicles. Early follicular development is primarily characterized by proliferation of granulosa cells and increasing numbers of layers of granulosa cells surrounding the oocyte. Based on the frequency of mitotic indices within the granulosa cell layer, Gougeon estimated that approximately 85—90 days are required for the growth of primordial follicle to a large preantral follicle [11]. Histological examination of ovaries throughout the menstrual cycle of both humans and macaques revealed the presence of all-sized preantral follicles regardless of the stage of the menstrual cycle [12,13]. These findings are interpreted as meaning that growth of preantral follicles does not require the fluctuations in gonadotropin secretion that are seen during the menstrual cycle. It is generally assumed that the process of preantral follicular development provides a continuous source of maturing follicles for final maturation to the preovulatory stage when appropriate gonadotropin concentrations are achieved.

Preantral follicle granulosa cells contain FSH receptors which, via a cAMP effector system, initiate the process of granulosa cell differentiation and preovulatory follicular development. Among many of the developmental modifications that granulosa cells undergo during preovulatory follicular development are the induction of LH receptors as well as the aromatase enzyme required for the conversion of thecally derived androgens to estrogen. In addition, FSH also induces enzymes responsible for progesterone production which enable the newly ovulated follicle to rapidly commence the secretion of progesterone as it is transformed into a corpus luteum [4]. The limiting factor in the continued maturation of follicles beyond the preantral stage to the preovulatory stage is FSH, as recent studies in women have shown that injection of pure recombinant FSH is able to stimulate preovulatory follicular development [14]. As described in the previous chapter, the role of LH in early preovulatory follicular development appears to be to supply androgen substrate to the follicle for adequate estrogen production. Evidence that the limiting factor in preovulatory follicular development is the absolute concentration of FSH derived from the observations that preovulatory follicular development can readily and rapidly be stimulated during the luteal phase of the menstrual cycle by the administration of exogenous gonadotropins [15].

Regulation of gonadotropin secretion during the follicular phase

Upon the regression of the corpus luteum at the termination of the nonfertile menstrual cycle there is an increase in the plasma concentration of FSH and LH [16]. As proposed by Baird, the production of estradiol by the primate corpus luteum results in a suppression of FSH secretion below concentrations necessary to initiate preovulatory follicular growth [17]. This is supported by the observations that administration of antiestradiol antibodies to monkeys during the latter portion of the menstrual cycle results in an increase in plasma FSH concentrations and a stimulation of follicular development [18]. Moreover, recent studies in humans have shown that administration of estrogen at the time of luteal regression prevents the perimenstrual rise in FSH concentrations [19]. The rise in FSH secretion during the early follicular phase is transient; as estrogen secretion commences during the midfollicular phase, plasma FSH concentrations decline [16]. The reciprocal relationship between FSH and estrogen concentrations during the follicular phase of the menstrual cycle constitutes an exquisitely sensitive feedback system which governs the selection of the preovulatory follicle. In response to the perimenstrual elevation in FSH concentrations, follicular growth beyond the early antral stage is stimulated. As mentioned previously, a hallmark of FSH action on the granulosa cell is the induction of aromatase which permits the thecally produced androgens to be further metabolized to estrogen. As sufficient aromatase is induced in a maturing follicle, plasma estrogen concentrations begin to rise. The rise in plasma estrogen concentrations, in addition to its effects on the developing endometrium, serves two paramount functions in the regulation of gonadotropin secretion. First, as a result of its negative feedback effects upon gonadotropin secretion, the secretion of estrogen by the maturing follicle suppresses FSH secretion and further maturation of preantral follicles to the preovulatory stage is prevented [20]. Second, as a result of its positive feedback effects on gonadotropin secretion, the continued rise in estrogen production by the maturing follicle triggers the midcycle gonadotropin surge which results in the ovulation of the Graafian follicle [21]. Thus, estrogen is a pivotal messenger that conveys information between the ovary and the hypothalamic pituitary axis. First, the early rise in estrogen production during the midfollicular phase is the mechanism by which the ovary informs the hypothalamic-pituitary axis that a follicle has been selected and the resultant suppression of FSH secretion prevents the maturation of additional preovulatory follicles. Second, the continuous increase in estrogen production by the maturing follicle is the mechanism by which the ovary tells the hypothalamic-pituitary axis that there is a mature follicle that is ready to ovulate and the resultant positive feedback stimulation in LH secretion results in the ovulation of the follicle and its transition into a corpus luteum.

The concept of an FSH threshold in the selection of a single preovulatory follicle

As mentioned previously, the studies of Brown and his co-workers demonstrated that the initiation of preovulatory follicular growth in humans occurs within a very narrow range in FSH concentrations, such that a 10—30% increment in the dosage of exogenous FSH is sufficient to initiate preovulatory follicular development. This "threshold" concept not only appears to explain the initiation of preovulatory follicular development, but also the physiological mechanism responsible for the selection of a single preovulatory follicle. The important concept regarding the threshold theory for follicular development is that the "threshold" FSH concentration is not a constant value, but rather the requirements of the maturing follicle for FSH changes as follicular development proceeds, such that the concentration of FSH required to maintain preovulatory follicular development is less than the concentration of FSH necessary to initiate follicular growth. This was demonstrated in cynomolgus monkeys in which plasma gonadotropin concentrations were regulated precisely by

---

Fig. 1. Demonstration of the threshold concept for gonadotropic stimulation of preovulatory follicular development in cynomolgus monkeys. The shaded areas depict serum concentrations of FSH, LH and estradiol in control animals which received pulsatile infusions of human FSH and LH on an hourly basis, calculated to yield plasma FSH and LH concentrations of 8—10 mIU/ml and 10—15 mIU/ml, respectively. When plasma FSH concentrations were kept at approximately 10 mIU/ml for a period of 14 days, there was no evidence of estrogen production and histological observation of ovaries at the termination of the experiment did not reveal the presence of any large antral follicles. In contrast, as shown by the line graph, in animals in which plasma FSH concentrations were progressively increased by increasing the concentration of FSH in the infusate, estrogen secretion became evident when plasma FSH concentrations were 15—20 mIU/ml. After estrogen production was evident, reducing plasma FSH concentrations by 12.5% per day over the next 5 days was associated with continued increases in estrogen secretion; at the termination of the experiment, histological examination of ovaries revealed the presence of large preovulatory follicles, the number of which was dependent on the duration that plasma FSH concentrations were maintained at 15—20 mIU/ml. These results demonstrate that the concentration of FSH necessary to initiate preovulatory follicular development is greater than that required to maintain preovulatory follicular growth and thus explains why the maturing follicle continues to develop in the presence of FSH concentrations that are insufficient to initiate the maturation of other follicles. This figure is reproduced from reference [22], which presents the complete details of the experiment.

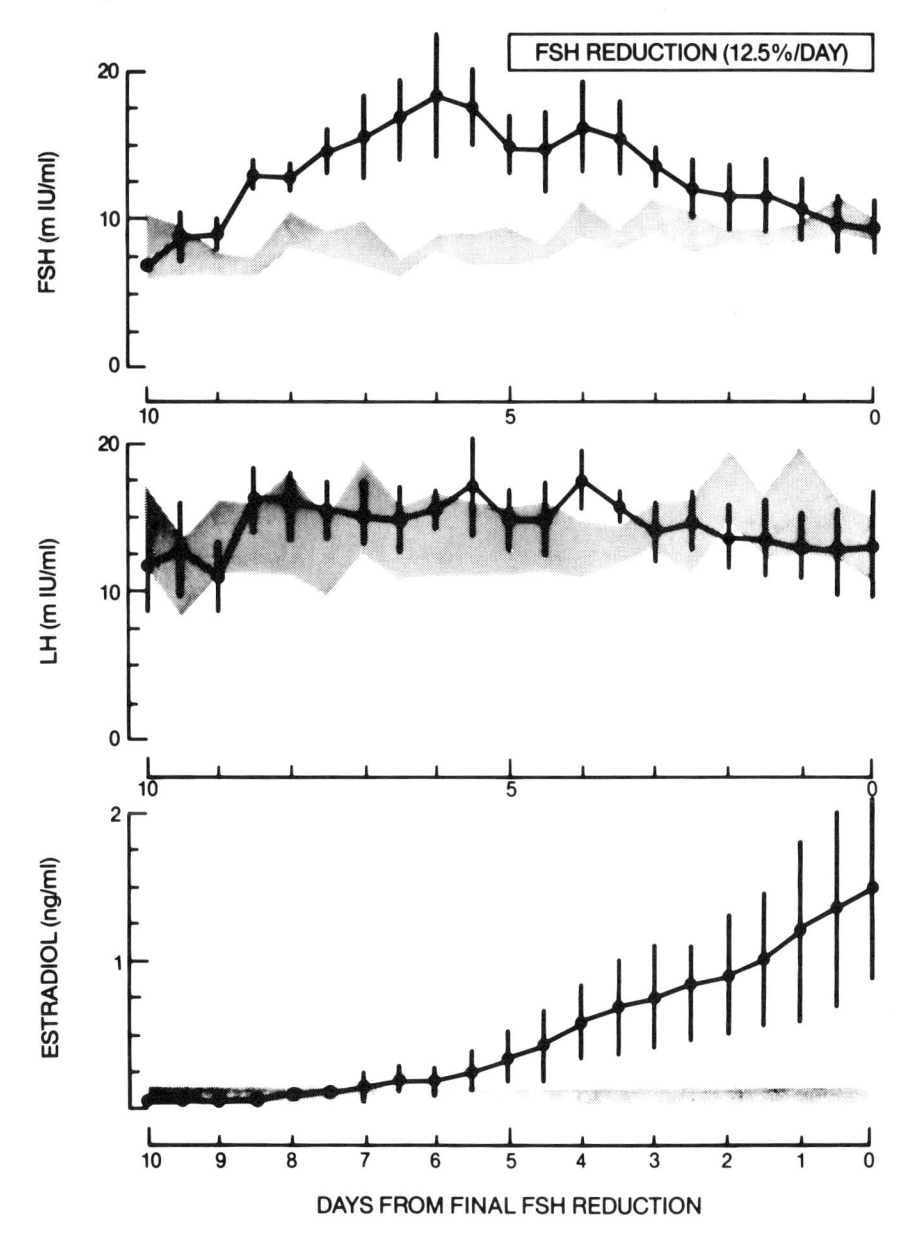

the pulsatile infusion of exogenous FSH and LH [22]. Results from these studies are reproduced in Fig. 1. The shaded areas depict results from control animals in which the absolute concentration of FSH was maintained at 8–10 mIU/ml and LH concentrations at 10–15 mIU/ml throughout a 14-day period. As can be seen, there was no evidence of estrogen secretion in the control animals, thus demonstrating that concentrations of FSH ≤10 mIU/ml are unable to initiate preovulatory follicular development. However, as shown by the solid lines, when FSH concentrations were elevated to 15—20 mIU/ml, preovulatory follicular development was initiated as reflected by increasing concentrations of estrogen. Moreover, once preovulatory follicular growth was stimulated by FSH, a 50% reduction of plasma FSH concentrations back to 8—10 mIU/ml over a 5-day period was associated with a continued rise in estrogen production. These data thus demonstrate that the concentration of FSH necessary to initiate follicular growth is greater than the concentration required to maintain preovulatory follicular growth. These data show that there is a threshold concentration of FSH (15—20 mIU/ml) that must be reached in order to initiate preovulatory follicle development. Once this threshold concentration is reached, follicles readily enter the final stages of preovulatory follicle growth and the number of follicles that reach maturity is dependent upon the duration that FSH concentrations are maintained above the threshold level, rather than the absolute concentration of FSH [22]. This experimentally determined threshold concentration of FSH is very close to the actual concentration of FSH measured during the early follicular phase of the human menstrual cycle when the initiation of preovulatory follicular development occurs [16].

Mechanisms by which the maturing follicle acquires increased sensitivity to FSH

The concept of a diminishing requirement for FSH as follicular development proceeds requires a physiological explanation that accounts for the mechanisms by which the maturing follicle becomes less dependent upon FSH. The answer to this problem likely involves one or more of the cellular changes that the follicle undergoes as a consequence of FSH stimulation. One possible explanation for this phenomenon is the FSH-mediated induction of LH receptors on granulosa cells [4]. As previously mentioned, one hallmark effect of FSH on the maturing follicle is to induce LH receptors on granulosa cells. Studies have shown that both FSH and LH act via the cAMP system and that granulosa cells with both FSH and LH receptors respond identically to both hormones [23]. Therefore, the acquisition of LH receptors on the granulosa cells of the maturing follicle would provide that follicle with the capacity to respond to both FSH and LH. Because the effects of FSH and LH at submaximal hormone concentrations are additive, granulosa cells with both FSH and LH receptors would have a greater number of "cAMP-generating" units than follicles of lesser maturity that only have FSH receptors. Moreover, the reduction in FSH secretion that occurs during the midfollicular phase as a result of the secretion of estrogen by the maturing follicle would deprive less mature follicles of their sole source of gonadotropic support (because they only have FSH receptors), while the maturing follicle may be spared from the reduced FSH concentrations by having developed the capacity to respond to LH. In addition to the induction of LH receptors, other changes such as increased vascularity as well as autocrine and paracrine agents could also increase the sensitivity of the maturing follicle to FSH [24,25].

Future investigation

The advent of pure gonadotropins by recombinant DNA technology will soon make it possible to directly test the hypothesis that the mature follicle is spared from the fall in FSH by developing the capacity to respond to LH. Should this prove to be a correct hypothesis, it is likely that novel regimens of gonadotropin treatment for induction of ovulation could be developed. In this regard, an important question that must be answered is at what size a follicle begins to exhibit a reduced requirement for FSH. Continued improvements in ovarian ultrasonography should provide this answer which may then make it possible to directly "select" the number of follicles that mature to the preovulatory stage. Lastly, the "threshold FSH concept" for follicular development may provide novel information on the pathophysiology of altered ovarian function such as polycystic ovarian disease. Careful dose/response studies in which the ovarian sensitivity to FSH is titrated by progressive increases in administration of FSH should answer the question if this disorder is caused by altered FSH responsiveness of early antral follicles.

References

1. Greep RO, van Dyke HB, Chow BF. Endocrinology 1942;30:635–649.
2. Armstrong DF, Papkoff H. Endocrinology 1976;99:1144–1151.
3. Hillier SG. In: Hillier SG (ed) Ovarian Endocrinology. Oxford: Blackwell Scientific Publications, 1991;25–72.
4. Zeleznik AJ, Midgley AR Jr, Reichert LE Jr. Endocrinology 1974;95:818–825.
5. Gemzell C. Recent Prog Horm Res 1965;21:179–204.
6. Knobil E, Kostyo JL, Greep RO. Endocrinology 1959;65:487–493.
7. Van Wagenen G. Fertil Steril 1968;19:15–29.
8. Brown JB. Aust NZ J Obstet Gynaecol 1978;18:46–54.
9. Zeleznik AJ. In: Adashi EY, Leung PCK (eds) The Ovary. New York: Raven Press, 1993;41–55.
10. Zeleznik AJ, Benyo DF. In: Knobil E, Neill JD (eds) The Physiology of Reproduction, 2nd Edn, vol 2. New York: Raven Press, 1993;751–782.
11. Gougeon A. Hum Reprod 1986;1:81–87.
12. Block E. Acta Endocrinol (Copenh) 1951;8:33–54.
13. Koering MJ. Am J Anat 1969;126:73–101.
14. Schoot DC, Coelingh Bennink HJT, Mannaerts BM, Lamberts SW, Bouchard P, Fauser BC. J Clin Endocrinol Metab 1992;74:1471–1473.
15. Zeleznik AJ, Resko JA. Endocrinology 1980;106:1820–1826.
16. Ross GT, Cargille CM, Lipsett MB, Rayford PL, Marshall JR, Strott CA, Rodbard D. Rec Prog Horm Res 1970;26:1–62.
17. Baird DT, Baker TG, McNatty KP, Neal P. J Reprod Fertil 1975;45:611–619.
18. Zeleznik AJ, Hutchison JS, Schuler HM. J Reprod Fertil 1987;80:403–410.
19. LeNestor E, Marraoui J, Lahlou N, Roger M, DeZeigler D, Bouchard P. J Clin Endocrinol Metab 1993;77:439–442.
20. Zeleznik AJ. Endocrinology 1981;109:352–355.
21. Knobil E. Rec Prog Horm Res 1974;30:1–46.
22. Zeleznik AJ, Kubik CJ. Endocrinology 1986;119:2025–2032.
23. Zeleznik AJ, Hillier SG. Clin Obstet Gynecol 1984;27:927–940.

24. Ravindranath N, Little-Ihrig LL, Phillips HS, Ferrara N, Zeleznik AJ. Endocrinology 1992;131:254–260.
25. Hillier SG. Sem Reprod Endocrinol 1991;9:332–340.

Nongonadotropic regulation of ovarian function

Nongonadotropic regulation of ovarian function: roles of follicular sex steroids

Stephen G. Hillier

Reproductive Endocrinology Laboratory, Department of Obstetrics and Gynaecology, University of Edinburgh, 37 Chalmers Street, Edinburgh EH3 9EW, UK

Abstract. The endocrine regulation of folliculogenesis is supported by nongonadotropic (paracrine) regulation. Follicle-stimulating hormone (FSH) stimulates granulosa cell proliferation and differentiation — hence follicular growth and estradiol synthesis. Response to FSH is subject to secondary regulation by androgens and nonsteroidal factors of LH-stimulated thecal origin. Factors like inhibin produced by FSH-stimulated granulosa cells exert reciprocal control over thecal androgen synthesis. Interfollicular differences in degree of paracrine signalling ultimately determine (select) the preovulatory follicle. Locally produced estrogen (during dominance) and progesterone (during luteinization) contribute to tertiary (autocrine) regulation of granulosa cell development in the preovulatory follicle, culminating in terminally differentiated functions in the corpus luteum.

The ovarian cycle — follicular maturation, ovulation and luteinisation — is fundamental to reproduction, and understanding its regulation is central to developing improved methods of enhancing (assisted reproduction) or suppressing (contraception) fertility. In the gonadotropic regulation of ovarian function, follicle-stimulating hormone (FSH) provides the primary endocrine drive to folliculogenesis through the activation of cyclic-AMP mediated postreceptor signalling in immature granulosa cells. However, there is increasing evidence that functional and morphological responses to FSH are also subject to secondary (paracrine) regulation by androgens and nonsteroidal factors produced by thecal cells in response to tonic stimulation by luteinizing hormone (LH). Conversely, steroids and growth factors originating in FSH-stimulated granulosa cells exert paracrine control of the theca. Interfollicular variations in the operation of this paracrine system seem likely to determine which follicle is selected to ovulate in each menstrual cycle. The emerging concept of nongonadotropic regulation of ovarian function is surveyed here, emphasizing roles for locally produced sex steroids [reviews: 1–4].

Theca-derived paracrine control

The theca interna produces various steroidal and nonsteroidal factors that are likely to influence granulosa cell function in vivo. The particular steroidogenic enzyme necessary for androgen synthesis is 17-hydroxylase/C_{17-20} lyase (cytochrome $P450_{C17}$), which is present and functionally coupled to LH receptors in thecal cells. $P450_{C17}$ is positively regulated by LH and modulated by paracrine factors produced by FSH-stimulated granulosa cells (see below). Besides serving as the obligatory precursor for estrogen synthesis, theca-derived androstenedione is locally metabolized to testosterone and other androgens able to augment the cytodifferentiative actions of FSH on granulosa cells [5]. This regulatory action is mediated via specific androgen receptors and entails amplification of cyclic AMP-mediated intracellular signalling leading to increased expression of various genes crucial to preovulatory follicular function. Aromatase (cytochrome $P450_{arom}$) activity and inhibin production are conspicuous among the FSH-inducible granulosa cell functions promoted by androgens in vitro. Conversely, and intriguingly, inhibin promotes LH-dependent thecal androgen synthesis in vitro. Thus the potential exists for a reciprocal interaction between granulosa-derived inhibin and theca-derived androgen, which may give rise to the development-related increases in estrogen biosynthesis that occur in the preovulatory follicle [6,7].

Many polypeptide growth factors are also produced by thecal-interstitial cells, including insulin-like growth factors (IGFs) and IGF-binding protein (IGF-BPs), transforming growth factor (TGF)-α and TGF-β [8—11]. It is not clear whether thecal production of such proteins is subject to endocrine control by LH, but they are inevitably part of the theca-granulosa dialogue that coordinates cellular proliferation and differentiation in the follicle wall.

Granulosa-derived paracrine control

The induction of granulosa cell differentiation by FSH is associated with increased production of diverse steroidal and nonsteroidal factors with putative paracrine and/or autocrine functions. Other than estrogen itself, relevant factors about which our knowledge has increased include IGFs [12], inhibin, activin and follistatin [4].

The raised follicular fluid estrogen level in the preovulatory follicle is generally assumed to contribute to the local mechanism whereby a single preovulatory follicle is selected to ovulate in the human menstrual cycle. However, this assumption is largely based on the evidence that estrogens augment FSH action in rat granulosa cells [2,3]. There is no direct evidence to support such an action of estrogen in human granulosa cells, and evidence to date that estrogen receptors are present in human and nonhuman primate granulosa cells has been unconvincing [13—15]. Granulosa-derived estrogen is, however, implicated as a negative regulator of thecal cell function and may be involved in the suppression of thecal androgen synthesis that occurs at the midcycle LH surge [16].

There is increasing evidence that stimulatory effects of FSH on granulosa cell growth and differentiation are augmented by locally produced IGFs [8,12]. The IGFs are low molecular weight single-chain peptides which share considerable structural and functional homologies with proinsulin. IGF-I and IGF-II each crossreact with the insulin receptor and receptors for insulin and both factors are present on most cells, including thecal and granulosa cells in the human ovary. Receptors for insulin and IGF-I also share structural and functional similarities, including intracellular signalling involving tyrosine kinases [17]. Both types of IGF exert endocrine effects on tissue growth throughout the body, being secreted by the liver under the control of growth hormone. IGFs are also synthesized and act locally in various tissues other than gonads, including muscle and bone.

Granulosa cells express IGF-I receptors that increase in number following treatment with FSH. Stimulation by FSH of steroidogenesis, LH-receptors, deposition of proteoglycans, and responsiveness to β-adrenergic agonists are all augmented by the presence of physiological concentrations of IGF-I or supraphysiological concentrations of insulin in granulosa cell culture medium. The action of IGF-I on FSH-induced cytodifferentiation entails amplification of intracellular cyclic AMP action by a mechanism which is not yet understood [8,12,16].

Granulosa cells also express IGF mRNA(s) and produce IGF protein(s) regulated by gonadotropins [8,12,18–20]. Specific IGF-binding proteins – thought likely to participate in local responses to IGF – are also produced in granulosa cells. Thus there is a wealth of experimental evidence to propose that granulosa cell growth and differentiation are subject to autocrine and/or paracrine control by IGFs [21,22].

Human thecal cells express IGF-I mRNA at low abundance but are richly endowed with insulin and IGF-type-I receptors [19,23]. Both basal and LH-stimulated synthesis of androgen in cultured thecal/interstitial cells are enhanced by the presence of insulin or IGF-I [24–26]. Under serum-free conditions of culture, IGF-I has a striking ability to enhance DNA synthesis as well androgen synthesis in human thecal cell monolayers [27]. Human granulosa cells do not appear to produce IGF-I. However, they may produce IGF-II, since the expression of IGF-II mRNA is upregulated by gonadotropins in vitro [28]. Preliminary studies indicate that IGF-I and IGF-II are similarly potent stimuli of human thecal androgen synthesis in vitro (S.G. Hillier et al., unpublished), in which case IGF-II of granulosa cell origin could exert positive paracrine control over the growth and steroidogenic function of the theca interna.

Inhibin/activin genes are developmentally regulated in granulosa cells in a manner that serves to coordinate and reinforce the endocrine functions of FSH and LH. In both primate [29] and rodent [30] ovaries, expression of inhibin/activin β-subunit mRNAs is relatively abundant in the granulosa cells of immature antral follicles as compared with the cells of larger, presumptive preovulatory follicles [31]. Conversely, inhibin α-subunit mRNA expression increases during preovulatory development, persisting at a relatively high level after ovulation in both human [32] and nonhuman [33] primate corpora lutea. This pattern of inhibin/activin gene expression would be expected to give rise to a relatively high level of ββ homodimeric protein (activin) formation in immature follicles with the heterodimeric αβ congener (inhibin) predominating in preovulatory follicles. It follows that the activin "tone" of the developing follicle declines as its inhibin "tone" increases. This has implications for the involvement of inhibin and activin in paracrine signalling, as considered below [6,29].

In vitro measurements of immunoactive inhibin protein confirm that human and nonhuman primate granulosa cells undertake development-related increases in α-inhibin subunit production [review: 34]. Secretion of inhibin protein by rat, bovine, human and nonhuman primate granulosa cells is regulated by gonadotropins and sex steroids in vitro. Immunoactive inhibin production by human granulosa cells is inducible by FSH and increases during preovulatory development. Onset of LH-responsive inhibin production coincides with increased granulosa cell aromatase activity, which has particular significance to the paracrine regulation of estrogen biosynthesis (see below). Development-related patterns of granulosa cell activin production have not been determined, due to the lack of suitably specific or sensitive assays.

There is in vitro experimental evidence that both inhibin and activin can act directly to modulate androgen synthesis in the theca interna. Treatment of cultured human thecal cells with recombinant activin-A potently inhibits stimulation of androgen (androstenedione, dihydroepiandrosterone and testosterone) production by LH and IGF-I [35]. Conversely, picomolar amounts of recombinant inhibin-A markedly augment LH/IGF-stimulated androgen production. Inhibin also dose-dependently overrides the inhibitory action of activin on androgen synthesis in rat and human thecal cells. The capacity of inhibin and activin to modulate C_{19} steroid production in vitro suggests action at the level of cytochrome $P450_{C17}$. Such experimental data support the concept of activin and inhibin as selective paracrine modulators of thecal androgen (and hence follicular estrogen) synthesis in the human ovary [34]. According to the paracrine inhibin hypothesis, increased production of inhibin accompanying FSH-induction of aromatase activity would provide a mechanism through which granulosa cells in the dominant follicle could locally up-regulate thecal androgen production, thereby sustaining the uniquely high rate of estrogen biosynthesis that occurs in the preovulatory follicle.

Activin is also a potential autocrine modulator of the aromatisation of androgen in granulosa cells. Potent augmentation by activin of FSH-inducible aromatase activity has been convincingly demonstrated both in rat [36] and nonhuman primate [37] granulosa cells in vitro. Stimulatory effects of activin on FSH receptor levels have also been reported [38,39]. Intriguingly, activin augments FSH-induced progesterone production in immature (i.e., LH-nonresponsive) granulosa cells, but in more mature, LH-responsive cells activin inhibits progesterone synthesis [36,37]. Activin also inhibits steroidogenesis in human granulosa-lutein cells [40,41]. The mechanism of this development-dependent switch from stimulation to inhibition of steroidogenesis by activin remains to be established, but these findings raise the possibility that activin has a physiological function in preventing premature luteinisation.

It is uncertain if inhibin is a physiologically relevant regulator of granulosa cell steroidogenesis. Studies on rat [38] and nonhuman primate [39] granulosa cell cultures showed no effect of recombinant human inhibin-A on basal or gonadotropin-responsive steroid synthesis at concentrations up to 10 ng/ml. At 100 ng/ml, weak (<10%) inhibition was occasionally observed. The ~25 kDa free inhibin α-subunit purified from bovine follicular fluid was similarly inactive (F. Miró and S.G. Hillier, unpublished).

Follistatin is an activin-binding protein that blocks activin action in vitro. This property qualifies follistatin as a potentially important intraovarian regulator along with activin and inhibin [reviews: 4,29]. Granulosa cell follistatin mRNA levels increase with preovulatory follicular development. Immunoactive follistatin production by rat and bovine granulosa cells is stimulated by FSH, but not LH, in vitro. The protein is expressed abundantly in the granulosa cells of healthy antral follicles, and the level of expression increases with preovulatory follicular development. Since follistatin functions as an activin-binding protein, this pattern of gene expression would be expected to bring about a progressive suppression of residual activin action within the preovulatory follicle. Consistent with its role as an activin-binding protein, follistatin inhibits the stimulatory action of activin on FSH-induced granulosa cell differentiation at all levels examined, including morphology, expression of FSH and LH receptors, and production of estradiol, progesterone and inhibin [4]. Effects of follistatin on thecal androgen synthesis have not been reported but blockade of the inhibitory action of activin is predictable.

Paracrine steroid action

Follicular steroids are prototypic ovarian paracrine regulators — long known to be present — are locally synthesized and have receptor-mediated effects within developing follicles [reviews: 1—3,5].

Cell-specific changes in steroid receptor expression may provide a mechanism through which granulosa and thecal cells respond differentially to follicular sex steroids. Steroid receptors are ligand-regulated transcription factors belonging to a nuclear receptor "superfamily", members of which have molecular structures that are organized into three functional domains comprising a variable N-terminal transactivation region, a highly conserved cysteine-rich DNA binding domain containing two zinc fingers, and a less well conserved C-terminal domain for steroid binding [reviews: 42,43].

Rat granulosa cells abundantly express androgen receptor mRNA (I.M.Turner, S.G. Hillier, unpublished), but contain little or no estrogen receptor mRNA [44]. Based on this and other evidence that nonhuman primate [45] and human granulosa cells possess androgen receptors [15], whereas estrogen receptors are absent or only weakly detectable [13,14], we propose that androgens are major paracrine regulators of granulosa cell function in the ovarian follicle [46]. Recent studies also point to an autocrine role for granulosa cell progesterone in mediating the luteotropic action of LH on the preovulatory follicle [47,48]. Because androgens and progestogens have intrafollicular regulatory functions and steroidal drugs that have syn/antiandrogenic or progestogenic properties are in widespread gynecological use it is of obvious importance to understand the molecular mechanisms through which these substances act within the ovaries.

Regulatory androgen

Androgens produced by thecal cells cross the lamina basalis, penetrate the granulosa cell layer and accumulate in follicular fluid. The granulosa cell layer is literally drenched in androgen throughout most of the preovulatory follicle's antral phase of development. Although there is experimental evidence for involvement of androgens in follicular atresia, androgen levels in follicular fluid of atretic follicles do not differ markedly from those in healthy follicles of a comparable size [reviews: 5,46]. Depending on the stage of development controlled by FSH, granulosa cells express enzymes which interconvert androstenedione and other steroids with potential regulatory functions in the follicle wall, including testosterone, 5α-reduced androgens, estradiol and catechol estrogens. FSH-induced differentiation of cultured granulosa cells is modulated by the presence of androgens at concentrations found in follicular fluid. Receptor-mediated androgen action in granulosa cells leads to increased generation of extracellular cyclic AMP and an attendant amplification of the cyclic AMP-dependent biochemical processes initiated by FSH. Androgens active in this regard include testosterone and androstenedione as well as their non-aromatizable 5α-reduced metabolites. The net effect is enhanced granulosa cell responsiveness to FSH, suggesting a role for locally produced androgens in modulating follicular threshold requirements for stimulation by FSH during preovulatory follicular selection.

Treatment with androgen in vitro has been shown to suppress the gonadotropin responsiveness of mature (LH-responsive) granulosa cells from nonhuman primate ovaries [50]. The mechanism of androgen action in granulosa cells at such advanced stages of differentiation is difficult to assess, since aromatization reduces the potential for direct effects of androgen. On the other hand, 5α-reduced androgen metabolites may be produced that are androgens in their own right as well as being competitive aromatase inhibitors [51]. Recent in vivo studies have shown that testosterone is metabolized to 5α-reduced androgens in human preovulatory follicles [52]. Two 5α-reductase isozymes encoded by two different genes, types 1 and 2, have been identified [53,54], which show different tissue-specific and developmental expression patterns in male secondary tissues. However, nothing is known of their temporal or spatial distribution in the ovary. Whether development-related changes in androgen action are due to changes in the expression of androgen receptors or alterations in the metabolism of Δ^4-3-oxo androgens such as testosterone and androstenedione to 5α-reduced compounds (e.g., 5α-dihydrotestosterone and androsterone) with different biological properties has yet to be resolved. Molecular techniques are now available to allow us to determine if androgen receptor expression in the ovary is granulosa cell specific, to determine how the androgen receptor is regulated in relation to follicular development, and to determine the exact contribution made by follicular androgen to the regultion of granulosa cell function.

Regulatory estrogen

Estradiol is the most abundant intrafollicular steroid for a brief period of time before the start of the LH surge when the preovulatory phase of development is being completed. For many years, estradiol has been regarded as "the" major local regulator of granulosa cell function [reviews: 2,3,5]. Treatment of hypohysectomized immature female rats with exogenous estrogen stimulates granulosa cell mitosis, raises gonadotropin receptor levels and amplifies follicular responsiveness to exogenous FSH. At the cellular level, estrogen augments FSH-induced expression of the regulatory subunit RIIβ of type II cyclic AMP-dependent protein kinase and the steroidogenic enzymes $P450_{arom}$ and $P450_{SCC}$. Estrogen also stimulates expression of inhibin α- and β-subunit mRNAs and augments FSH-induced inhibin production by cultured rat granulosa cells. Although rodent granulosa cells contain proteins with ligand-binding properties similar to estrogen receptors [reviews: 2,55], it is not clear that the estrogen receptor gene is expressed, based on Northern analysis of granulosa cell total RNA [44]. Estrogen action in granulosa cells could at least partly be explained by crossreaction of estrogen with the androgen receptors present in these cells [5]. Moreover, estrogens may be metabolized to catechol estrogens in granulosa cells, and estradiol metabolites such as 2-hydroxyestradiol potently augment FSH action on rodent immature granulosa cells in vitro [review: 46]. It is of interest that regulatory actions of catechol estradiol in rat granulosa cells are susceptible to antiandrogenic blockade [46] — further implicating the androgen receptor system in mediating regulatory actions of estrogen.

Raised estrogen levels in follicular fluid are thought to be part of the local mechanism governing preovulatory follicular selection [review: 1]. Although there is no direct evidence to support regulatory estrogen action in human granulosa cells based on an absence of measurable estrogen receptor mRNA [16] and lack of measurable estrogen effect in vitro [56], aromatase activity and follicular fluid estradiol levels increase during preovulatory follicular development and correlate positively with with follicular "health" [57]. Once selected, the preovulatory follicle is presumed to be developmentally favored through a local positive feedback loop by which estrogen promotes granulosa cell proliferation and responsiveness to FSH and LH. Granulosa-derived estrogen is also implicated as a paracrine negative regulator of thecal cell function and may be involved in the suppression of thecal androgen synthesis in response to the midcycle LH surge. Although estrogen receptor mRNA transcripts in human granulosa-lutein cells were undetectable after reverse transcriptase and amplification by polymerase chain reaction [16], low abundance estrogen receptor mRNA transcripts were revealed in cumulus/oocyte masses and isolated oocytes [16]. Estrogen may therefore directly influence oocyte maturation in the human ovary. However, it may not be essential, since stimulation of multiple preovulatory follicular development with exogenous gonadotropins, collection of mature ooocytes and fertilisation in vitro have been achieved in a woman congenitally deficient in 17-hydroxylase, and hence unable to biosynthesise estrogens [58].

Regulatory progesterone

The life cycle of a preovulatory follicle terminates in a hyperprogestogenic state when C_{21} compounds are quantitatively the most important class of sex steroid that is synthesized, accumulated and secreted [5]. Several lines of evidence suggest that locally produced progesterone affects ovulation and luteinization through influencing prostaglandin production and activating proteases that digest the follicle wall prior to its rupture [review: 59]. Recently, it was shown that rat granulosa cells express increased levels of progesterone receptor coincident with increased expression of prostaglandin synthase in response to an ovulation-inducing injection of human chorionic gonadotropin (HCG) [49]. Progesterone receptors have also been demonstrated immunocytochemically in nonhuman primate granulosa-lutein cells [60]. Autocrine action via progesterone receptors may be a crucial component of the ovulatory response to LH/HCG, since functional and morphological luteinization in vitro can be blocked by the presence of antiprogestins such as RU486 [47–49]. At least three types of signal transduction system (protein kinase-A, protein kinase-C and tyrosine kinase) mediate LH action on granulosa-lutein cells, and all three have been implicated in progesterone action [61]. Development-related changes in the expression of receptors for progesterone and any other regulatory factor(s) utilizing these signal transduction pathways could therefore be integral to luteinization. The corpus luteum also contains progesterone receptors [13], however, a specific progesterone-regulated luteal cell function has not been described. Paradoxically, since the life span of the corpus luteum is thought to be defined by subcellular events set in motion at the ovulation-inducing LH surge [62], regulatory progesterone action could ultimately explain the initiation of luteolysis.

References

1. Hsueh AJW, Adashi EY, Jones PBC, Welsh Jr TJ. Endocrine Rev 1984;5:76–126.
2. Richards JS, Jahnsen T, Hedin L, Lifka J, Ratoosh SL, Durica JM, Goldring, NB. Recent Prog Horm Res 1987;43:231–270.
3. Hillier SG. In: Hillier SG (ed) Ovarian Endocrinology. London: Blackwell Scientific Publications, 1991;73–106.
4. Findlay JK. Biol Reprod 1993;48:15–23.
5. Hillier SG. Oxford Rev Reprod Biol 1985;7:168–222.
6. Hillier SG. J Endocrinol 1991;131:171–175.
7. Hillier SG, Turner IM. In: Gibori G (ed) Signaling Mechanisms and Gene Expression in the Ovary (proceedings of the VIIIth ovarian workshop). New York: Springer-Verlag, 1991;84–96.
8. Adashi EY, Resnick CE, Hurwitz A, Ricciarelli E, Hernandez ER, Roberts CT, Leroith D, Rosenfeld R. Hum Reprod 1991;6:1213–1219.
9. Kudlow JE, Kobrin MS, Purchio AF, Twardzik DR, Hernandez ER, Asa SL, Adashi EY. Endocrinology 1987;121:1577–1579.
10. Chegini N, Flanders KC. Endocrinology 1992;130:1707–1715.
11. Sakal E, Gertler A, Aflalo L, Meidan R. Mol Cell Endocrinol 1992;90:39–46.
12. Hammond JM, Hsu C-J, Mondschein JS, Canning SH. J Anim Sci. 1988;66(suppl 2):21–31.
13. Hild-Petito S, Stouffer RL, Brenner RM. Endocrinology 1988;123:2896–2905.

14. Horie K, Takakura K, Fujiwara H, Suginami H, Liao S, Mori T. Hum Reprod 1992;7:184–190.
15. Wu T-CJ, Wang L, Wan Y-JY. Fertil Steril 1993;59:54–59.
16. Erickson GF, Magoffin DA, Dyer CA, Hofeditz C. Endocrine Rev 1985;6:371–399.
17. Giudice LC. Endocrine Rev 1992;13:641–669.
18. Oliver JE, Aitman TJ, Powell JF, Wilson CA, Clayton RN. Endocrinology 1989;124:2671–2679.
19. Hernandez ER, Hurwitz A, Vera A, Pellicer A, Adashi EY, LeRoith D, Roberts Jr, CR. J Clin Endocrinol Metab 1992;74:419–425.
20. Zhou J, Bondy C. Biol Reprod 1993;48:467–482.
21. Adashi EY, Resnick CE, Hernandez E, Hurwitz A, Ricciarelli E, Hernandez ER, Rosenfeld RG. Endocrinology 1991;128:754–760.
22. Samaras SE, Hagen DR, Shimasaki S, Ling N, Hammond JM. Endocrinology 1992;130:2739–2744.
23. Bergh C, Olsson JH, Carlsson B, Selleskog U, Hillensjö T. Fertil Steril 1992;59:323–331.
24. Barbieri RL, Makris A, Randall RW, Daniels G, Kistner RW, Ryan KJ. J Clin Endocrinol Metab 1986;62:904–910.
25. Hernandez ER, Resnick CE, Svoboda ME, Van Wyk JJ, Payne DW, Adashi EY. Endocrinology 1988;122:1603–1612.
26. Cara JF, Rosenfield RL. Endocrinology 1989;123:733–739.
27. Hillier SG, Yong EL, Illingworth PI, Baird DT, Schwall RH, Mason AJ. J Clin Endocrinol Metab 1991;72:1206–1211.
28. Voutilainen R, Miller WL. Proc Natl Acad Sci USA 1987;84:1590–1594.
29. Hillier SG. In: Findlay JK (ed) Molecular Biology of the Female Reproductive System. New York: Academic Press, 1994;1–37.
30. Schwall RH, Mason AJ, Wilcox JN, Bassett SG, Zeleznik AJ. Mol endocrinol 1990;4:75–79.
31. Meunier H, Cajander SB, Roberts HJ, Rivier C, Sawchenko P, Hsueh AJW, Vale W. Mol Endocrinol 1988;2:1352–1363.
32. Davis SR, McLachlan RI, Burger HG. J Endocrinol 1987;115:R21–R23.
33. Hillier SG, Wickings EJ, Saunders PTK, Shimasaki S, Reichert Jr LE, McNeilly AS. J Endocrinol 1989;123:65–73.
34. Hillier SG, Miró F. Ann NY Acad Sci 1993;687:29–38.
35. Hillier SG, Yong EL, Illingworth PI, Baird DT, Schwall RH, Mason AJ. Mol Cell Endocrinol 1991; 75:R1–R6 (corrigendum 79:177).
36. Miró F, Hillier SG. J Clin Endocrinol Metab 1992;75:1556–1561.
37. Miró F, Smyth CD, Hillier SG. Endocrinology 1991;129:3388–3394.
38. Xiao S, Robertson DM, Findlay JK. Endocrinology 1992;131:1009–1016.
39. Nakamura M, Minegishi T, Hasegawa Y, Nakamura K, Igarishi S, Ito I, Shinozaki H, Miyamoto K, Eto Y, Ibuki Y. Endocrinology 1993;133 538–544.
40. Li W, Yuen BH, Leung PCK. J Clin Endocrinol Metab 1992;75:285–289.
41. Rabinovici J, Spencer S, Doldi N, Goldsmith PC, Schwall R, Jaffe RB. J Clin Invest 1992;89:1528–1536.
42. Evans RM. Science 1988;240:889–895.
43. Freedman LP. Endocrine Rev 1992;13:129–145.
44. Hillier SG, Saunders PTK, White R, Parker MG. J Mol Endocrinol 1989;2:39–45.
45. Hild-Petito S, West NB, Brenner RM, Stouffer RL. Biol Reprod 1991;44:561–568.
46. Hillier SG. J Steroid Biochem 1987;27:351–357.
47. Iwai M, Yasuda K, Fukuoka M, Iwai T, Takahura K, Taii S, Nakanishi S, Mori T. Endocrinology 1991;129:1621–1627.
48. Park O-K, Mayo K. Mol Endocrinol 1991;5:967–978.
49. Natra U, Richards JS. Endocrinology 1993;133:761–769.
50. Harlow CR, Shaw HJ, Hillier SG, Hodges JK. Endocrinology 1988;122:2780–2787.
51. Hillier SG, van den Boogaard AJM, Reichert Jr LE, van Hall EV. J Clin Endocrinol Metab 1980; 50:640–647.

52. Haning Jr RV, Hackett RJ, Flood CA, Loughlin JS, Zhao QY, Longcope C. J Clin Endocrinol Metab 1993;77:710—715.
53. Normington K, Russell DW. J Biol Chem 1992;267:19548—19554.
54. Thigpen AE, Silver RI, Guileyardo JM, Casey ML, McConnell JD, Russell DW. J Clin Invest 1993; 92:903—910.
55. Richards JS. Physiol Rev 1980;60:51—69.
56. Hillier SG, Wickings EJ, Illingworth PJ, Yong EL, Reichert Jr LE, Baird DT, McNeilly AS. Clin Endocrinol 1991;35:71—78.
57. McNatty KP. Aust J Biol Sci 1981;34:249—268.
58. Rabinovici J, Blankstein J, Goldman B, Rudak E, Dor Y, Pariente C, Geier A, Lunenefeld B, Mashiach S. J Clin Endocrinol Metab 1989;68:693—697.
59. Brannstrom M, Janson PO. In: Hillier SG (ed) Ovarian Endocrinology. London: Blackwell Scientific Publications, 1991;132—166.
60. Zelinski-Wooten MB, Hess DL, Baughman WL, Molskness TA, Wolf DP, Stouffer RL. J Clin Endocrinol Metab 1993;76:988—995.
61. Morris JK, Richards JS. Endocrinology 1993;133:770—779.
62. Fisch B, Margara RA, Winston RLM, Hillier SG. J Endocrinol 1989;122:303—311.

The effect of exogenous recombinant human activin A on pituitary and ovarian hormone secretion and ovarian folliculogenesis in female rats and monkeys

Teresa K. Woodruff[1*], Theodore A. Molskness[2], Kristine D. Dahl[3], Jennie P. Mather[1] and Richard L. Stouffer[2]

[1]*Department of Cell Biology, Genentech, Inc., South San Francisco, CA 94080;* [2]*Division of Reproductive Sciences, Oregon Regional Primate Research Center, Beaverton, OR 97006; and* [3]*Department of Medicine, Veterans Administration Medical Center and University of Washington, Seattle, WA 98108, USA*

Abstract. The process of follicular maturation was explored using rh-activin A administered to rats and monkeys at various times during the reproductive cycle. In both species, the pituitary or ovarian response depends on the hormonal milieu. In the rat, local injection of recombinant human activin A (rh-activin A) results in follicular atresia, while systemic injection results in an increase in circulating follicle-stimulating hormone (FSH). In the monkey, activin injected systemically during the follicular phase causes a rise in LH. However, coincident with rh-activin A administration in the luteal phase, LH falls. This paper will explore the unifying themes which have resulted from our experiments and delineate areas for future study.

Introduction

Activin, a TGF-β superfamily member, participates in the endocrine, paracrine, and autocrine regulation of cellular growth and differentiation as well as hormone secretion [review: 1]. The activity originally assigned to activin was the stimulation of follicle-stimulating hormone (FSH) release from anterior pituitary cells. Further investigation with purified and recombinant activin and in situ mRNA localization studies implicated activin in embryonic development, neuronal survival, ovarian folliculogenesis, steroidogenesis, and hematopoiesis [review: 2]. The ability of activin to modulate multiple activities in many organs led to the hypothesis that the physiological role(s) of activin, like TGF-β, may be confined within the tissues that synthesize activin. The absence of detectable activin in serum samples during the normal ovarian cycle supports this hypothesis [3]. However, activin may circulate at levels less than the detectable limit of current immunoassays and/or may circulate in a binding protein:hormone complex.

The principal activin-binding protein is called follistatin [review: 2]. Follistatin is a single-chain, glycosylated molecule that bioneutralizes activin activity in a pituitary

---

Address for correspondence: Dr T.K. Woodruff, Genentech, Inc., 460 Pt. San Bruno Blvd., South San Francisco, CA 94080, USA

cell FSH-release bioassay and a hematopoietic cell differentiation bioassay [4]. Based on these findings, it is proposed that activin-follistatin complexes in the circulation are similarly bioinactive. This hypothesis has yet to be confirmed experimentally. In addition to its role as a bioinhibitor, follistatin may aid in the rapid elimination of activin from the circulation.

Conflicting with the local regulatory hypothesis of activin action is the presence of activin A in the maternal serum during pregnancy. Activin A is initially detected during the first trimester of pregnancy and serum concentrations reach peak levels coincident with parturition [3]. The binding protein-free activin may participate in re-establishing the nonpregnant hypothalamic-pituitary-ovarian axis, aiding in parturition or both. Elevated serum activin suggests that mechanisms of tissue-specific targeting must be in place to permit appropriate hormone activity. The presence of activin within the circulation does not preclude autocrine or paracrine mechanisms from predominating within specific tissues. It does, however, place activin in a unique subclass of the TGF-β superfamily.

Our laboratory groups have used activin, its binding protein follistatin, and the functional antagonist, inhibin, as tools of investigation. The focus of our research is to understand follicular growth dynamics, mechanisms of aberrant ovulation, and the role of ovarian and pituitary hormones in the maintenance of reproductive cyclicity. These goals have been aided by the availability of recombinant human activin A (rh-activin A) for in vitro studies and systemic and local administration to female rodents and monkeys. The present paper reviews the results of several studies designed to evaluate the effects of activin on the pituitary and ovary in two species, rats and monkeys. Perhaps not surprisingly, activin effects are dependent on the species, dose, route of administration, and time of the cycle that the hormone is delivered. Because addition of activin A in the intact animal is, by definition, pharmacological dosing, the studies described in this communication address questions of "what activin can do", but do not specifically address what activin "does" physiologically. It is hoped, however, that through these investigations additional insight will be gained about reproductive cyclicity and unifying themes uncovered regarding follicular dynamics.

Activin as a modulator of pituitary gonadotropins, ovarian steroids, and follicular maturation in the rat

In vitro, activin stimulates rat granulosa cells to produce estradiol and cAMP and rat pituitary cells to produce FSH. In an extensive review, Findlay describes the known responses of granulosa cells, in various stages of differentiation, to activin [5]. Importantly, the effect of activin on granulosa cell function depends on the stage of granulosa cell differentiation paralleling the stage-specific sequelae of events in vivo.

The effects of exogenous rh-activin A on pituitary and ovarian hormones were investigated in the rat during the estrous cycle [6]. Serum gonadotropins and ovarian steroids were monitored at frequent intervals on proestrus and metestrus, and 24 h after hormone administration on diestrus and estrus. Rh-activin A induced an increase in circulating FSH within 6 h of drug administration on both proestrus and metestrus. These data suggest that activin A is capable of modulating both basal and GnRH-stimulated FSH release in vivo. LH was unaffected on proestrus; however, a slight but significant rise in LH was noted on metestrus. The increase in LH resulted in a delay in the fall of progesterone levels on metestrus. The proestrus estradiol surge was greater following activin administration but unaffected on metestrus. These results confirm that activin stimulates ovarian estradiol and progesterone in a cycle-dependent manner. Moreover, the steroid observations suggest a requirement for signals, in addition to activin, to achieve the noted effect.

In other studies, intrabursal injection of rh-activin A resulted in widespread follicular atresia in PMSG-treated, immature rats [7]. While initially this finding seemed to contradict the in vitro results, further studies validate activin as a modulator of apoptosis (a reported means for cell death in atretic follicles [8]) and suggest potential mechanisms whereby in vitro and in vivo experimental results overlap. Schwall et al. demonstrated that high doses of rh-activin A stimulate liver apoptosis [9]. Likewise, TGF-β is known to participate in cellular apoptosis in several tissues, suggesting that the superfamily modulates cellular function in a fundamental way including decision cues for growth or death [10]. TGF-β and activin interact with highly homologous receptors generically labeled type I and type II [11,12]. The signaling pathways for the family may be quite similar and work is ongoing to delineate specific signaling pathways.

It is clear that apoptosis occurs in vivo following activin administration and that activin causes an estrogenic state in vitro. In culture, theca cells are not present, whereas a highly interregulated theca-granulosa-stroma cell consortium exists in vivo. It is likely that the cell-to-cell interactions in the ovary reflect an integrated effect of hormone. Specifically, Hillier et al. observed that activin decreases androgen production in cultured human theca cells [13]. Additionally, the primary site of iodinated activin accumulation is in the theca cells. With time (1 h) the labeled ligand does diffuse into the granulosa cells, but the major site of accumulation is retained in the theca [14]. Coupled with experimental data that activin stimulates granulosa cell estradiol production, a unifying hypothesis can be suggested. It is plausible that exogenous activin binds the theca cell and rapidly depletes the available androgen precursor by inhibiting its synthesis and turning it over to estradiol, thereby creating two cells depleted of precursor and product. Cellular death thus ensues. Studies using whole ovarian or cell cocultures may be illuminating in this regard.

Activin stimulates pituitary LH and FSH secretion, yet inhibits follicular maturation during the follicular phase of monkeys

The effect of activin on gonadotropins and steroids in the early follicular phase of the menstrual cycle immediately following menses was studied in the adult female rhesus monkey [15]. Rh-activin A was administered intravenously using two different injection schemes: twice a day for 1 day or twice a day for 7 days. Following a single activin injection, serum LH increase rapidly (within 8 h) and robustly (273% over baseline), while estradiol increased later (in 24 h) and FSH remained unchanged. Continued stimulation of the system with activin resulted in a second LH plateau at 4 days, estradiol circulating concentrations similar to midcycle levels (peaks at 2 days and 5 days) and a progressive rise in FSH (peak at 4 days) coincident with a second LH peak. Follicular development was inhibited for the course of the ensuing menstrual cycle in both dose regimens. Our in vivo data in the rat suggests that the activin may be suppressing follicular development directly; however, the increase in LH and estradiol is also likely to quell the maturation process. The enhancement of both LH and FSH was not predicted by previous studies either in culture or in the rat. One study in the male monkey, however, reported that activin A enhanced GnRH-stimulated LH and FSH release [16]. The biphasic nature of the LH response to rh-activin A may reflect an initial direct effect of activin on pituitary LH secretion, followed by a rise in LH due to the indirect interaction of other feedback hormones (e.g., estradiol).

The absence of observable follicular maturation was further investigated by direct intraovarian administration of activin into the ovary (Figs. 1A and 1B). Activin infusion for 7 days resulted not only in a hiatus in follicular maturation, but also disrupted the normal profile of pituitary gonadotropins and ovarian steroid in serum samples. In this paradigm, neither LH nor estradiol is a negative regulator of follicular maturation. This suggests that activin can participate, in a pharmacological way, in the suppression of follicular maturation. The effect appears independent of local stress, because rh-inhibin A and vehicle, administered in an identical fashion, did not disrupt the gonadotropin or steroid serum profiles (Fig. 2).

Activin suppresses LH and progesterone secretion during the luteal phase in monkeys

Luteal phase pituitary gonadotropin response was evaluated in a similar paradigm to that described above: activin was administered systemically during the midluteal phase to three adult female monkeys [17]. In all animals serum progesterone concentration immediately fell commensurate with a decrease in circulating LH, followed by an early menses. FSH was not changed under these experimental conditions. These events are likely the result of a pituitary effect or factor, since activin administered directly into the corpus luteum did not have any effect on pituitary or steroid hormones. In fact, these animals exhibited timely menses. However, activin does directly inhibit progesterone production by luteal cells in vitro which suggests that under some conditions activin may participate in ovarian function during the luteal phase [18].

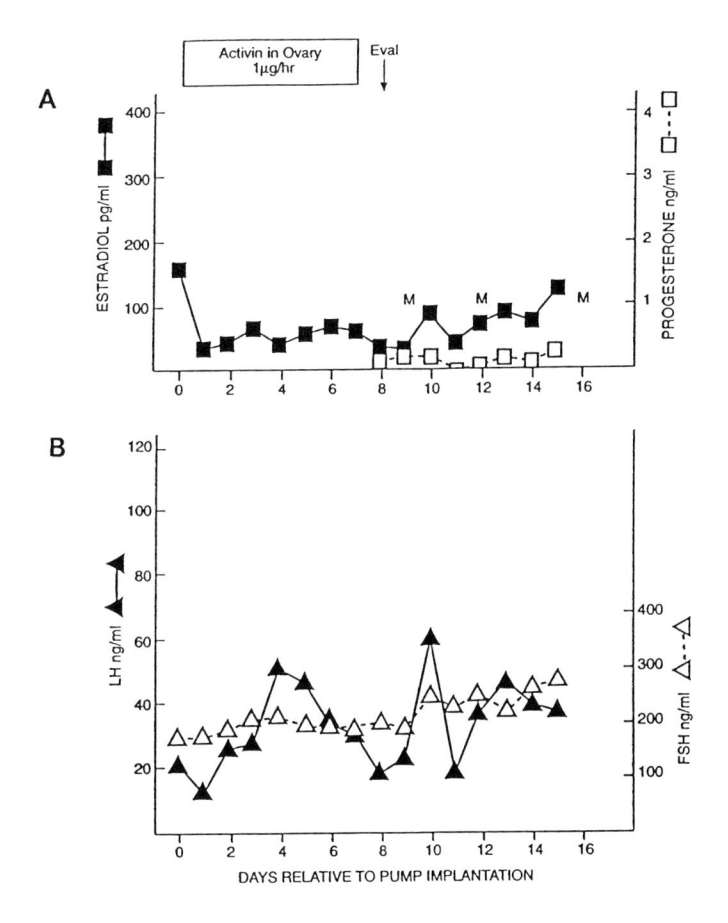

Fig. 1. Effect of rh-activin A infusion into the adult female rhesus monkey. Two normally cycling adult female rhesus monkeys were administered rh-activin A via a miniosmotic pump and the pattern of one representative monkey is shown here. Hormone was delivered at a rate of 1 µg/10 µl/h. Serum steroids (A) and gonadotropins (B) were measured as previously described [15] and follicular maturation was evaluated. Estradiol and progesterone, as well as FSH and LH, were suppressed in both animals and there was no evidence of follicular maturation.

Discussion

The fundamental difference in activin activity achieved in the monkey vs. that now accepted as represented by the rat data, leaves us with a new set of paradigms to explore. The presence and circulating levels of the binding protein follistatin, circulating levels of endogenous activin and alternate targets (such as adrenal, bone marrow, or kidney) which may produce additional factors influencing the hypothalamic-pituitary gonadal axis remain to be investigated. Further studies on the ability of activin to modulate gonadal and pituitary function in hypophysectomized or

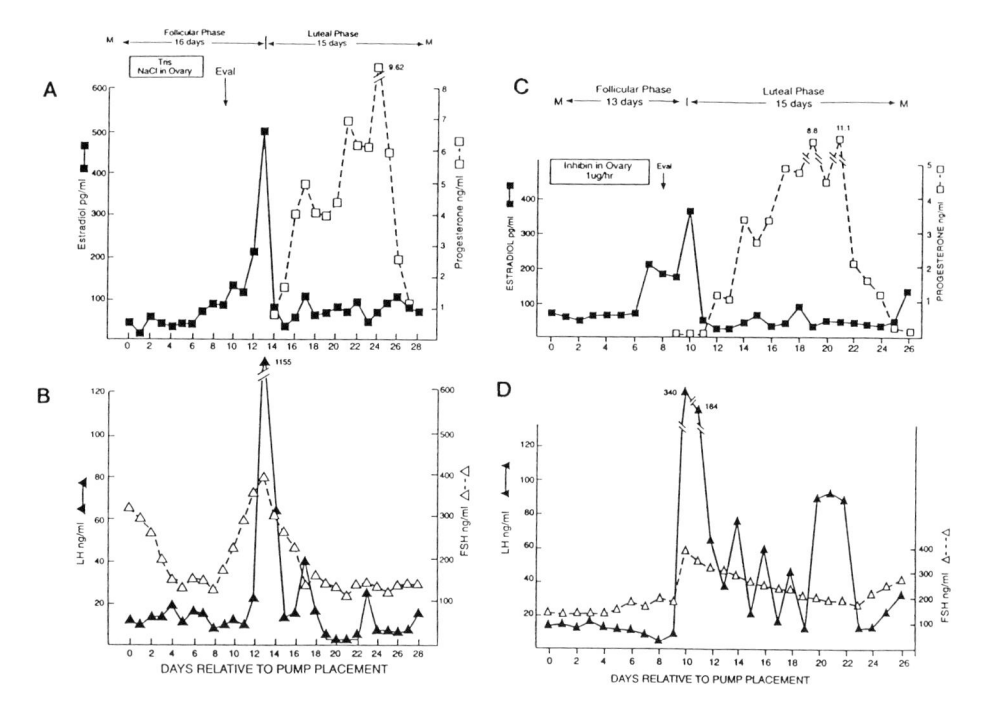

Fig. 2. Effect of vehicle (Tris:NaCl) or rh-inhibin A infusion into the adult female rhesus monkey. Two normally cycling adult female rhesus monkeys were administered the test compounds via a miniosmotic pump and the pattern of one representative monkey is shown here. Hormone was delivered at a rate of 1 µg/10 µl/h. Serum steroids (A and C) and gonadotropins (B and D) were measured as previously described [15] and follicular maturation appeared normal in all animals.

ovariectomized primates will increase our understanding of the role this molecule plays in regulating cyclicity in the female.

Acknowledgements

The assistance of the Animal Care Technicians and the Surgical Department at ORPRC in performance of the animal protocols is recognized. Special thanks goes to the technical assistants within the Assay Laboratories in Seattle and Beaverton for performing the gonadotropin and steroid assays. This project was supported by Genentech, Inc. and NIH Grant RR-00163 (R.L.S., T.A.M.) and Office of Research Development, Medical Research Service, Department of Veterans Affairs (K.D.D.).

References

1. Vale W, Rivier C, Hsueh A, Campen C, Meunier H, Bicsak T, Vaughan J, Corrigan A, Bardin W, Sawchenko P, Petraglia F, Yu J, Plotsky P, Spiess J, Rivier J. Recent Prog Horm Res 1988;44:1–34.

2. DePaulo L, Bicsak T, Erickson G, Shimasaki S, Ling N. Soc Exp Med Biol 1991;198:500—512.
3. Petraglia F, Garg S, Florio P, Sadick M, Gallinelli A, Wong W-L, Krummen L, Comitini G, Mather J, Woodruff T. Endocrine J 1993;1:323—327.
4. Krummen L, Woodruff T, DeGuzman L, Cox E, Baly D, Mann E, Garg S, Cossum P, Mather J. J Endocrinol 1993;132:431—443.
5. Findlay J. Biol Reprod 1993;48:15—23.
6. Woodruff T, Krummen L, Lyon R, Stocks D, Mather J. Endocrinology 1993;132:2332—2341.
7. Woodruff T, Lyon R, Hansen S, Rice G, Mather J. Endocrinology 1990;127:3196—3205.
8. Tilly J, Kowalski K, Johnson A, Hsueh A. Endocrinology 1991;129:2799—2801.
9. Schwall R, Robbins K, Jardieu P, Chang L, Lai C, Terrell T. Hepatology 1993;18:347—356.
10. Tenniswood M, Guenette R, Lakins J, Mooibroek M, Wong P, Welsh J. Cancer Metastasis Rev 1992; 11:197—220.
11. Mathews L, Vale W. Cell 1991;65:1—20.
12. Ebner R, Chen R, Shum L, Lawler S, Zioncheck T, Lee A, Lopez A, Derynck R. Science 1993;260: 1344—1347.
13. Hillier S, Yong E, Illingworth P, Baird D, Schwall R, Mason A. J Clin Endocrinol Metab 1991; 72:1206—1211.
14. Woodruff T, Krummen L, Chen S, Lyon R, Hansen S, DeGuzman L, Covello R, Mather J, Cossum P. Endocrinology 1993;132:725—734.
15. Stouffer R, Woodruff T, Dahl D, Hess D, Mather J, Molskness T. J Clin Endocrinol Metab 1993; 77:241—248.
16. McLachlan R, Dahl D, Bremner W. Endocrinology 1989;125:2787—2789.
17. Stouffer R, Dahl K, Hess D, Woodruff T, Mather J, Molskness T. Biol Reprod 1994;50:888—895.
18. Brannian J, Woodruff T, Mather J, Stouffer R. J Clin Endocrinol Metab 1992;75:756—761.

Nongonadotropic regulation of ovarian function: insulin

José F. Cara

Division of Pediatric Endocrinology, University of Chicago Pritzker School of Medicine, Chicago, Illinois, USA

Abstract. Accumulating evidence indicates that insulin plays an important role in modulating ovarian function. Insulin receptors are present in all ovarian cell types, indicating that the ovary is a target for the actions of this peptide. In vivo, insulin increases androgen levels and suppresses SHBG and IGFBP-1 concentrations. In vitro, insulin acts synergistically with the gonadotropins to enhance both granulosa and theca-interstitial cell differentiation. The actions of insulin appear to be mediated by its interaction with both insulin and insulin-like growth factor-1 receptors, or potentially with "hybrid" receptors present on these cells.

Background

Normal ovarian function is dependent of the coordinated interaction of two cellular compartments within the ovary, the theca-interstitial cell and the granulosa cell compartments. The two-cell, two-gonadotropin model of ovarian function states that normal follicular development depends on LH-induced theca-interstitial cell androgen production with subsequent aromatization of androgenic precursors by FSH-induced granulosa cell aromatase activity, to form estrogens [1,2]. Estrogens, acting in concert with FSH, stimulate follicular growth and maturation, inhibit androgen production, and help maintain secondary sexual development. Androgens, in turn, induce follicular atresia and may help in the selection of a single follicle for ovulation [2].

Accumulating information indicates that the actions of the gonadotropins on the ovary are modulated by intra- and extraovarian factors, including insulin and the insulin-like growth factors. This manuscript will review the role of insulin in ovarian function, especially with regard to its modulation of ovarian granulosa and theca-interstitial cell function. For a discussion of the pathophysiology of insulin resistance and ovarian hyperandrogenism, the reader is referred to the corresponding manuscript in this collection, as well as to several recent reviews of the subject [3–5].

Insulin and the IGFs

Insulin, together with insulin-like growth factor-I (IGF-I), and insulin-like growth factor-II (IGF-II), forms part of a family of serum proteins with similar structural characteristics and overlapping biological activities [6,7]. These hormones are all formed by an "A" and a "B" peptide chain loosely joined by disulfide bonds. IGF-I and IGF-II also contain a "D" extension peptide chain that is absent in insulin, as well as a "C" or connecting peptide chain that is cleaved from proinsulin during the proteolytic processing of the peptide to yield the two-chained insulin molecule. The overall sequence homology between insulin and the IGFs suggest that these hormones have a very similar tertiary structure [7].

Insulin initiates its biological actions by binding to a specific, high affinity cell surface receptor [8]. The insulin receptor is a heterotetramer composed of two α subunits of approximately 135,000 kDa containing the hormone binding domain, and two β subunits of approximately 95,000 kDa containing the tyrosine kinase domain. The gene for the insulin receptor is located on chromosome 19, contains 22 exons, and codes for a single proreceptor molecule that requires glycosylation, cleavage, and final assembly to form the mature receptor. Ligand binding to the insulin receptor results in phosphorylation of tyrosine residues on the insulin receptor molecule [9–11]. This, in turn, leads to phosphorylation of specific intracellular proteins, believed to be important components of insulin's intracellular signaling mechanism [9–11]. The insulin receptor can also bind IGF-I, although with about 100- to 1,000-fold lower affinity than insulin.

The IGF-I receptor, like the insulin receptor, contains two α and two β subunits of 130,000 kDa and 90,000 kDa which contain the hormone binding and tyrosine kinase domains, respectively [12]. The gene for the IGF-I receptor is located on chromosome 15 and codes for a proreceptor molecule that, like the insulin receptor, requires proteolytic cleavage and final assembly before giving rise to the mature receptor. The IGF-I receptor shares nearly 60% overall sequence homology with the insulin receptor. Because of this homology, it binds IGF-I with high affinity and also binds insulin, but with approximately 500-fold lower affinity than IGF-I [12].

Because of the overlapping structural characteristics and binding affinities of insulin, IGF-I, and their corresponding cell surface receptors, the biological actions mediated by each ligand and receptor type have been difficult to delineate. Traditionally, the insulin receptor has been viewed as mediating primarily metabolic actions, including glucose uptake and inhibition of gluconeogenesis and lipolysis, while the IGF-I receptor has been seen as stimulating mitogenic responses, including cellular replication and differentiation [9]. It is now clear that ligand binding to the insulin receptor can stimulate DNA and RNA synthesis and cellular replication and differentiation, while hormone binding to the IGF-I receptor can mediate metabolic actions, including glucose uptake and inhibition of lipolysis [9,13–15]. The overlapping actions of the insulin and IGF-I receptor systems may be accounted for, in part, by the presence of "hybrid" receptors, composed of both insulin and IGF-I heterodimers. Ligand binding to such "hybrid" receptors may account for both metabolic and mitogenic actions in target cells [16].

Unlike insulin, IGF-I and IGF-II circulate bound to plasma and tissue binding proteins that, like the IGFs themselves, have important biological functions [17]. Six plasma and tissue IGF binding proteins (IGFBPs) have been described to date, designated IGFBP-1 through IGFBP-6. These binding proteins bind IGF-I and/or IGF-

II with high affinity, but do not bind insulin. The IGFBPs modify the binding and/or biological activities of IGF-I and IGF-II, enhancing or suppressing the actions of these peptides. Insulin plays a primary role in the regulation of one of these binding proteins, IGFBP-1; IGFBP-1 levels increase in insulin deficiency states, such as fasting, untreated diabetes, and growth hormone deficiency, and are quickly suppressed by insulin treatment [17]. The regulation of IGFBP-1 may represent an important mechanism by which free IGF levels, and consequently IGF action, are modified by insulin.

Insulin and the ovary

Clinical evidence suggests that insulin plays an important role in ovarian function. Insulinopenic states are often associated with sexual infantilism and/or amenorrhea [18,19], which are generally reversed with exogenous insulin therapy [19]. Congenitally hyperinsulinemic infants, born of diabetic mothers [20] or those with Beckwith-Wiedemann syndrome [21], have hyperplasia of testicular Leydig cells, the male homologue of ovarian theca-interstitial cells. Congenital and acquired disorders of insulin action, such as those resulting from point mutations of the insulin receptor (as has been postulated to occur in leprechaunism) or from other pre- and post-receptor defects, are accompanied by compensatory hyperinsulinism and are often complicated by hyperplasia of ovarian theca-interstitial cells and hyperandrogenism [22–28]. In effect, every form of insulin resistance described to date has been associated with functional ovarian hyperandrogenism and polycystic ovary syndrome (PCOS), highlighting the potential significance of altered insulin secretion and/or action in the pathophysiology of ovarian dysfunction [3–5].

The frequent association of insulin resistance, hyperinsulinism, and ovarian hyperandrogenism has prompted substantial interest in the role of insulin in ovarian function, especially with regard to ovarian androgen production. Considerable disagreement has arisen as to whether hyperinsulinemia causes hyperandrogenism, or whether elevated androgen concentrations lead to insulin resistance. Whereas some investigators have suggested the latter, studies by Geffner et al. [29], Dunaif et al. [30], Stuart et al. [31], and Micic et al. [32], among others, indicate that hyperinsulinemia itself results in ovarian hyperandrogenism. Geffner and co-workers [29] and Dunaif et al. [30] independently found that suppression of androgen production following LHRH agonist therapy or oophorectomy failed to produce a fall in insulin concentrations and reverse insulin resistance. Stuart et al. [31] and Micic et al. [32] utilized a euglycemic clamp technique to show that androgen production was directly increased by the infusion of insulin to normal women and women with polycystic ovary syndrome, even in those with insulin resistance. Nestler and his colleagues [33] demonstrated that decreasing insulin levels with diazoxide therapy reduced serum concentrations of androgens in women with PCOS. More recently, Velazquez et al. [34] demonstrated that treatment with metformin, a biguanide that improves insulin action without affecting insulin secretion, reduced insulin concentrations, reversed hyperandrogenism, and facilitated normal menses and pregnancy in women with PCOS. Taken together, these studies indicate that hyperandrogenism is the result, rather than the cause of insulin resistance.

Insulin's role in ovarian function has been examined more directly in vitro using primary cultures of human, bovine, and rat ovarian cells. Specific high affinity binding sites for insulin, and the related peptides IGF-I and IGF-II, have been identified in animal and human ovarian tissue, suggesting that the ovary is a target site for the actions of these hormones. Rein and Schomberg [35], using standard competitive binding techniques, characterized the insulin binding site of porcine granulosa cells and observed that insulin binding was saturable, dependent on temperature and pH, and was constant throughout follicular development. Veldhuis et al. [36,37] found insulin and IGF-I receptors in swine granulosa cells while Davoren and co-workers [38] and Adashi's group [39] identified IGF-I receptors in rat granulosa cells. In rat ovarian theca-interstitial cells, Hernandez et al. [40,41] and our group [42] independently identified specific, high affinity binding sites for both insulin and IGF-I. Molecular biology studies by Adashi's group [43,44] have documented the presence of IGF-I and IGF-II receptor mRNA in these cells, suggesting that rat theca-interstitial cells express both IGF-I and IGF-II receptors.

Comparable studies with human ovarian tissue indicate that the human ovary also contains binding sites for insulin and the IGFs, and is a target for the actions of these hormones. Poretsky et al. [45] reported finding insulin receptors in stromal tissue from normal women, in stromal tissue from women with PCO, in follicular tissue from normal women and in purified human granulosa cells. Insulin binding to human ovarian plasma membranes was documented by Jarrett et al. [46]. Bergh et al. [47] recently identified both insulin and IGF-I receptor transcripts in human thecal cells, while Hernandez et al. [48] observed expression of both IGF-I and IGF-II receptor mRNA in human granulosa and thecal cells. In situ hybridization and immunohistochemistry studies by El-Roeiy and his colleagues [49] documented the presence of insulin receptor mRNA and mature protein in all cell types of dominant follicles and in thecal, granulosa, and stromal cells of small antral follicles. Further, IGF-I receptor mRNA was expressed only in granulosa cells, while IGF-II receptor mRNA was found in both granulosa and thecal cells of human ovaries. Whereas insulin and insulin mRNA were not evaluated in these studies, both IGF-I and IGF-II mRNA were found in human ovarian tissue, indicating their potential paracrine and/or autocrine role in ovarian function.

Insulin, like the IGFs, stimulates specific biological actions in both ovarian granulosa and theca-interstitial cells. In cultured bovine and porcine ovarian granulosa cells, insulin has been found to change cellular morphology and viability as well as stimulate cellular growth and proliferation [50,51]. As shown by the studies of Poretsky et al. [52], Channing et al. [53], Veldhuis et al. [36,37] and Adashi et al. [39], steroidogenesis is enhanced by insulin in human, bovine, porcine, and rat granulosa cells, in some cases through its synergistic interaction with FSH. Adashi et al. [39] reported finding that insulin enhanced the FSH-mediated induction of LH receptors and increased aromatase activity in rat ovarian granulosa cells. Aromatase activity was found to be increased by insulin in human granulosa cells but inhibited by insulin in swine granulosa cells [54]. Recent studies by Romero, Garney and Veldhuis [55] suggest that the insulin-mediated increase in granulosa cell steroidogenesis in cultured swine granulosa cells follows an autocrine model involving, in part, the release of inositol phosphoglycan mediators into the cell culture medium. Botero et al. [56] have shown that insulin helps prevent the decline in IGF-I gene expression in cultured rat ovarian cells, perhaps by increasing the rate of transcription of the IGF-I gene or by stabilizing the IGF-I message. An increase in IGF-I expression and release into the culture medium may represent a potential mechanism by which insulin mediates granulosa cell differentiation.

Insulin has also been found to modulate the differentiation of human and animal theca-interstitial cells. Barbieri et al. [57,58] observed that high concentrations of insulin stimulated androgen production in incubations of human stroma and theca obtained from women with insulin resistance and hyperandrogenism. Using cultured thecal cells from normal women, Bergh et al. [47] showed that insulin acted synergistically with LH to increase androgen production in these cells. Adashi's group [40] found that insulin amplified the effect of human chorionic gonadotropin (hCG) in rat ovarian theca-interstitial cell differentiation; whereas insulin alone had little effect on androgen production, the combination of insulin with hCG increased androsterone production 6-fold above levels seen with the gonadotropin alone. Comparable results were reported by Magoffin and Erickson [59], and our group [42]. More recently, studies in our laboratory [60] have shown that the increase in androgen production stimulated by insulin and LH is due, in part, to an increase in LH binding capacity stimulated by insulin; preincubation of rat ovarian theca-interstitial cells with 1, 10, 100, and 1,000 ng/ml insulin increased LH binding to 102%, 112%, 137%, and 152% of control values, respectively. Additional studies by Magoffin and his colleagues [61–63] have provided indirect evidence to suggest that insulin may synergyze with LH to increase androgen production by increasing the expression of several enzymes in the steroidogenic cascade.

It remains to be determined conclusively whether the actions of insulin on ovarian function are mediated through its own or other receptor types. The high concentrations of insulin needed to stimulate granulosa and theca-interstitial cell differentiation suggest that many of the actions of insulin are mediated through the IGF-I receptor [39–41,57–59]. However, dose-response data from Hernandez et al. [40], from Magoffin and Erickson [59], and from our group [42] suggest that insulin, at low doses, mediates theca-interstitial cell responses by binding to its own receptor, whereas at high concentrations its actions are mediated by its binding to the IGF-I receptor. Another possibility is that the actions of insulin are mediated by its binding to hybrid insulin/IGF receptors. These receptors are composed of insulin and IGF-I dimers (or "halves") and appear to bind both peptides. Whereas the properties and tissue expression of these receptors remain to be fully examined, their presence may help explain the paradox of insulin-induced hyperandrogenism in insulin resistant states [4,16].

In addition to its direct effects on the ovary, insulin has biological actions which

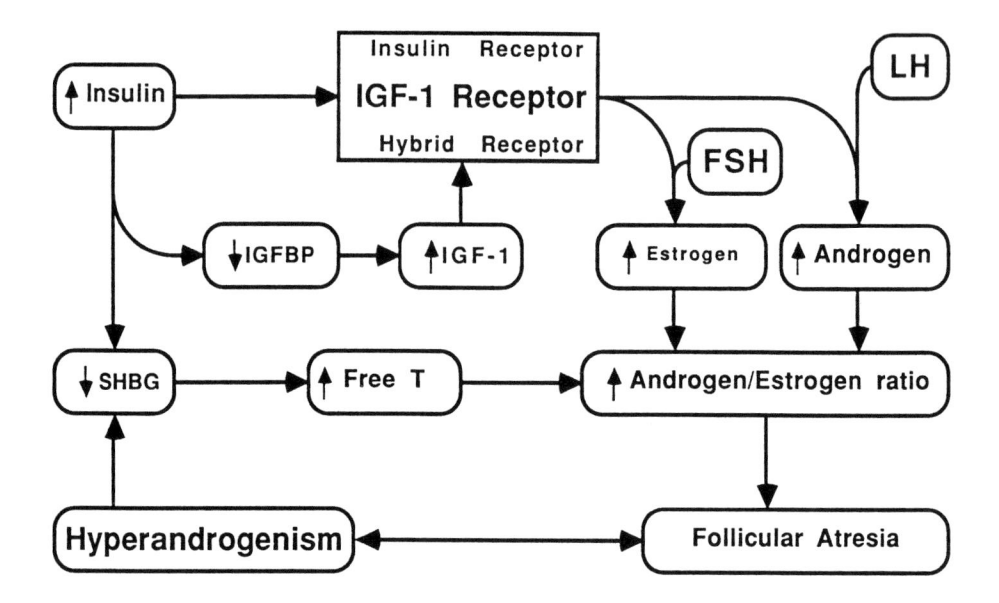

Fig. 1. Hypothetical mechanisms by which insulin modulates ovarian function and leads to ovarian hyperandrogenism.

may indirectly modulate ovarian function. For example, insulin has a direct effect on IGFBP-1 expression, decreasing the levels of this binding protein [17]. Whereas IGFBP-1 expression has not been identified in the ovary to date, Nobels and Dewailly [64] have suggested that an insulin-mediated decrease in IGFBP-I may result in an increase in the free intraovarian concentration of IGF-I, with subsequent potentiation of gonadotropin-mediated theca-interstitial cell androgen production [41]. Insulin has also been found to suppress circulating levels of sex hormone binding globulin (SHBG), the principal plasma androgen binding protein [65,66]. A decrease in SHBG would result in an increase in the free, and biologically available, androgen concentration. Because androgens are atretogenic in nature, an increase in the level of androgens would lead to follicular atresia and increased androgen output by the ovary [1,2].

Taken together, these observations suggest that the actions of insulin on the ovary may be represented by the sum of both direct and indirect biological actions which work in a complex manner to modulate ovarian function. Further, they support the concept that insulin, acting directly on the ovary and indirectly through its modulation of IGFBP-1 and SHBG expression, plays a role in the pathophysiology of ovarian hyperandrogenism, as shown in Fig. 1.

References

1. Liu Y-X, Hsueh AJW. Biol Reprod 1986;35:27–36.
2. Richards JS, Hedin L. Ann Rev Physiol 1988;50:441–463.

3. Poretsky L, Kalin M. Endocrine Rev 1987;8:132—141.
4. Poretsky L. Endocrine Rev 1991;12:3—13.
5. Dunaif A. Endocrinologist 1992;2:248—260.
6. Blundell TL, Humbel RE. Nature 1980;287:781—787.
7. Blundell TL, Bedarkar S, Rinderknecht E, Humbel RE. Proc Natl Acad Sci USA 1978;75:180—184.
8. Ullrich A, Bell JR, Chen EY, Herrera R, Petruzzelli LM, Dull TJ, Gray A, Coussens L, Liao Y-C, Tsubokawa M, Mason A, Seeburg PH, Grunfeld C, Rosen OM, Ramachandran J. Nature 1985;313: 756—761.
9. Rosen OM. Science 1987;237:1452—1458.
10. Kahn CR, White MF. J Clin Invest 1988;82:1151—1156.
11. Sun XJ, Rothenberg P, Kahn CR, Backer JM, Araki E, Wilden PA, Cahill DA, Goldstein BS, White MF. Nature 1991;352:73—77.
12. Ullrich A, Gray A, Tam AW, Yang-feng T, Tsubokawa M, Collins C, Henzel W, Le Bon T, Kathuria S, Chen E, Jacobs S, Francke U, Ramachandran J, Fujita-Yamaguchi. EMBO J 1986;5:2503—2512.
13. Czech MP. Cell 1989;59:235—238.
14. Froesch ER, Schmid C, Schwander J, Zapf J. Ann Rev Physiol 1985;47:443—467.
15. Hill DJ, Milner RDG. Pediatr Res 1985;19:879—886.
16. Moxham CP, Duronio V, Jacobs S. J Biol Chem 1989;264:13238—13244.
17. Rechler MM, Brown AL. Growth Reg 1992;2:55—68.
18. Bestetti G, Locatelli V, Tirone F, Rossi GL, Muller EE. Endocrinology 1985;117:208—216.
19. Levitsky L. Sem Adolesc Med 1987;3:233—239.
20. Nistal M, Gonzalez-Peramato P, Paniagua R. Histopathology 1988;12:307—317.
21. Smith DW. Recognizable Patterns of Human Malformation, 3rd edn. Philadelphia: WB Saunders Company, 1982;130—132.
22. Summitt R. Leprechaunism. In: Bergsma D (ed) Birth Defects Compendium. New York: Alan R. Liss, 1979;644—645.
23. Yoshimasa Y, Seino S, Whittaker J, Kakehi T, Kosaki A, Kuzuya H, Imura H, Bell G, Steiner DF. Science 1988;240:784—787.
24. Kadowaki T, Bevins CL, Cama A, Ojamaa K, Marcus-Samuels B, Kodawaki H, Beitz L, Mckeon C, Taylor SI. Science 1988;240:787—790.
25. Moller DE, Flier JS. N Engl J Med 1988;319:1526—1529
26. Kahn CR, Flier SJ, Bar RS, Archer JA, Gorden D, Martin MM, Roth J N. Engl J Med 1976;294: 739—745.
27. Taylor SI. Clin Res 1987;35:459—472.
28. Taylor SI, Cama A, Accili D, Barbetti F, Imano E, Kadowaki H, Kadowaki T. J Clin Endocrinol Metab 1991;73:1158—1163.
29. Geffner ME, Kaplan SA, Bersch N, Golde DW, Landaw EM, Chang RZ. Fertil Steril 1986;45:327—333.
30. Dunaif A, Green G, Futterweit W, Dobrjanski A. J Clin Endocrinol Metab 1990;70:699—704.
31. Stuart CA, Prince MJ, Peters EJ, Meyer III WJ. Obstet Gynecol 1987;69: 921—925.
32. Micic D, Popovic V, Nesovic M, Sumarac M, Dragasevic M, Kendereski A, Markovic D, Djordjevic P, Manojlovic D, Micic J. J Steroid Biochem 1988;31:995—999.
33. Nestler JE, Barlascini CO, Matt DW, Steingold KA, Plymate SR, Clore JN, Blackard WG. J Clin Endocrinol Metab 1989;68:1027—1032.
34. Velazquez EM, Mendoza S, Hamer T, Sosa F, Glueck CJ. Metformin therapy in polycystic ovary syndrome reduces hyperinsulinemia, insulin resistance, hyperandrogenemia, and systolic blood pressure, while facilitating normal menses and pregnancy. Metabolism 1994 (in press).
35. Rein MS, Schomberg DW. Biol Reprod 1982;26(suppl 1):113.
36. Veldhuis JD, Tamura S, Kolp L, Furlanetto RW, Larner J. Biochem Biophys Res Comm 1984;120: 144—149.
37. Veldhuis JD, Furlanetto RW, Juchter D, Garmuy J, Veldhuis P. Endocrinology 1985;116:1235—1242.
38. Davoren JB, Kasson BG, Li CH, Hsueh AJW. Endocrinology 1986;119:2155—2162.

39. Adashi EY, Resnick CE, D'Ercole AJ, Svoboda ME, Van Wyk JJ. Endocrine Rev 1985;6:400–420.
40. Hernandez ER, Resnick CE, Holztclaw WD, Payne DW, Adashi EY. Endocrinology 1988;122:2034–2043.
41. Hernandez ER, Resnick CE, Svoboda ME, Van Wyk JJ, Payne DW, Adashi EY. Endocrinology 1988;122:1603–1612.
42. Cara JF, Rosenfield RL. Endocrinology 1988;123:733–739.
43. Hernandez ER, Hurwitz A, Botero L, Ricciarelli E, Werner H, Roberts CT Jr, LeRoith D, Adashi EY. Mol Endocrinol 1991;5:1799–1805.
44. Hernandez ER, Roberts CT, Hurwitz A, LeRoith D, Adashi EY. Endocrinology 1990;127:3249–3251.
45. Poretsky L, Grigorescu F, Seibel M, Moses AC, Flier JS. J Clin Endocrinol Metab 1985;61:728–734.
46. Jarrett JC, Ballejo G, Tsibris JCM, Spellacy WN. J Clin Endocrinol Metab 1985;60:460–463.
47. Bergh C, Carlsson B, Olsson J-H, Selleskog U, Hillensjö T. Fertil Steril 1993;59:323–331.
48. Hernandez ER, Hurwitz A, Vera A, Pellicer A, Adashi EY, LeRoith D, Roberts CT. J Clin Endocrinol Metab 1992;74:419–425.
49. El-Roeiy A, Chen X, Roberts VJ, LeRoith D, Roberts CT, Yen SSC. J Clin Endocrinol Metab 1993;77:1411–1418.
50. Baranao JLS, Hammond JM. Biochem Biophys Res Commun 1984;124:484–490.
51. Davoren JB, Hsueh AJW. Mol Cell Endocrinol 1984;35:97–105.
52. Poretsky L, Smith D, Seibel M, Pazianes A, Moses AC, Flier JS. J Clin Endocrinol Metab 1984;59:809–811.
53. Channing CP, Tsai V, Sachs D. Biol Reprod 1976;15:235–247.
54. Garzo VG, Dorrington JH. Am J Obstet Gynecol 1984;148:657–662.
55. Romero G, Garmey JC, Veldhuis JD. Endocrinology 1993;132:1561–1568.
56. Botero LF, Roberts CT Jr, LeRoith D, Adashi EY, Hernandez ER. Endocrinology 1993;132:2703–2708.
57. Barbieri RL, Makris A, Ryan KJ. Obstet Gynecol 1984;64(supp):73s–80s.
58. Barbieri RL, Makris A, Ryan KJ. Endocrinology 1985;116(suppl):204.
59. Magoffin DA, Erickson GF. In Vitro Cell Dev Biol 1988;24:862–870.
60. Cara JF, Fan J, Azzarello J, Rosenfield RL. J Clin Invest 1990;86:560–565.
61. Magoffin DA, Kurtz KM, Erickson GF. Mol Endocrinol 1990;4:489–496.
62. Magoffin DA, Weitsman SR. Biol Reprod 1993;48:1166–1173.
63. Magoffin DA, Weitsman SR. Endocrinology 1993;132:1945–1951.
64. Nobels F, Dewailly D. Puberty and the polycystic ovarian syndrome: the insulin/insulin-like growth factor I hypothesis. Fertil Steril 1992;58:655–666.
65. Plymate SR, Matej LA, Jones RE, Friedl KE. J Clin Endocrinol Metab 1988;67:460–464.
66. Nestler JE, Powers LP, Matt DW, Steingold KA, Plymate SR, Rittmaster RS, Clore JN, Blackard WG. J Clin Endocrinol Metab 1991;72:83–89.

Nongonadotropic regulation of ovarian function: growth hormone and IGFs

Gregory F. Erickson
Department of Reproductive Medicine, University of California at San Diego, La Jolla, CA 92093-0947, USA

The ability of the ovary to secrete an egg into the oviduct to be fertilized is one of the bases of fertility in the female mammal. In order for this to occur, the egg, granulosa and theca cells must express a developmental program that generates a dominant follicle. This developmental program consists of a precise quantitative and temporal pattern of expression of a large number of genes that ensure the proper growth and differentiation of the follicle cells. Follicle-stimulating hormone (FSH) is obligatory for evoking the program, and no other ligand, by itself, can serve in this regulatory capacity. It follows, therefore, that any ligand (hormone or growth factor) that inhibits FSH receptor signal transduction would compromise the expression of this developmental program, thus causing the follicle to proceed along the atretic pathway. Conversely, if a ligand amplifies the FSH signal, the expression of the developmental program would be enhanced and the follicle would differentiate along a preovulatory pathway. The current problem is to understand the mechanisms by which specific GF-FSH interactions regulate follicle development and atresia. Here, we summarize the recent advances in the function of one GF family in regulating FSH action, namely the IGF family.

The growth factor concept

It is clear that dominant follicle development is determined by the endocrine hormones FSH and LH. These ligands interact with transmembrane receptors, and the binding events are transduced via the G proteins into intracellular signals that coordinate the expression of those genes that specify a preovulatory follicle. One of the most important concepts to evolve in recent years is that proteins with growth factor (GF) activity modulate either amplify or attenuate the follicle responses to FSH and LH. All GF are ligands that interact with receptors to activate different mechanisms of signal transduction. Because GF are produced locally, they act in an autocrine/paracrine fashion to stimulate or inhibit follicle growth and development. This is the growth factor concept (Fig. 1). There are five different classes of GF, and all five classes have been identified in developing follicles of rat and human ovaries [1–11] (Table 1). The conclusion emerging from this large body of evidence is that

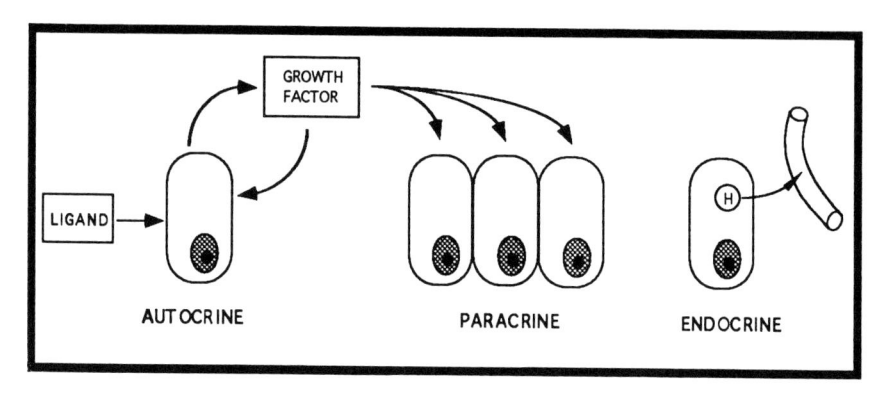

Fig. 1. The growth factor concept.

GF, which are themselves the product of follicle cells, act to modulate the FSH and LH signals. We do not yet understand the nature of the specific GF interactions; however, the theory has emerged that GF may serve as mediators of hormone action in target cells (Fig. 2).

The granulosa IGF system

One of the most thoroughly studied ovarian GF families, and one that has received clinical attention in recent years, is the IGF family [12,13]. Results from studies on the rat suggest that a GHRH/GH/IGF-I axis, complete with their negative regulatory proteins, exists within the granulosa cells (GC). The major lines of evidence supporting this concept are as follows.

First, a GHRH-like protein and its mRNA are expressed in GC of the immature estrogen-primed rat ovary [14]. What controls the production of the GHRH is unknown. Each GC contains 4,600 high-affinity GHRH receptors, and FSH up-regulates the number of GHRH receptors to 12,000 sites/cell [15]. Interaction of GHRH with its receptor generates a modest increase in cAMP, but coincubation of GHRH with FSH causes a synergistic increase in cAMP, as well as estradiol (E_2), LH receptor, and progesterone (P^4) production [16]. These observations support the idea

Table 1. The five classes of follicular growth factors

Growth factors	References	
	Rat	Human
IGF	[1]	[2–4]
TGF-β	[5,6]	[7]
TGF-α/EGF	[5]	[8]
FGF	[9]	[9]
Cytokine	[10,11]	[10,11]

ENDOCRINE SYSTEM

$[H] + [R] \longrightarrow [H \bullet R]^* \xrightarrow{\text{SIGNAL TRANSDUCTION}}$ EXPRESSION OF INTRINSIC GROWTH FACTORS (GF) AND GF RECEPTORS

INDUCTION OF PHYSIOLOGIC BIOLOGICAL RESPONSES $\xleftarrow{\text{SIGNAL TRANSDUCTION}} [GF \bullet R]^* \xleftarrow{} [GF] + [R]$

AUTOCRINE AND PARACRINE SYSTEM

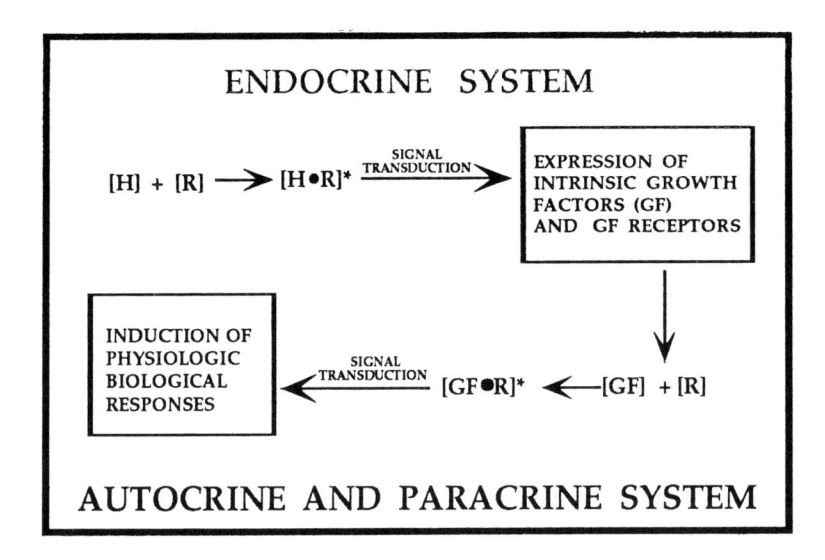

Fig. 2. The concept that growth factors (GF) act as mediators of hormone-induced biological responses in target cells. H: hormone; R: receptor; *: active HR complex after allosteric shape change. In rat granulosa cells, there is evidence that intrinsic IGF-I is an obligatory mediator of FSH action.

that intrinsic GHRH may play a role in determining maximal FSH activity in rat GC.

Second, the GH receptor protein [17] and its 4.5 kb mRNA [18] are expressed in GC of adult cycling rats [19]. The questions of how the GH receptor is regulated and whether the GH ligand is actually produced in the GC, have yet to be answered. Significantly, when GC are incubated with GH in vitro, they become much more sensitive to FSH with respect to cAMP, LH receptor, and P^4 production [20,21]. No effect of GH on FSH-induced E_2, 20α dihydroprogesterone [20,21], or mitosis [22], is observed. Thus, GH-FSH interactions appear to be positively coupled to the acquisition of the ovulation/luteinization potential of rat GC.

Third, high levels of IGF-I mRNA are produced in granulosa cells of healthy, but not atretic follicles [23,24]. In vitro, the level of GC IGF-I mRNA is stimulated by E_2, GH, dexamethasone and insulin, but FSH has little effect [25,26]. Interestingly, exogenous GH causes a dramatic increase (3.6- to 6.4-fold) in immunoreactive ovarian IGF-I in vivo [27]. The GC also express IGF-I receptor mRNA [22,24,27] and the amount of message is increased dramatically by FSH and E_2 [24,27]. That the receptor message is translated into protein is demonstrated by binding studies [28]. Considerable effort has been devoted to the analysis of biological responses of IGF-I at the level of the GC [29]. The results demonstrate that nM amounts of IGF-I act synergistically with FSH to markedly enhance cAMP, E_2, P^4, LH receptor, proteoglycan [29], and inhibin [30] production. IGF-I does not influence FSH receptor levels [31]. Except for inhibin [30], proteoglycan [29] and DNA [32] synthesis which are stimulated by IGF-I in a dose-dependent manner, IGF-I by itself has little or no effect on GC.

An important consideration in the overall activity of the system is the concept that GHRH, GH and IGF-I can be modulated by negative regulatory molecules. A hormone that is capable of inhibiting GHRH activity is somatostatin (GHIH). McIntyre et al. [33] recently showed that immature rat ovaries contain immunoreactive GHIH and that pM amounts of GHIH induce biological responses on GC/oocyte complexes. The question of whether GHIH interferes with the GHRH responses in GC has yet to be answered. Tiong and Herington [18] identified GH binding protein (GHBP) mRNA in rat ovaries. The functional role of the GHBP is unknown, but it would be expected to negate the potentiating effects of GH on GC. Further work is needed to investigate possible interactions between GH, GHBP and FSH in the ovary. Finally, IGFBPs are potent modulators of IGF-I activity [34]. The dramatic evidence demonstrating the ability of IGFBPs to inhibit FSH action has led to the concept that IGFBPs play a crucial role in modulating GC differentiation [13].

In summary, the proposition which emerges is that the mechanism by which FSH evokes GC differentiation involves the activation of an intrinsic GHRH/GH/IGF-I system which is necessary for maintaining and enhancing FSH activity; inhibition of this activity by GHIH, GHBP, and/or IGFBPs would perturb FSH action and send the follicle along the atretic pathway (Fig. 3).

IGFBPs are FSH antagonists

In 1989, Drs Ling and Shimasaki purified a novel protein from porcine follicular fluid that could inhibit almost completely the ability of FSH to stimulate E_2 and P^4 produc-

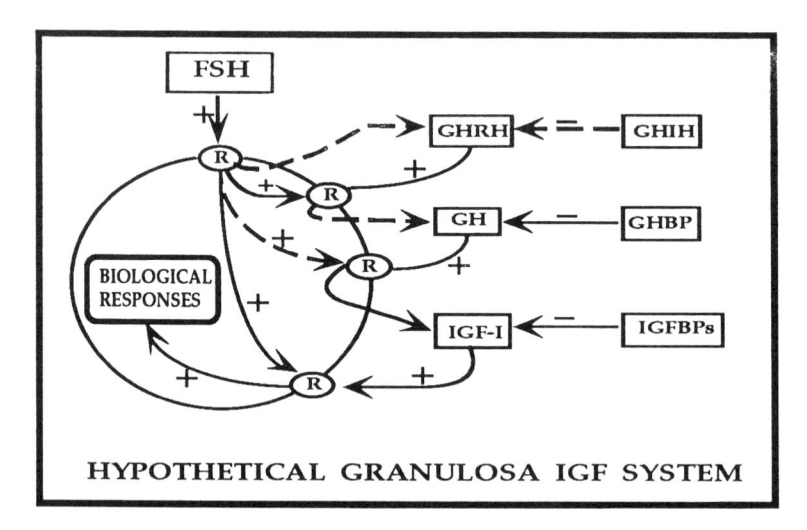

Fig. 3. The intrinsic GHRH/GH/IGF-I axis in rat granulosa cells (GC). The proposition is that the regulated production of GHRH, GH and IGF-I in GC is required for FSH to evoke dominant follicle formation, perhaps via an autocrine/paracrine cascade mechanism. Locally produced inhibitors that interfere with ligand action, e.g., somatostatin (GHIH) and binding proteins (GHBP, IGFBPs) would act as FSH antagonists. Broken line: unproven.

tion by cultured rat GC [35,36]. The FSH antagonist proved to be IGFBP-3 [37]. In 1990, their laboratory showed that the IGFBP inhibition was mimicked by a specific IGF-I antibody [38]. Consequently, they concluded that the mechanism by which IGFBP-3 (and -2) antagonize FSH is by binding intrinsic IGF-I, thereby negating its activity. Collectively, these results suggested the exciting proposition that IGF-I is an obligatory mediator of FSH-induced biological responses in rat GC and that IGFBPs, if present, are highly potent in antagonizing IGF-I activity. Accordingly, IGFBPs are FSH antagonists. Then, Drs Ling and Shimasaki discovered three new IGFBPs and cloned and sequenced their cDNAs in the rat and human [39]. Now, six different IGFBPs are known to exist: 1) rIGFBP-1, 247aa, Mr 26,801; 2) rIGFBP-2, 270aa, Mr 29,564; 3) rIGFBP-3, 265aa, Mr 28,856; 4) rIGFBP-4, 233aa, Mr 25,681; 5) rIGFBP-5, 252aa, Mr 28,428; and 6) rIGFBP-6, 201aa, Mr 21,461 [39]. The amino acid sequences are highly homologous and the location of the cysteines in the molecules are conserved. By virtue of their structure, all IGFBPs bind IGF-I and -II, but not insulin [34,39]. Because the IGFBPs are potentially important in the regulation of FSH action, it was of great interest to know their cellular localization in the ovary.

Expression of IGFBP-1 to -6 in rat ovaries

Using in situ hybridization techniques, we found that the genes encoding the six IGFBPs are expressed in a highly tissue-specific manner in adult rat ovaries. Further, the stage in the reproductive cycle dramatically effects the levels of the mRNA transcripts [13]. These findings support the concept that ovarian IGFBP gene activity is under hormone and/or GF control. In regard to the cellular localization of the IGFBPs in the ovary, it can be seen (Table 2) that IGFBP-2 is expressed in the interstitial (theca and secondary) and surface epithelial cells [40,41]; IGFBP-3 is expressed in corpora lutea during luteolysis [42]; IGFBP-4 is strongly expressed in

Table 2. Cellular localization of mRNAs for the family IGFBPs in adult rat ovary tissue (modified from [13])

Tissue	IGFBP-1	IGFBP-2	IGFBP-3	IGFBP-4	IGFBP-5	IGFBP-6
Granulosa cells:						
Healthy	–	–	–	–	–	–
Atretic	–	–	–	+	+	–
Theca interstitial cells	–	+	–	–	–	–
Secondary interstitial cells	–	+	–	–	+/–	–
Corpora lutea	–	–	+/–	+/–	+/–	–
Oocyte	–	–	–	–	–	–
Theca externa	–	–	–	–	–	+
Surface epithelium	–	+	–	–	+	–

–: mRNA was undetectable; +: mRNA was detectable and the hybridization signal was strong; +/–: there was heterogeneity in mRNA expression, i.e., some of the histological units contained the mRNA, others did not.

some atretic GC and in some corpora lutea, interstitial and stromal cells [43]; IGFBP-5 is strongly expressed in some atretic GC, secondary interstitial, corpora lutea, and surface epithelial cells [44]; IGFBP-6 is expressed in some theca externa smooth muscle cells [13]; IGFBP-1 is undetectable [40]. These new findings led to the concept that the physiological mechanisms of folliculogenesis and luteogenesis involve the regulation of inducible and tissue-specific IGFBP-2 to -6 expression. Although the physiological function of the ovarian IGFBPs is unknown, it is clear that IGFBP-4 and -5 (mRNA and protein) are strongly expressed in rat GC during atresia. By contrast, no IGFBP mRNAs are evident in GC of dominant follicles as they grow and develop to the preovulatory stage (Fig. 4). Thus, it can be concluded that inducible IGFBP-4 and -5 may play a central role in the physiological mechanism of atresia in the rat ovary. Indeed, the in vitro data (discussed below) suggest that these pathways are linked.

IGFBP-4 and -5 are FSH antagonists

We have shown that IGFBP-4 or -5 are potent inhibitors of FSH-stimulated E_2 and P^4 production by rat GC in vitro [45,46]. As seen in Fig. 5, coincubation of a

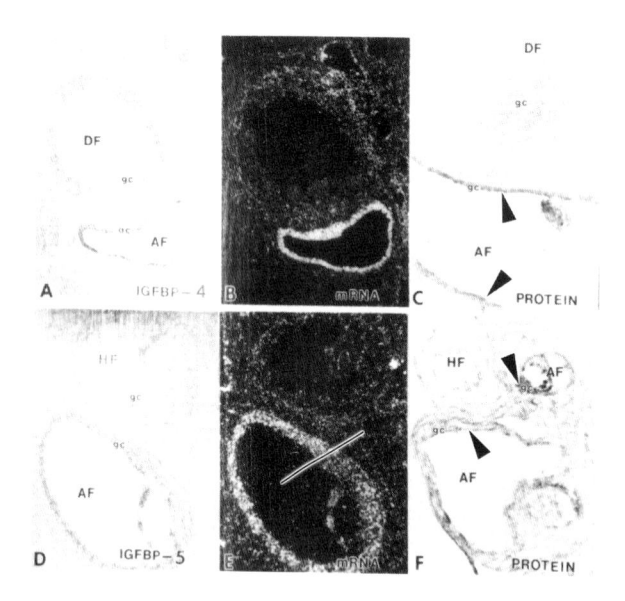

Fig. 4. Tissue-specific expression of IGFBP-4 and -5 mRNA and protein in rat granulosa cells during atresia. AF: atretic follicle; DF: dominant follicle; HF: healthy preantral follicle; gc: granulosa cells. Arrowheads: IGFBP protein. A and D: bright field; B and E: dark field after hybridization with IGFBP-4 and -5 antisense cRNA probes. C and F: sections immunostained by the avidin-biotin immunoperoxidase technique using a specific antiserum to rIGFBP-4 and -5 (1:1,000 dilution). The slides were counterstained lightly with hematoxylin. The conclusion is that IGFBP-4 and -5 mRNA is translated into protein during physiological atresia in vivo.

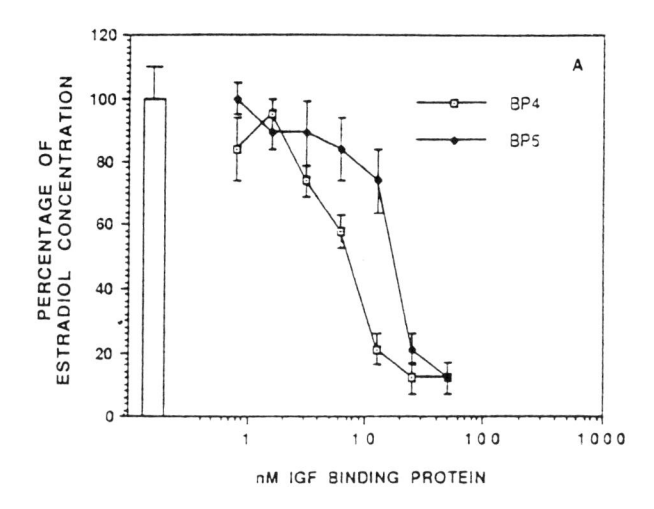

Fig. 5. FSH antagonist activity of IGFBP-4 and -5 in cultured rat granulosa cells (from [30], with permission).

maximally effective dose of FSH (30 ng/ml) with increasing concentrations of IGFBP-4 and -5 inhibited E_2 in a dose-dependent manner. The inhibitory doses are in the nM range and the maximally effective doses (~30 nM) caused ~90% inhibition of FSH action (Fig. 5). How IGFBP-4 and -5 antagonize FSH action is unknown. We presume the inhibiting mechanisms involve binding of intrinsic IGF-I, but further work is necessary to prove this point. It should be noted that although the IGFBP-4 and -5 effects are similar, they are not identical. This raises the possibility that IGFBP-4 and -5 might possess different potencies and different functional activities as the GC express their developmental program during folliculogenesis. For instance, some of the IGFBP effects might be positive, particularly with respect to IGFBP-5, since in other systems IGFBP-5 has been found to potentiate IGF-I action [34]. Nevertheless, based on these in vitro data, we conclude that IGFBP-4 and -5 are potent FSH antagonists. If our in vitro data can be extrapolated to the in vivo situation, then it seems reasonable to assume that GC express two FSH antagonists, IGFBP-4 and -5, when undergoing atresia in vivo. Because FSH is obligatory for folliculogenesis, the expression of FSH antagonists by the follicle cells themselves could have important negative consequences for follicle survival.

Regulation of IGFBP-4 and -5 by FSH

Evidence that GC from immature DES primed rats produce IGFBPs in vitro was initially provided by Adashi and workers [47,48]. Two general principles emerge from their work: 1) rat GC produce relatively large amounts of the 28,000–29,000 Mr and 23,000 Mr IGFBP proteins spontaneously in vitro; and 2) FSH via the cAMP/PKA signal transduction pathway [49] dramatically effects the levels of

IGFBPs in a time-dependent (high doses of FSH initially increase IGFBPs above controls, but then the levels decrease to undetectable levels), and dose-dependent manner (low FSH doses stimulate, while high doses inhibit IGFBP production). These observations led to the proposition that rat GC synthesize several types of IGFBPs and their production is tightly regulated by FSH [47,48]. What types of IGFBPs were synthesized by the GC was, however, not clear.

A major impediment to the study of IGFBP production by GC was removed when Liu et al. [45] developed specific antisera to the IGFBPs known to be produced in the rat ovary (IGFBP-2, -3, -4, -5, -6). Using a battery of specific IGFBP antisera [45], it was established that the IGFBPs reported by Adashi using ligand blotting were actually IGFBP-4 and -5. Because there was no detectable staining with the other antisera (raised against IGFBP-2, -3 and -6), it was clear that IGFBP-4 and -5 are the only IGFBPs produced by untreated rat GC in vitro. The physiological significance of this result is emphasized by our data (Fig. 4), showing that IGFBP-4 and -5 proteins are strongly expressed in rat GC during physiological atresia in situ. An intriguing implication of these observations is that these GC undergo spontaneous atresia in vitro. We do not know what controls the spontaneous expression of IGFBP-4 and -5 by control GC, but it may be related to decreased E_2 stimulation since E_2/DES withdrawal leads to atresia in this animal model [50].

Confirming and extending the work of Adashi [47–49], we also found that FSH exerts biphasic effects of IGFBP-4 production, e.g., the major 24,000 and minor 28,000 Mr IGFBP-4 proteins are stimulated and inhibited by low (<3 ng/ml) and high (>10 ng/ml) concentrations of FSH respectively (Fig. 6). Interestingly, these bands are reduced/absent when cells are treated with >30 ng/ml of FSH, but the 17,500 and

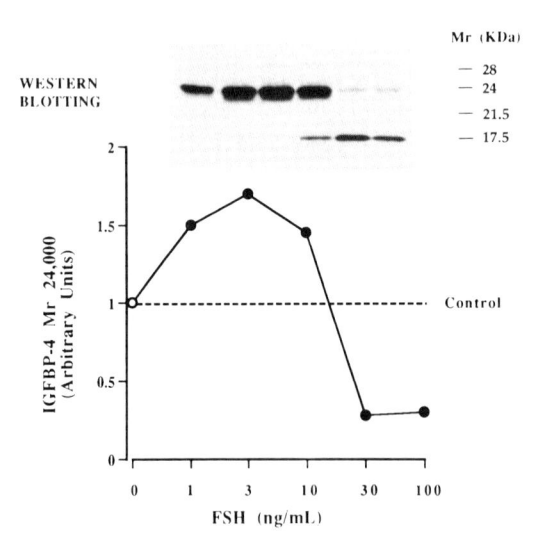

Fig. 6. Biphasic effects of FSH on the accumulation of the 24,000 and 28,000 Mr IGFBP-4 proteins in conditioned medium of rat granulosa cells cultured for 48 h under serum-free conditions. Note that high doses of FSH (>10 ng/ml) induced a protease that hydrolyzed the mature proteins with smaller 21,000 and 17,500 Mr fragments (modified from [53]). Importantly, the smaller fragments do not bind IGF-I [45].

21,500 Mr bands were induced (Fig. 6). These smaller fragments are formed by the hydrolysis of the 24,000 and 28,000 proteins by an FSH-induced protease. The importance of the protease is emphasized by the fact that the fragments no longer bind IGF-I [45]. Thus a major mechanism by which FSH controls IGFBP-4 (and -5) activity appears to be at the level of a specific protease that destroys its IGF-I binding potential.

What might this mean physiologically? NcNatty [51] discovered that FSH levels in the microenvironment of healthy and atretic follicles are high and low respectively. Further, we have found that IGFBP-4 and -5 (mRNA and protein) are likely to play a role in physiological mechanisms of atresia (Figs. 4 and 5). Thus, we might predict that a high concentration of FSH in follicular fluid prevents atresia by destroying intrinsic IGFBP-4 and -5 and any other IGFBPs that might enter the follicle from the outside. Such an action by FSH would promote dominant follicle formation. At the opposite extreme, one would predict that a low concentration of FSH in the microenvironment might actually enhance IGFBP-4 (and -5) production and inhibit protease induction. Such an action by FSH would promote atresia. Thus, these observations are consistent with the notion that the physiological processes of both selection and atresia could be controlled by FSH alone. Further, they suggest that the mechanism might involve the concentration-dependent regulation of the genes encoding IGFBP-4 and -5 and their specific proteases.

Stimulation of IGFBP-4 and atresia

Given the nature of ovarian regulation, it is possible that other hormones, GF, or neuromodulators effect the IGFBP responses to FSH. In this regard, we reported previously that GnRH induces meiotic maturation in oocytes in subpopulations of atretic preantral follicles of the immature, hypophysectomized DES primed rat [52]. This led us to postulate that ovarian GnRH might be involved in atresia. To test this possibility, we used the GC tissue culture model to determine the effects of GnRH on the expression of IGFBP-4 protein. We found that GnRH has a marked stimulatory effect (up to 4-fold) on IGFBP-4 production in vitro, and totally inhibited the FSH responses on IGFBP-4 and its protease [53]. These GnRH actions are time- and dose-dependent and blocked by an GnRH-antagonist. This evidence suggests a relationship between GnRH and atresia. In these experiments, we also found that GnRH inhibited mitosis and induced pyknosis in rat GC in vivo. Because reduced mitosis and induction of pyknosis are classic markers of physiologic atresia, our results argue that a major extrapituitary action of GnRH in the rat is to induce atresia. Although not conclusive, these data strongly suggest that GnRH-induced atresia is mediated by increases in IGFBP-4 production; however, further work is necessary to prove this theory.

Conclusions and implications

In conclusion, there is no doubt that the concentration of FSH in the microenvironment is of utmost importance in determining whether or not a Graafian follicle expresses its preovulatory or atretic potential (Fig. 7). Recent evidence has been obtained which supports the concept that FSH-induced growth and development of preovulatory follicles are mediated, at least in part, by the stimulation of the production of IGF-I and IGFBP proteases by the GC. The IGF-I ligand interacts with transmembrane receptors and the binding event is transduced into signals that evoke granulosa proliferation and differentiation. The protease would inactivate IGFBPs, such as IGFBP-4 and -5, in follicular fluid, thereby ensuring sufficient free IGF-I to express the developmental program of FSH. Questions concerning GHRH and GH are of particular interest in this model, because of their ability to amplify GC responses to FSH; however, the answers to these questions remain to be found. In this model, we would propose that the entry of an atretogenic molecule, such as GnRH, into the microenvironment would increase the level of IGFBP-4 and -5 (mRNA and protein) and block protease activity. The consequence would be a reduction in free IGF-I. In the absence of IGF-I stimulation, the GC would be committed to apoptosis and the follicle would die by atresia. In this context, our data argue that a major site of control of selection and atresia is at the level of FSH-induced IGFBP protease.

We have concentrated in this discussion on a single GF system, the IGF family. It should be kept in mind that all GF families are able to modulate FSH action.

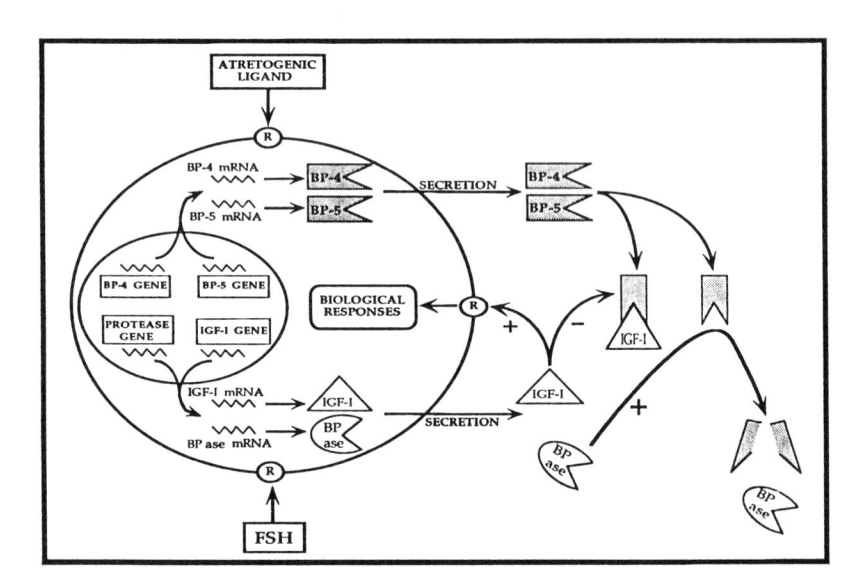

Fig. 7. Diagram showing how FSH-induced granulosa cytodifferentiation is mediated by intrinsic IGF-I and an IGFBP protease (BPase). High concentrations of FSH in follicular fluid (FF) stimulate IGF-I and BPase gene transcription and translation. IGF-I-bound receptor then causes cytodifferentiation and the BPase hydrolyzes any FF IGFBPs. Atretogenic ligands, like GnRH, trigger IGFBP-4 and -5 gene transcription and translation and the secreted BPs reduce free IGF-I, thereby dampening FSH action.

Therefore, one might predict that the same concepts are also important in determining how other GF act and interact with FSH to control folliculogenesis. There is little doubt that we are entering into a new era in ovulation induction and that the era is deeply rooted in the GF concept (Fig. 2). The author predicts that knowledge of the GF concept will continue to improve ovulation induction protocols and perhaps someday will replace current methods within the field.

Acknowledgements

The author thanks his co-workers Drs Ling, Shimasaki and Nakatani for their invaluable contributions to this work; Danmei Li and Stephanie Kokka for excellent technical assistance; Ali Sadighian for preparing the figures; and Marta Murray for typing. This work was supported by NICHD grants HD09690, HD29008 and P50-HD12303-15.

References

1. Adashi EY. In: Adashi EY, Leung PCK (eds) The Ovary. New York: Raven Press, 1993;319–335.
2. Giudice LC. Endocrine Rev 1992;13:641–669.
3. Zhou J, Bondy C. Biol Reprod 1993;48:467–482.
4. El-Roeiy A, Chen K, Roberts VJ, LeRoith D, Roberts CT, Yen SSC. J Clin Endocrinol Metab 1993;77:1411–1418.
5. Mulheron GW, Schomberg DW. In: Adashi EY, Leung PCK (eds) The Ovary. New York: Raven Press, 1993;337–362.
6. Findlay JK, Xiao S, Shukovski L, Michel U. In: Adashi EY, Leung PCK (eds) The Ovary: New York: Raven Press, 1993;413–432.
7. Hillier SG. J Endocrinol 1991;131:171–175.
8. Chegini N, Williams RS. J Clin Endocrinol Metab 1992;74:973–980.
9. Gospodarowitz D, Ferrara N, Schweigere L, Neufeld G. Endocrine Rev 1987;8:95–114.
10. Kokia E, Adashi EY. In: Adashi EY, Leung PCK (eds) The Ovary. New York: Raven Press, 1993:383–394.
11. Terranova PF, Sancho-Tello M, Hunter VJ. In: Adashi EY, Leung PCK (eds). The Ovary. New York: Raven Press, 1993:395–411.
12. Katz E, Ricciarelli E, Adashi EY. Fertil Steril 1993;59:8–34.
13. Erickson GF, Nakatani A, Shimasaki S, Ling N. In: Findlay JK (ed) Cellular and Molecular Mechanisms in Female Reproduction. New York: Academic Press (in press).
14. Bagnato A, Moretti C, Ohnishi J, Frajese G, Catt KJ. Endocrinology 1992;130:1097–1102.
15. Bagnato A, Moretti C, Frajese G, Catt KJ. Endocrinology 1991;128:2889–2894.
16. Moretti C, Bagnato A, Solum N, Frajese G, Catt KJ. Endocrinology 1990;127:2117–2126.
17. Lobie PE, Breipohl W, Aragon JC, Waters MJ. Endocrinology;1990;126:2214–2221.
18. Tiong TK, Herington AC. Endocrinology 1991;129:1628–1634.
19. Carter-Su C, Stubbart JR, Wang K, Stred SE, Argetsginer LS, Shafer JA. J Biol Chem 1989;264:18654–18661.
20. Jia X-C, Kalmijn J, Hsueh AJW. Endocrinology 1986;118:1401–1409.
21. Hutchinson LA, Findlay JK, Herington AC. Mol Cell Endocrinol 1988;55:61–69.
22. Usuki S, Shioda M. Horm Metab Res 1989;21:455–456.
23. Oliver JE, Aitman TJ, Powell JF, Wilson CA, Clayton RN. Endocrinology 1989;124:2671–2679.

24. Zhou J, Chin E, Bondy C. Endocrinology 1991;129:3281—3288.
25. Hernandez ER, Roberts CT, LeRoith D, Adashi EY. Endocrinology 1989;125:572—574.
26. Botero LF, Roberts CT, LeRoith D, Adashi EY, Hernandez ER. Endocrinology 1993;132:2703—2708.
27. Daveron JB, Hsueh AJW. Endocrinology 1986;118:888—890.
28. Adashi EY, Resnick CE, Hernandez ER, Svoboda ME, VanWyk JJ. Endocrinology 1988;122:1388—1389.
29. Adashi EY, Resnick CE, De'Ercole AJ, Svoboda M, VanWyk JJ. Endocrine Rev 1985;6:400—420.
30. Zhiwen Z, Carson RS, Herington AC, Lee VWK, Burger HG. Endocrinology 1987;120:1633—1638.
31. Tilly JT, LaPolt PS, Hsueh AJW. Endocrinology 1992;130:1296—1302.
32. Bley MA, Simon JC, Estevez AG, Asua LJ, Barano JL. Endocrinology 1992;1223—1229.
33. McIntyre HD, Marechal DJ, Deby GP, Mathieu AG, Hezec-Hagelstein M-T, Franchimont PP. Acta Endocrinol 1992;126:553—558.
34. Rechler MM. Vitamins Horm 1993;47:1—114.
35. Ling N, Ui M, Shimonaka M, Shimasaki S, Bicsak T. In: Yen SSC, Vale W (eds) Neuroendocrine Regulation of Reproduction. New York: Serano Symposia Publ, 1990;207—215.
36. Ui M, Shimonaka M, Shimasaki S, Ling N. Endocrinology 1989;125:912—916.
37. Shimasaki S, Shimonaka M, Ui M, Inouye S, Shibata F, Ling N. J Biol Chem 1990;265:2198—2202.
38. Bicsak TA, Shimonaka M, Malkowski M, Ling N. Endocrinology 1990;126:2184—2189.
39. Shimasaki S, Ling N. Prog Growth Factor Res 1991;3:243—266.
40. Nakatani A, Shimasaki S, Erickson GF, Ling N. Endocrinology 1991;129:1521—1529.
41. Erickson GF, Mitchell C, Nakatani A, Ling N, Shimasaki S. Ovarian insulin-like growth factor binding protein-2 mRNA levels change over the estrous cycle. Endocrine J 1994 (in press).
42. Erickson GF, Nakatani A, Ling N, Shimasaki S. Endocrinology 1993;133:1147—1157.
43. Erickson GF, Nakatani A, Ling N, Shimasaki S. Endocrinology 1992;130:625—636.
44. Erickson GF, Nakatani A, Ling N, Shimasaki S. Endocrinology 1992;130:1867—1878.
45. Liu X-J, Malkowski M, Guo Y-L, Erickson GF, Shimasaki S, Ling N. Endocrinology 1993;132:1176—1183.
46. Ling NC, Liu X-J, Malkowski M, Guo Y-L, Erickson GF, Shimasaki S. Growth Reg 1993;3:7074.
47. Adashi EY, Resnick CE, Hernandez ER, Hurwitz A, Rosenfeld RG. Endocrinology 1990;126:1305—1307.
48. Adashi EY, Resnick CE, Hurwitz A, Ricciarelli E, Hernandez ER, Rosenfeld RG. Endocrinology 1991;128:754—760.
49. Adashi EY, Resnick CE, Tedeshi C, Rosenfeld RG. Endocrinology 1993;132:1463—1468.
50. Hillier SG, Ross GT. Biol Reprod 1979;20:261—268.
51. McNatty KP, Smith DM, Dsathanondh R, Ryan KJ. Ann Biol Biochem Biophys 1979;19:1547—1558.
52. Sadrkhanloo R, Hofeditz C, Erickson GF. Endocrinology 1987;120:146—155.
53. Erickson GF, Li D, Sadrkhanloo R, Liu X-J, Onoda N, Shimasaki S, Ling N. Endocrinology 1994;133:1147—1157.

Nongonadotropic regulation of ovarian function: interleukin-1

Eli Y. Adashi

Division of Reproductive Endocrinology, Departments of Obstetrics and Gynecology, University of Maryland School of Medicine, 405 West Redwood Street, Baltimore, MD 21201, USA

While most attention has been directed thus far at the somatic cellular components of the ovary, the potential role(s) and relative importance of the resident ovarian white blood cell and its cytokine product(s) have received relatively limited attention. Efforts are currently underway to reconcile traditional ovarian physiology with observations relevant to intraovarian components of the white blood cell series.

Interleukin-1 (IL-1), a polypeptide cytokine (previously referred to as lymphocyte activating factor) predominantly produced and secreted by activated macrophages, has been shown to possess a wide range of biological functions as well as to play a role as an immune mediator [1]. Although the relevance of IL-1 to ovarian physiology remains uncertain, an increasing body of evidence supports such a possibility. First, measurable amounts of IL-1-like activity have been documented in both porcine [2] and human [3] follicular fluid. Second, in vitro studies at the level of the murine and porcine ovary revealed IL-1 to possess antigonadotropic [4–9] or steroidogenic [10] properties contingent upon the experimental circumstances under study. Accordingly, it is tempting to speculate that locally-derived IL-1, possibly originating from somatic ovarian cells or resident ovarian macrophages, may be the centerpiece of an intra-ovarian regulatory loop. Since IL-1 is an established mediator of inflammation [1] and since ovulation may constitute an inflammatory-like reaction [11], consideration may be given to the possibility that IL-1 may play an intermediary role in the preovulatory developmental cascade and the terminal ovulatory process. Such speculation is supported by the recognition that IL-1 has been shown in multiple (nonovarian) tissues to promote several ovulation-associated phenomena such as prostaglandin biosynthesis, plasminogen activator production, glycosaminoglycan generation, collagenase activation, and vascular permeability enhancement [1].

To begin to evaluate the above hypothesis, we have set out to evaluate rat ovarian IL-1β gene expression, to determine its cellular localization, and to study its modulation by key endocrine and autocrine regulatory signals [12]. To this end, use was made of a solution hybridization/RNase protection assay in which rat ovarian total RNA (20 µg) was hybridized with a [^{32}P]-labeled 272 base rat IL-1β antisense riboprobe. To assess rat ovarian IL-1β gene expression under in vivo circumstances, use was made of an established experimental model capable of simulating naturally-occurring follicular maturation, ovulation, and corpus luteum formation. Specifically, a single subcutaneous injection of PMSG (151 U/rat) was followed (48 h) later by an ovulatory dose (151 U) of human chorionic gonadotropin (hCG). A faint protected fragment 222 bases long corresponding to the IL-1β message was detectable in whole ovarian material prior to gonadotropic stimulation. Treatment with PMSG for 48 h resulted in a modest, albeit measurable increase in the densitometrically-quantified steady-state levels of the ovarian IL-1β message. Most striking, however, were the increments noted in the relative abundance of ovarian IL-1β transcripts following a 6 h exposure to hCG producing a 4- to 5-fold increase ($p < 0.05$) over the untreated state at a time point approximately 6 h prior to projected follicular rupture. Subsequent evaluation of ovarian IL-1β transcripts, 24 and 48 h following hCG administration, revealed significant ($p < 0.05$) decrements (relative to the 6 h peak) to a level comparable to that seen at the conclusion of 48 h of treatment with PMSG. Cellular localization studies revealed the gonadotropin-dependent IL-1β mRNA to be theca-interstitial cell-exclusive. To assess rat ovarian IL-1β gene expression under in vitro circumstances, we have set out to determine whether IL-1 itself may influence the relative level of its own message. Treatment of whole ovarian dispersates with rhIL-1β (10 ng/ml) for 4 and 24 h resulted in a marked ($p < 0.05$) time-dependent increase (up to 12-fold) in the relative abundance of IL-1β transcripts when compared with untreated controls. Taken together, these observations establish the rat ovarian theca-interstitial cell as a site of IL-1β gene expression, the preovulatory acquisition of which is gonadotropin-dependent. In addition, our present findings document the ability of IL-1β to exert a positive upregulatory effect on its own expression, an autocrine action potentially concerned with self-amplification. As such, this temporal (potentially self-amplifying) sequence of events provides strong indirect support for the proposal that intraovarian IL-1β may play an intermediary role in the preovulatory developmental cascade.

To delineate the scope of the human intraovarian IL-1 system we have undertaken to explore the possibility that the genes encoding IL-1, its receptor, and its receptor antagonist are expressed at the level of the human ovary [13]. To this end, use was made of solution hybridization/RNase protection assays in which total RNA (20 μg) was hybridized with the corresponding [^{32}P]-labeled riboprobes. No detectable IL-1 signal was evident in whole ovarian material from days 4 or 12 of an unstimulated menstrual cycle. However, as in the epidermal carcinoma cell line A431, used herein as a positive control, expected protected fragments corresponding to IL-1α (670 bp) and IL-1β (175 bp) transcripts (IL-1β>>IL-1α) were detected in preovulatory follicular aspirates secured in the course of a gonadotropin-stimulated cycle. Given that preovulatory follicular aspirates may constitute a complex mix of somatic ovarian and circulating cellular elements we have undertaken to further identify the cell type responsible for IL-1 gene expression. In this connection, preovulatory peripheral monocytes obtained at the time of oocyte retrieval proved negative thereby effectively eliminating the possibility that contaminating peripheral monocytes contribute to IL-1 transcripts detected in preovulatory follicular aspirates. Moreover, IL-1β transcripts were detected in cultured forskolin (25 μM)-treated (macrophage-poor) granulosa (but not theca-interstitial) cells suggesting (but not conclusively proving) that the granulosa cell may be a site of IL-1β gene expression. That this is indeed may be the case was further documented by observing IL-1β transcripts in macrophage-depleted follicular aspirates prepared by magnetically-driven immune sorting and validated by flow cytometry analysis. A single protected fragment (projected to be 477 bases long) corresponding to type I IL-1 receptor transcripts was detected in whole ovaries from days 4 and 12 of an unstimulated menstrual cycle, in preovulatory follicular aspirates, and in term placenta used herein as a positive control. Type I IL-1 receptor transcripts were also detected in cultured granulosa and theca-interstitial cell preparations but not in preovulatory peripheral monocytic cells obtained at the time of oocyte retrieval. Treatment of cultured granulosa or theca-interstitial cells with forskolin (25 μM) resulted in a 2- to 3-fold increase in the steady-state levels of type I IL-1 receptor transcripts. A single protected fragment (147 bases long) corresponding to IL-1 receptor antagonist transcripts was detected in whole ovarian material from day 4 of an unstimulated menstrual cycle as well as in macrophage-free preovulatory follicular aspirates. No detectable signal was noted in granulosa or theca-interstitial cells cultured in the absence or presence of forskolin. Taken together, these findings reveal the existence of a complete, highly compartmentalized, hormonally-dependent intraovarian IL-1 system replete with ligands, receptor, and receptor antagonist. The apparent midcycle induction of ovarian IL-1 gene expression and the reported ability of IL-1 to promote a host of ovulation-associated phenomena (in multiple nonovarian tissues) gives rise to the speculation that locally-derived IL-1 may be the centerpiece of an intraovarian regulatory loop concerned with the genesis and maintenance of the preovulatory cascade of follicular events.

In a recent report, we also examined the possibility that the theca-interstitial (androgen-producing) cell may also be a site of IL-1 reception and action [14]. The basal accumulation of androsterone, the major androgenic steroid synthesized by whole ovarian dispersates from immature rats, in the presence of insulin (1 μg/ml), increased 8- to 9-fold after treatment with hCG (1 ng/ml). Although IL-1α or IL-1β (10 ng/ml) by themselves were without effect on basal androsterone accumulation, both cytokines (IL-1β>IL-1α) inhibited hCG hormonal action (in the presence of insulin) in a dose-dependent manner, the maximal inhibitory effect being 75%. Similar results were obtained when using highly purified theca-interstitial cells derived from the same animal model suggesting that IL-1-attenuated androgen biosynthesis is due, at least in part, to IL-1 acting directly at the level of the theca-interstitial cell. The IL-1 effect proved relatively specific since all other known interleukins (IL-2, IL-3, IL-4, IL-5, and IL-6) were without effect. Moreover, IL-1β action was effectively immunoneutralized when concurrently applied with anti-IL-1β (but not nonimmune) sera. Significantly, the antigonadotropic action of IL-1 could not be accounted for by a decrease in the viable cell mass. Tracer studies with radiolabeled steroid substrates suggested that IL-1-attenuated ovarian androsterone accumulation is due, if only in part, to inhibition of transformations catalyzed by (theca-interstitial) 17α-hydroxylase/17:20 lyase, stimulation of theca-interstitial (or granulosa) 20α-hydroxysteroid dehydrogenase-mediated conversions, or both. Taken together, these findings indicate that relatively low concentrations of IL-1, possibly originating from somatic ovarian cells or resident ovarian macrophages, are capable of exerting an inhibitory effect upon gonadotropin-supported androgen production. As such, these and previous observations suggest that intraovarian IL-1 may play a dual regulatory role in the developing ovarian follicle by targeting both the granulosa and theca-interstitial cells as its sites of action.

While the rudimentary nature of current observations is clearly apparent, there is every reason to believe that continued investigation will provide new and meaningful insight relevant to the understanding of the complex interactions between the various cellular components of the ovary. Now that the necessary tools are available, additional efforts in this area are to be anticipated. If progress to date is any indication, odds are that the next decade will reveal the resident ovarian white blood cell and its cytokine messengers to play major roles throughout the ovarian life cycle.

References

1. Dinarello CA. FASEB J 1988;2:108–115.
2. Takakura K, Taii S, Fukuoka M, Yasuda K, Tayaga Y, Yodoi J, Mori T. Endocrinology 1989;125: 618–623
3. Khan SA, Schmid K, Hallin P, Paul RD, Geyter CD, Nieschlag E. Mol Cell Endocrinol 1988;58: 221–230.
4. Gottschall PE, Uehara A, Hoffman ST, Arimura A. Biochem Biophys Res Commun 1987;149:502–509.
5. Gottschall PE, Katsuura G, Arimura A. Biochem Biophys Res Commun 1989;163:764–770.
6. Gottschall PE, Katsuura G, Arimura A. J Reprod Immun 1989;15:281–290.
7. Kasson BG, Gorospe WC. Mol Cell Endocrinol 1989;62:103–111.
8. Yasuda K, Fukuoka M, Taii S, Takakura K, Mori T. Biol Reprod 1990;43:905–912.
9. Fukuoka M, Taii S, Yasuda K, Takakura K, Mori T. Endocrinology 1989;125:136–143.
10. Nakamura Y, Kato H, Terranova PF. Biol Reprod 1990;43:169–173.
11. Espey L. Biol Reprod 1980;22:73–106.
12. Hurwitz A, Ricciarelli E, Botero L, Rohan RM, Hernandez ER, Adashi EY. Endocrinology 1991; 129:3427–3429.
13. Hurwitz A, Loukides J, Ricciarelli E, Botero L, Katz E, McAllister JM, Garcia JE, Rohan RM, Adashi EY, Hernandez ER. J Clin Invest 1992;89:1746–1754.
14. Hurwitz A, Payne DW, Packman JN, Andreani CL, Resnick CE, Hernandez ER, Adashi EY. Endocrinology 1991;129:1250–1256.

Pathophysiology of anovulation

LH-dependent polycystic ovary syndrome

Sarah L. Berga

Division of Reproductive Endocrinology, Departments of Obstetrics, Gynecology, and Reproductive Sciences and of Psychiatry, University of Pittsburgh School of Medicine, Pittsburgh, PA 15213, USA

Introduction

Polycystic ovary syndrome (PCOS) is a heterogeneous disorder of ovarian cyclicity, the central pathognomonic features of which are still open to debate. For instance, if PCOS is defined strictly on the basis of ultrasonically-derived criteria, the population selected for study may differ substantially from that selected on the basis of biochemical features, such as elevated peripheral LH or insulin concentrations [1–3]. For purposes of this presentation, a somewhat reductionistic definition of PCOS will be used. PCOS will be defined as oligo-ovulation not due to any known cause of ovarian dysfunction and associated with hyperandrogenism, as determined by an elevated serum androstenedione and/or testosterone, that is likely to be derived from the ovarian compartment (i.e., recognizable adrenal sources excluded) and not due to a discrete ovarian neoplasm. Menstrual irregularities would be a certain feature of this subgroup, but ultrasonic features such as multiple cysts or increased ovarian stroma would not necessarily be, nor would hyperinsulinemia, acanthosis nigricans, acne, or hirsutism. In order to distinguish this group from that subgroup which displays polycystic ovaries by ultrasonography but may lack classical biochemical features, it has been suggested that the former subgroup be referred to as hyperandrogenic anovulation (HAA).

Although some investigators have not found a clear-cut association between hyperandrogenic anovulation and altered gonadotropin secretory dynamics [3], we recently found that women with HAA not only express characteristic aberrant gonadotropin secretory patterns, with LH levels increased relative to FSH, but also increased LH and free α-subunit pulse frequency when compared to eumenorrheic women studied in the midfollicular phase as shown in Fig. 1 and Table 1 [4]. The discrepancy between our findings and those which found that women with ovarian features such as multiple small cysts, increased stroma, or increased volume, did not consistently display increased LH and androgen concentrations [1–3] may reflect ascertainment bias inherent in obtaining single blood specimens, as both LH and testosterone are secreted into the peripheral compartment in a pulsatile fashion. On the other hand, we did not ascertain ovarian morphology by ultrasonography in our study. Thus, while our data demonstrate an association between anovulation due to ovarian hyperandrogenism and altered gonadotropin release, they do not permit us to

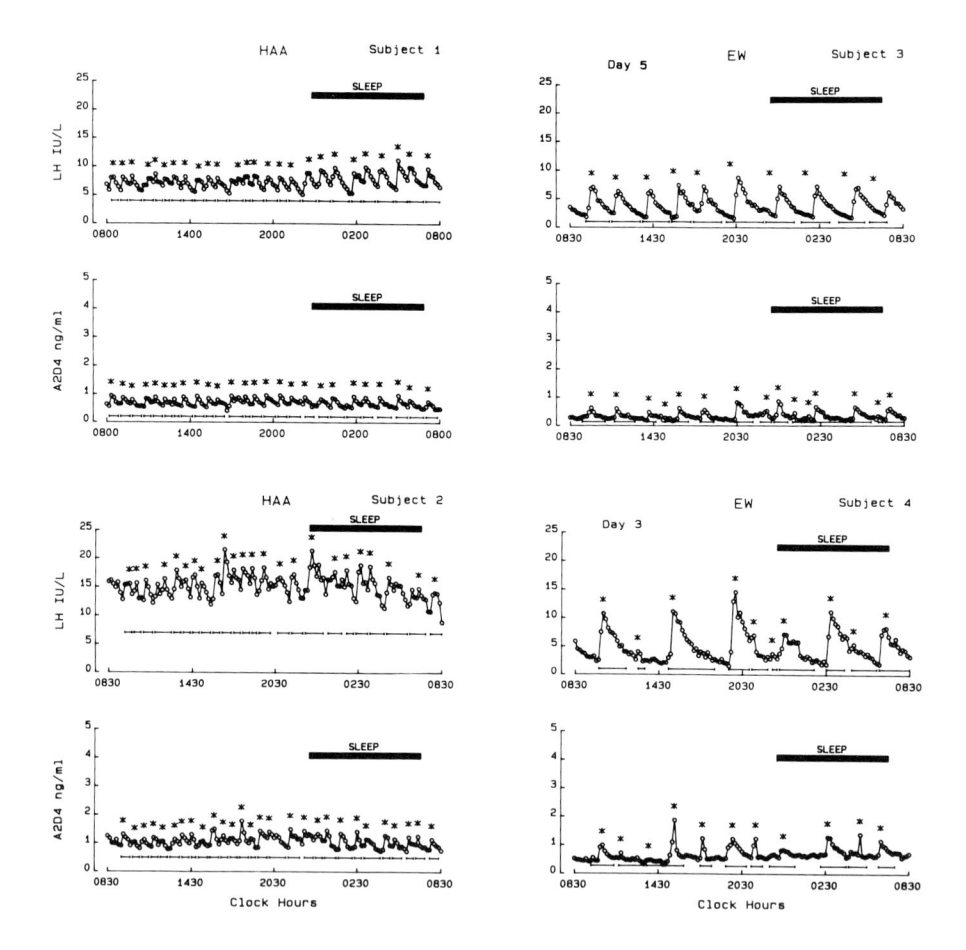

Fig. 1. Twenty-four-hour concentration profiles of LH (top) and α-subunit (bottom) in two eumenorrheic women (EW, right) studied in the follicular phase and in two women with hyperandrogenic anovulation (HAA, left).

discern if the above features are also associated with altered ovarian morphology.

The present aim is to consider whether alterations in gonadotropin secretion characteristic of PCOS or HAA are primary and therefore etiologic, or secondary and therefore a consequence of some other derangement. While elucidation of the pathogenesis of PCOS or HAA is interesting for its own sake, such an understanding also has implications for the clinical management of women with this disorder.

Gonadotropin secretory derangements in PCOS

In 1970, Yen and colleagues described an elevation of serum LH relative to FSH in women with PCOS [5]. Interestingly, the diagnosis of PCOS was made on the basis

Table 1. Individual and mean LH pulse frequency and LH pulse amplitude in nine women with hyperandrogenic anovulation (HAA) and nine eumenorrheic women (EW) [4]

Cycle day		LH pulse no./24 h	LH pulse amplitude (IU/l)
EW	5	10	4.6
	5	24	1.1
	2	12	2.7
	4	21	2.1
	7	18	1.8
	5	14	1.0
	6	13	2.2
	8	19	2.3
	4	23	0.9
Mean ± SEM		17.1 ± 1.7	2.1 ± 0.4
HAA		19	1.9
		25	4.6
		22	2.7
		24	3.4
		24	3.1
		25	2.6
		23	2.2
		25	5.6
		20	2.4
Mean ± SEM		23.0 ± 0.7	3.2 ± 0.4
p value		0.002	0.07

of ovarian morphology observed by culdoscopy or wedge resection. Blood samples were obtained daily on a longitudinal basis. LH levels were found to be higher, and FSH levels lower, than those observed in women studied in the early follicular phase (Fig. 2).

The above observation [5] has fueled considerable investigative attention regarding the proximate cause of the altered gonadotropin patterns. The increase in LH levels could be due to GnRH hypersecretion, increased pituitary responsiveness to GnRH, stimulatory factors other than GnRH, or any combination of these possibilities. In theory, our recent observation that women with HAA had an increase in LH and free α-subunit pulse frequency when compared to eumenorrheic women studied in the midfollicular phase (Fig. 1 and Table 1) would indicate GnRH hypersecretion. Some studies [6–9], but not all [10–12], have observed a similar increase in LH pulse frequency. Although an increase in LH pulse frequency is consistent with GnRH hypersecretion, an increase in pituitary sensitivity to GnRH, a consistent finding in women with PCOS, would facilitate the detection of GnRH pulses. On the other hand, increased GnRH secretion is a potential determinant of increased pituitary responsivity. Thus, without direct measurements of GnRH, the issue of whether LH hypersecretion is a consequence and reflection of GnRH hypersecretion cannot be

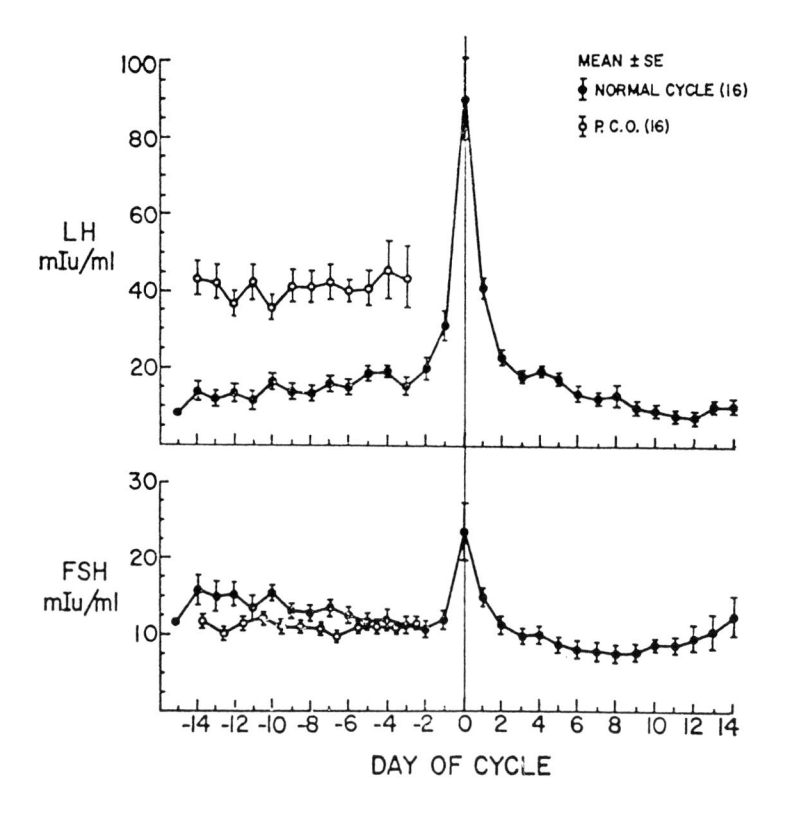

Fig. 2. Daily concentrations of LH and FSH (mean ± SE) in 16 patients with PCO are plotted against the daily FSH and LH concentrations (mean ± SE) observed in 16 normal menstrual cycles. (From Ref. [5], reprinted with permission.)

confirmed. A considerable body of data are consistent, however, with the premise that GnRH hypersecretion occurs in HAA.

Could GnRH hypersecretion account for PCOS?

Assuming it exists, the question remains as to whether sustained GnRH hypersecretion could cause PCOS. As shown in Fig. 4, there are several hypothetical mechanisms by which it could. *First*, GnRH hypersecretion could elicit LH excess which, in turn, could induce theca cell hyperplasia and secondary hyperandrogenemia. *Second*, persistent hyperandrogenemia could alter metabolism, including insulin action, which could directly or indirectly disrupt folliculogenesis. *Third*, sufficient hyperandrogenemia could disrupt folliculogenesis directly at the ovarian level [13]. A *fourth* possibility is that the gonadotropin response to increased GnRH pulse frequency prevents FSH from exceeding for a sufficient duration the threshold needed to initiate and/or sustain folliculogenesis [14,15]. The exogenous administration of

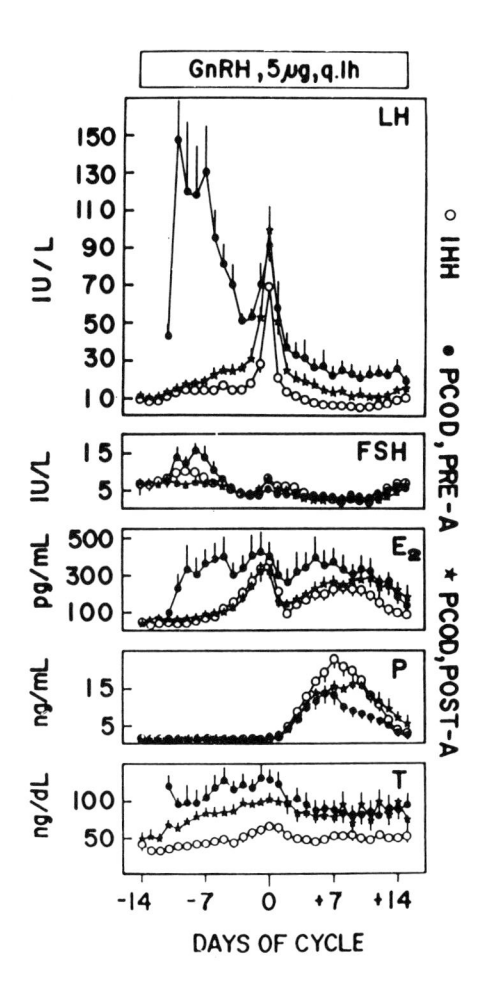

Fig. 3. Daily serum gonadotropin and gonadal steroid concentrations (mean ± SE) during pulsatile GnRH administration in ovulatory cycles of patients with primary hypogonadotropic hypogonadism (IHH) and polycystic ovarian disease (PCOD), before (pre-A) and after (post-A) GnRH analog suppression. (From Ref. [42], reprinted with permission.)

pulsatile GnRH during a single cycle with either a rapid [16] or a slow [17] pulse frequency has been shown to induce corresponding changes in the LH:FSH ratio and luteal phase insufficiency in women with presumably normal ovaries. Also, the exogenous administration of estradiol and progesterone to women with PCOS reduced LH pulse frequency, normalized the LH:FSH ratio, and promoted follicular development, but not to the point of ovulation [18]. *Alternatively* or *additionally*, FSH levels could be suppressed relative to those of LH by the conversion of excess androgens to estrogens. *Sixth*, excess LH could directly disturb and arrest folliculogenesis and/or ovulation [19]. In summary, sustained GnRH hypersecretion theoretically could induce theca cell hyperplasia, hyperandrogenism, gonadotropin

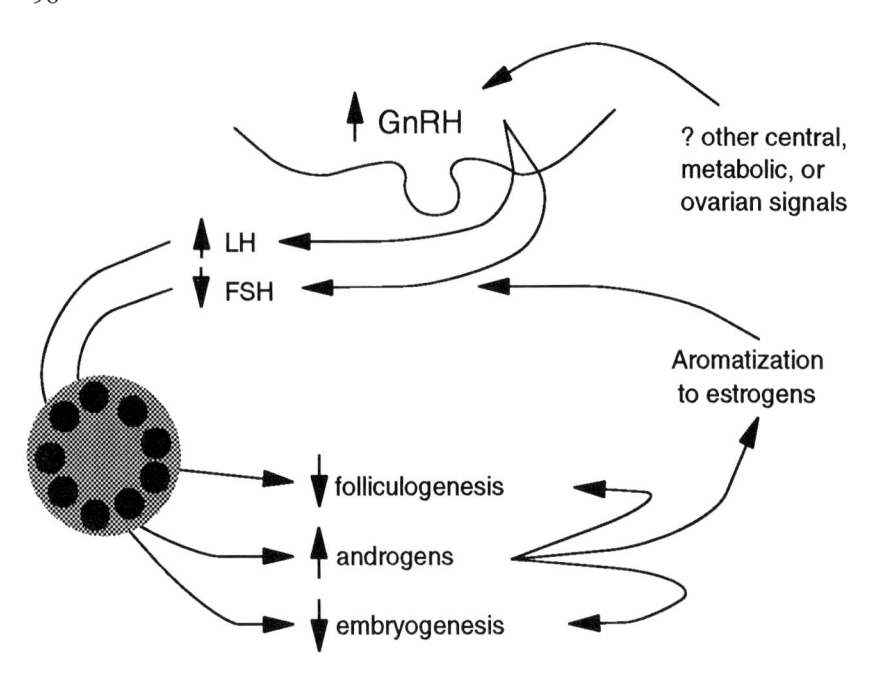

Fig. 4. A proposal for the pathogenesis of polycystic ovary syndrome (PCOS).

derangements, and anovulation. The recent finding that women with adrenal hyperandrogenism display insulin resistance [20] and that prolonged androgen administration decreased insulin sensitivity in Turner's girls [21] lends credence to the concept that, rather than being an independent or primary derangement, the hyperinsulinemia frequently observed in women with PCOS could be at least partially the consequence of long-term hyperandrogenism (which itself could be a manifestation of GnRH hypersecretion).

The potential origins of gonadotropin derangements

Assuming GnRH hypersecretion exists, another query is whether its origin is primarily hypothalamic or central. LH, and presumably GnRH, pulse frequency is slowed in women with PCOS by progesterone [24], an endogenous inhibitor of GnRH pulsatility in primates [22]. We previously showed that progestin exposure not only slows LH pulse frequency, but also induces endogenous opioidergic neuroregulation of GnRH in PCOS, as evidenced by a reversal of the progestin-induced slowing of LH pulse frequency by naloxone [23]. While these data demonstrate that the central neuroregulation of GnRH is preserved in PCOS, the data do not exclude a primary hypothalamic acceleration of GnRH secretion. These data [23], like others [18,24], also demonstrate that a primary determinant of GnRH pulse frequency is the steroidal milieu.

Other data support the hypothesis that the gonadotropin aberrations seen in PCOS are a consequence, rather than a cause, of abnormal steroidal secretion, particularly androgen excess. Dunaif observed that the LH:FSH ratio and the LH, but not FSH, responsivity to exogenous GnRH were increased in a woman with a virilizing ovarian tumor (luteinized thecoma). These gonadotropin derangements were reversed following surgical removal [25]. Similarly, we observed a suppression of FSH and an increase of LH concentrations in a woman rendered amenorrheic for 9 months by a right ovarian arrhenoblastoma. Surgical removal restored LH and FSH levels and the LH:FSH ratio (Table 2). Interestingly, the LH pulse frequency observed 9 weeks postoperatively (2 days following her second menses) was comparable to that observed preoperatively. As noted in Table 1, the postoperative decrease in circulating testosterone concentrations was accompanied by a decline in estrogen levels and a corresponding increase in FSH. These data from women with relatively acute exposures to high androgen levels due to ovarian tumors demonstrate that the LH:FSH ratio may be altered by androgen excess, possibly by conversion to estrogens, but these observations do necessarily account for the acceleration of GnRH-LH pulse frequency observed in PCOS. However, androgen exposure at critical developmental stages might if such an exposure imprinted the GnRH pulse generator (i.e., had an impact upon neural organization and connections). Data from neonatal rhesus primates revealed that castrate males had a circhoral LH pulse frequency whereas castrate females displayed a slower LH pulse frequency of one pulse/3—4 h [26]. Recently, Knobil and colleagues suggested that GnRH activity varies in response to hypothalamic remodelling induced by steroid exposure or withdrawal [27]. In a similar fashion, data suggest that excess androgen exposure alters ovarian morphology, producing features found in PCOS. In a study of female to male transsexuals, exogenous androgen therapy for 21 months resulted in an increase in cystic and atretic follicles, a thickened and collagenized cortex, and hyperplasia of the theca internal and stromal compartments [28]. Unfortunately, the impact of this prolonged androgen exposure upon gonadotropins was not reported. In

Table 2. Biochemical data from a 20-year-old primiparous woman before and after removal of a virilizing right ovarian arrhenoblastoma present for 9 months. Serum samples were obtained at 20-min intervals for 24 h, 2 days before surgery and about 9 weeks after surgery on day 3 following her second postoperative menses.

	Testosterone (pg/ml)	Androstenedione (pg/ml)	Estrone (pg/ml)	Estradiol (pg/ml)
Before	2871	1360	37	50
After	210	856	28	23

	LH (IU/l)	FSH (IU/l)	LH/FSH ratio	LH pulse no./24 h (Q 20 min)	LH pulse amplitude (IU/l)
Before	17.2	5.1	3.4	10	9.2
After	12.36	13.8	0.9	11	7.7

short, prolonged or timely exposure to excess androgen levels could mimic the derangements characteristic of PCOS, i.e., it could accelerate GnRH pulse frequency, increase LH levels, decrease FSH levels, and alter ovarian morphology.

Other factors that might play a role in the genesis of PCOS include estrogens, inhibin, follistatin, GH, insulin, insulin-like growth factors (IGFs), and IGF binding proteins. While any of these substances might regulate FSH levels or alter ovarian function, to date there is no evidence to suggest that these factors could account for LH hypersecretion in PCOS [27,29]. A primary ovarian defect in FSH responsivity is also unlikely because exogenously administered FSH generally results in an augmented ovarian response in women with PCOS when compared to that of eumenorrheic women given a comparable dose [30–32]. While weight loss has been shown to reduce insulin and androgen levels, LH pulse frequency was not changed [33]. In an experimental paradigm in which insulin levels were decreased acutely for 10 days with diazoxide in women with PCOS, gonadotropin secretion, including LH pulse frequency, was unaltered, although serum testosterone levels fell [34]. An acute insulin elevation for 6 h altered steroid metabolism, but not gonadotropin secretion, in women with PCOS [35]. Although short-term (3–6 months) ovarian suppression achieved with GnRH agonist therapy in women with PCOS decreased androgen levels [36,37], it did not alter insulin sensitivity. As noted earlier, however, more chronic androgen exposure may [20,21]. Not all investigators have found that insulin insensitivity is a common characteristic of PCOS [2]. It may be a consequence of obesity [38] and/or androgen excess. Certainly, in the absence of LH stimulation, insulin resistance alone is unlikely to elicit a PCOS-like picture. Thus, of the factors identified and investigated, only androgens seem to have the potential to cause GnRH-LH hypersecretion. However, if excess androgen exposure is not the cause, another possibility is that GnRH-LH hypersecretion is an endowed hypothalamic attribute.

Implications of treatment interventions

If GnRH hypersecretion and LH-induced hyperandrogenemia are etiologic features of PCOS, then those interventions which slow LH pulsatility by about 30% ought to restore normal ovarian function. Unfortunately, there is no therapy presently available that will cause a graded slowing of GnRH pulse frequency. In theory, the slowing of GnRH and accompanying decrements in LH would have to be sustained long enough for LH-induced thecal hyperplasia and its consequence, hyperandrogenism, to regress [18]. Although the perfect agent does not appear to presently exist, there are lessons to be learned from existing interventions.

If the anovulation associated with PCOS is due to the conversion of androgens to estrogens and secondary suppression of FSH, then an antiestrogen or aromatase inhibitor ought to restore ovulation. This, in fact, appears to be the mechanism by which clomiphene acts [39]. Unfortunately, as clomiphene does not slow LH pulsatility, hyperandrogenism persists and it may account for the compromised folliculogenesis often associated with its use [19]. Other methods that increase FSH, such as exogenously-administered gonadotropins and the exogenous delivery of GnRH also do not interrupt LH-induced excess androgen secretion [40,41]. Interestingly, pretreatment with a GnRH-agonist did suppress androgen levels and acutely improved rates of ovulation and conception [42]. As shown in Fig. 3, GnRH agonist pretreatment followed by pulsatile GnRH therapy produced estradiol and progesterone excursions identical to that produced in women with normal ovaries, but unfortunately androgen levels were suppressed for only two out of the 4 weeks and high rates of miscarriage followed [42]. These observations demonstrate that merely correcting the FSH deficit is insufficient to confer reproductive success and suggest that elevated LH and/or LH-induced hyperandrogenemia are fundamental to the pathophysiology of PCOS and the reproductive impairment associated with it.

Summary

Women with PCOS display deranged gonadotropin secretion, particularly increased LH and free α-subunit pulsatility, increased basal LH and free α-subunit levels, and a suppression of FSH levels. Hyperandrogenemia and chronic anovulation are primary manifestations of PCOS, whereas insulin resistance varies [2] and is exacerbated by obesity [38]. The finding of LH hypersecretion, particularly the increase in LH pulse frequency (Fig. 1 and Table 1), suggests that there is altered neuroendocrine regulation of gonadotropin secretion in PCOS. An acceleration of GnRH pulsatility potentially could explain both the LH hypersecretion and the decreased FSH levels. Although GnRH hypersecretion could be a primary hypothalamic attribute, the central neuroregulation of GnRH appears to be largely intact in PCOS.

Chronic GnRH hypersecretion could induce hyperandrogenism, or vice versa. If the latter pertains, PCOS could be due to an ovarian or adrenal diathesis toward excess androgen production. If this diathesis were expressed during fetal, neonatal, or pubertal development, it might imprint the GnRH pulse generator and cause an increase in its pulsatility. The chronic anovulation characteristic of PCOS is most likely attributable to relative FSH insufficiency, but other reproductive consequences such as increased miscarriage rates following ovulation induction are more likely to be due to altered hormonal relationships, including hyperandrogenism or increased LH [19]. In turn, FSH insufficiency may be due directly to increased GnRH pulse frequency and/or may be a consequence of hyperandrogenism. Chronic hyperandrogenism also may contribute directly to follicular arrest.

There is no evidence to date that the insulin resistance commonly associated with PCOS causes LH or GnRH hypersecretion. However, hyperinsulinemia, either congenital or acquired, may directly or indirectly potentiate the actions of LH upon the ovary. By promoting the ovarian secretion of excess androgens or other factors, hyperinsulinemia may perpetuate gonadotropin aberrations, particularly the suppression of FSH, but hyperinsulinemia in the absence of LH hypersecretion is unlikely to lead to PCOS. Furthermore, the androgen excess caused by LH hypersecretion may also serve to exacerbate insulin resistance.

In short, although PCOS is a disorder of ovarian cyclicity associated with metabolic aberrations, as illustrated in Fig. 4, the possibility remains that a primary hypothalamic event, GnRH hypersecretion, is one of the etiologic derangements necessary for the development or expression of this disorder. If so, clinical success in the treatment of PCOS awaits the availability on an agent that can slow the GnRH pulse generator directly without having unwanted consequences upon other organs, such as the endometrium in the case of progesterone. A better understanding of the intrinsic and central regulation of GnRH pulse generator will likely aid in the quest to develop better clinical interventions for PCOS.

Acknowledgements

The author is grateful for the dedicated secretarial support of Ms Pat Baeslach and the technical expertise of Ms T.L. Daniels.

References

1. Pache TD, de Jong FH, Hop WC, Fauser BJCM. Fertil Steril 1993;59:544—549.
2. Conway GS, Jacobs HS, Holly JMP, Wass JAH. Clin Endocrinol 1990;33:593—603.
3. Conway GS, Honour JW, Jacobs HS. Clin Endocrinol (Oxford) 1989;30:459—470.
4. Berga SL, Guzick DS, Winters SJ. J Clin Endocrinol Metab 1993;77:895—901.
5. Yen SSC, Vela P, Rankin J. J Clin Endocrinol Metab 1970;30:435—442.
6. Burger CW, Korsen T, van Kessel H, van Dop PA, Caron FJM, Schoemaker J. J Clin Endocrinol Metab 1985;61:1126—1132.
7. Waldstreicher J, Santoro NF, Hall JE, Filicori M, Crowley WF, Jr. J Clin Endocrinol Metab 1988; 66:165—172.
8. Imse V, Holzapfel G, Hinney B, Kuhn W, Wuttke W. J Clin Endocrinol Metab 1992;74:1053—1061.
9. Venturoli S, Porcu E, Fabbr R, Magrini O, Gammi L, Paradisi R, Forcacci M, Bolzani R, Flamigni C. Clin Endocrinol 1988;28:93—107.
10. Dunaif A, Mandeli J, Fluhr H, Dobrjansky A. J Clin Endocrinol Metab 1988;66:131—139.
11. Kazer RR, Kessel B, Yen SSC. J Clin Endocrinol Metab 1987;65:233—236.
12. Couzinet B, Brailly S, Thomas G, Schaison G, Thalabard JC. Fertil Steril 1989;52:42—50.
13. Louvet J-P, Harman SM, Schreiber JR, Ross GT. Endocrinology 1975;97:366—372.
14. Zeleznik AJ. Endocrinology 1981;109:352—355.
15. Le Nestour E, Marraoui J, Lahlou N, Roger M, DeZiegler D, Bouchard Ph. J Clin Endocrinol Metab 1993;77:439—442.
16. Soules MR, Clifton DK, Bremmer WJ, Steiner RA. J Clin Endocrinol Metab 1987;65:457—464.
17. Filicori M, Flamigni C, Campaniello E, Ferrari P, Merriggiola MC, Michelacci L, Pareschi A, Valdiserri A. Am J Physiol 1989;257:E930—936.
18. Christman GM, Randolph JF, Kelch RP, Marshall JC. J Clin Endocrinol Metab 1991;72:1278—1285.
19. Shoham Z, Jacobs HS, Insler V. Fertil Steril 1993;59:1153—1161.
20. Speiser PW, Serat J, New MI, Gertner JM. J Clin Endocrinol Metab 1992;75:1421—1424.
21. Wilson DM, Frane JW, Serhman B, Johanson AJ, Hintz RL, Rosenfeld RG. J Pediatr 1988;112:210—217.
22. Van Vugt DA, Lam NY, Ferin M. Endocrinology 1984;115:1095—1101.
23. Berga SL, Yen SSC. Clin Endocrinology 1989;30:177—184.

24. Malloy BG, El Shekh MAA, Chapman O, Oakley RE, Hancoc RW, Glass MR. Br J Obstet Gynaecol 1984;9:457–465.
25. Dunaif A, Scully RE, Andersen RN, Chapin DS, Crowley Jr. WF. J Clin Endocrinol Metab 1984; 59:389–393.
26. Plant TM. Endocrinology 1986;119:539–545.
27. O'Byrne KT, Chen MD, Nishihara M, Williams CL, Thalabard JC, Hotchkiss J, Knobil E. Neuroendocrinology 1993;57:588–592.
28. Pache TD, Chadha S, Gooren LJ, Hop WC, Jaarsma KW, Dommerholt HBR, Fauser BCJM. Histopathology 1991;19:445–452.
29. Buckler HM, McLachlan RI, MacLachlan VB, Healy DL, Burger HG. J Clin Endocrinol Metab 1988; 66:798–803.
30. Buvat J, Vuvat-Herbaut M, Marcolin G, Dehaene JL, Verbecq P, Renouard O. Fertil Steril 1989;2: 553–559.
31. Anderson RE, Cragun JM, Chang RJF, Stanczyk FZ, Lobo RA. Fertil Steril 1989;52:216–220.
32. McClamrock HD, Miller Bass K, Adashi EY. Fertil Steril 1991;55:73–79.
33. Guzick DS, Wing R, Smith D, Berga SL, Winters SJ. Endocrine consequences of weight loss in obsese, hyperandrogenic, anovulatory women. Fertil Steril (in press).
34. Nestler JE, Barlascini CO, Matt DW, Steingold KA, Plymate SR, Clore JN, Blackard WG. J Clin Endocrinol Metab 1989;68:1027–1032.
35. Dunaif A. Graf M. J Clin Invest 1989;83:23–29.
36. Geffner ME, Kaplan SA, Bersch N, Golde DW, Landaw EM, Chang RJ. Fertil Steril 1986;45: 327–333.
37. Dunaif A, Green G, Futterweit W, Dobrjansky A. J Clin Endocrinol Metab 1990;70:699–704.
38. Weber RFA, Pache TD, Jacobs ML, Docter R, Loraux DL, Fauser BCJM, Birkenhager JC. Clin Endocrinol 1993;38:295–300.
39. Kettel LM, Roseff SR, Berga SL, Mortola JF, Yen SSC. Fertil Steril 1993;59:532–538.
40. Homburg R, Armar NA, Eshel A, Adams J, Jacobs HS. BMJ 1988;297:1024–1026.
41. Burger CW, Hompes PGA, Korsen TJM, Schoemaker J. Fertil Steril 1989;51:20–29.
42. Filicori M, Flamigni C, Campaniello E, Valdiserri A, Ferrari P, Meriggiola C, Michelacci L, Pareschi A. J Clin Endocrinol Metab 1989;69:825–831.

Role of obesity and insulin in the development of anovulation

John E. Nestler

Medical College of Virginia, Department of Internal Medicine, Division of Endocrinology and Metabolism, MCV Station, Box 111, Richmond, VA 23298-0111, USA

Abstract. Obesity is an insulin-resistant state accompanied by hyperinsulinemia. Hyperinsulinemic insulin resistance has been shown to be an integral feature of women with the polycystic ovary syndrome (PCO), and obesity likely contributes to the development of PCO in some women by exacerbating pre-existing insulin resistance.

Hyperinsulinemia can produce hyperandrogenism in PCO women via two independent mechanisms: 1) by increasing circulating ovarian androgens, and 2) by directly reducing serum SHBG. The net result is a reduction in circulating free testosterone. An inherent (genetically determined) ovarian defect appears likely in women with PCO, which makes the ovary susceptible to insulin's stimulation of androgen production.

Classically, the polycystic ovary syndrome (PCO) has been defined clinically by hyperandrogenism and anovulation. In addition, obesity has always been a prominent feature of this disorder. Between 50–80% of women with PCO are obese [1,2], and many women with PCO have a history of weight gain immediately prior to the onset of oligomenorrhea.

Obesity is characterized by insulin resistance accompanied by a compensatory hyperinsulinemia (i.e., hyperinsulinemic insulin resistance). Recently, it has become apparent that hyperinsulinemic insulin resistance is also a prominent and integral feature of women with PCO. Even nonobese women with PCO manifest hyperinsulinemic insulin resistance, and evidence suggests that hyperinsulinemia plays a pivotal role in the pathogenesis of this disorder [3]. Hence, hyperinsulinemic insulin resistance is a feature common to both obesity and PCO. Furthermore, as will be discussed subsequently, it seems likely that obesity contributes to the development of PCO in some women by exacerbating pre-existing insulin resistance [4,5].

In the following pages, we will review evidence indicating that insulin contributes to the hyperandrogenism of PCO by both increasing serum levels of ovarian androgens and decreasing circulating sex hormone-binding globulin (SHBG) levels. In addition, the possible effects of insulin on pituitary secretion of gonadotropins and follicular development will also be discussed.

Insulin resistance: an integral feature of PCO

There is now overwhelming evidence that PCO is a disorder characterized by insulin resistance and hyperinsulinemia. In multiple studies both obese and nonobese women with PCO have been shown to be more insulin-resistant and hyperinsulinemic than age- and weight-matched normal women [6–19]. To note, insulin resistance and hyperinsulinemia have been shown to be features of PCO not only in the USA, but in other societies as well. In a recent study by Carmina and colleagues [20], women with PCO from the USA, Japan and Italy were compared to their respective normal counterparts. Clinical differences existed among these women. Women with PCO from the USA were significantly more obese than Japanese women with PCO. Moreover, women with PCO from the USA and Italy were hirsute, whereas women with PCO from Japan were not. Nonetheless, regardless of these differences, women with PCO from all three countries manifested insulin resistance, as determined by an insulin tolerance test, and hyperinsulinemia. This common finding across multiple ethnic groups suggests that insulin resistance and hyperinsulinemia represent universal features of PCO.

It is unlikely that the hyperinsulinemic insulin resistance of PCO occurs as a result of hyperandrogenism for the following reasons. Insulin resistance persists in women with PCO who have undergone either subtotal [21] or total [22] removal of the ovaries, or in whom ovarian androgen production has been suppressed with the use of a long-acting gonadotropin hormone-releasing hormone (GnRH) agonist [11,14,23]. Prepubertal women with acanthosis nigricans (a clinical marker for insulin resistance [24]) are hyperinsulinemic, yet elevated serum androgen levels do not appear until several years following the diagnosis of insulin resistance [25]. Some women with point mutations in the insulin receptor gene causing hyperinsulinemic insulin resistance have been shown to have PCO [26,27]. Finally, normal men have androgen levels 10- to 30-fold higher than women, yet they do not demonstrate insulin resistance. Collectively, these observations support the notion that the hyperinsulinemia of PCO is a causal factor in the accompanying hyperandrogenism.

Insulin and ovarian androgens

Effects of insulin on ovarian androgen metabolism

Human ovaries possess insulin receptors [28–30], suggesting a role for this peptide in the regulation of ovarian function. This idea is supported by the in vitro studies of Barbieri and colleagues [31]. These investigators obtained ovarian stroma from both women with PCO and normal women, and incubated the stroma in the presence of vehicle, luteinizing hormone (LH), or insulin. After 24 h, the amount of testosterone released into media was determined. While LH stimulated testosterone release by ovarian tissue from women with PCO, insulin also stimulated testosterone release to an equal or even greater extent. To note, insulin did not stimulate testosterone release by ovarian stroma obtained from normal healthy women. These findings suggested 1) that insulin is capable of directly stimulating ovarian androgen production in women with PCO; and 2) in contrast, ovaries of normal women are not susceptible to this action of insulin.

It has been substantially more difficult to demonstrate an effect of insulin on ovarian androgens in vivo. Multiple studies have been conducted where serum testosterone was monitored in women during an acute elevation of circulating insulin, and the results in women with PCO appeared to be confusing and conflicting. Serum testosterone either rose, did not change, or fell in the women with PCO [32–36]. In contrast, serum testosterone did not change in the normal women [32,33,35,36]. Again, these observations suggest a disparity between women with PCO and normal women in that women with PCO appear to be susceptible to insulin's actions on ovarian steroids, whereas normal women are not.

There are several problems associated with insulin infusion studies that may account for the conflicting results reported in the literature. First of all, the very nature of these studies dictates that the duration of insulin elevation be brief, lasting only a few hours. Furthermore, in many studies the degree of insulin elevation was far above the physiologic range. Finally, several of these studies did not control for the volume of fluids infused, diurnal and day-to-day variations in steroid levels, or for unmeasured perturbations such as the well-described increase in catecholamines that accompanies insulin infusions [37].

Perhaps the single situation in which investigators induced long-term hyperinsulinemia while monitoring serum androgen levels was the case study reported by DeClue and co-workers [38]. These investigators cared for a young woman with PCO who was diabetic and manifested a high degree of insulin resistance. High-dose insulin therapy was started, and marked hyperinsulinemia was maintained over several months. During this period of insulin elevation, circulating testosterone levels progressively rose and ovarian volume, as measured by ultrasound, increased 2-fold. When the insulin infusion was discontinued and serum insulin levels began to fall, serum testosterone levels fell as well, eventually falling into the normal range. A clear concordance existed between serum insulin and testosterone levels, suggesting a cause-and-effect relationship. These findings strongly suggested that insulin stimulated ovarian androgen production in this woman, and was directly responsible for the observed hyperandrogenism.

In order to study the role of physiologic elevations of insulin in PCO, and at the same time avoid problems associated with insulin infusions, we recently utilized the drug diazoxide to suppress insulin release from the pancreas. Simply put, diazoxide was used as a tool to lower insulin levels in women with PCO while monitoring serum androgens.

When five obese women with PCO were administered diazoxide for 10 days, the fasting serum insulin level was suppressed, serum glucose rose, and the insulin response to an oral glucose challenge decreased markedly [39]. More importantly, serum total testosterone levels fell in all five women with PCO during this period of insulin suppression by diazoxide. Mean serum total testosterone fell by 17% from 2.5 ± 0.4 nmol/l to 2.1 ± 0.3 nmol/l ($p < 0.007$). Moreover, serum SHBG levels rose during diazoxide administration from a mean value of 13.2 ± 1.0 nmol/l to 21.7 ± 4.1 nmol/l, but this elevation did not attain statistical significance ($p = 0.09$). Because of the concurrent fall in serum total testosterone and rise in SHBG levels, serum-free (i.e., non-SHBG-bound) testosterone levels fell by 28% from 0.19 ± 0.03 nmol/l to 0.14 ± 0.02 nmol/l (p < 0.01).

To make certain that this decline in circulating testosterone was not due to diazoxide itself, as well as to determine whether insulin regulates ovarian androgens in normal women, a control group of five nonobese healthy women was studied subsequently in an identical manner [40]. In marked contrast to the obese women with PCO, diazoxide treatment altered neither serum testosterone (p = 0.71) nor SHBG (p = 0.24) concentrations in the nonobese healthy women with normal levels of circulating insulin.

Lack of effect of insulin on ovarian androgens in normal women: evidence for a PCO gene?

At least two possible interpretations exist for the disparate results obtained in women with PCO [39] versus normal women [40] during insulin suppression with diazoxide. First of all, insulin levels are not elevated in normal women. Serum insulin in normal women may simply not be sufficiently high to stimulate ovarian androgen biosynthesis, and hence insulin may not regulate ovarian androgens under physiologic conditions.

However, an alternate and more attractive explanation is that normal women lack a genetic predisposition to insulin's stimulatory action on ovarian androgens. That is, it seems likely that there exists a PCO gene or combination of genes, which makes the ovaries of a woman with PCO susceptible to insulin's stimulation of androgen production. This hypothesis would explain not only the experimental data from our laboratory. It is also consistent with the in vitro studies of Barbieri et al. [31], which showed that insulin stimulates testosterone release by ovarian stroma of women with PCO but not by ovarian stroma of normal women, and with the results of in vivo insulin infusion studies, which showed no effect of acute hyperinsulinemia on circulating testosterone in normal women [32,33,35,36]. This hypothesis is further supported by the observation that there is familial clustering of PCO [41], which suggests genetic inheritance. This inheritance is probably polygenic in nature [42]. Finally, this hypothesis would also explain why every woman who is obese, and is therefore by definition hyperinsulinemic, does not develop PCO.

As discussed previously [4,43], this hypothesis suggests that the predisposition to PCO may be more widespread than presently appreciated. As long as a woman who possesses the PCO gene does not develop the requisite degree of insulin resistance and hyperinsulinemia, she does not manifest her underlying tendency to PCO. However, if that genetically susceptible woman should gain weight, the acquired obesity would exacerbate any pre-existing insulin resistance and cause increased hyperinsulinemia. Heightened insulin levels would then act to increase circulating ovarian androgens and yield the phenotypic woman with PCO, who suffers from hyperandrogenism and anovulation. It should be emphasized that this hypothesis is also consonant with the anecdotal observation of many gynecologists that women with PCO frequently give a history of substantial weight gain immediately prior to the clinical development of PCO.

Mechanisms by which insulin could affect ovarian androgen metabolism

On the surface, it may seem paradoxical that insulin should stimulate ovarian androgen production in a woman who is otherwise "resistant" to insulin. Heterogeneity in severity of insulin resistance may exist among different tissues, and insulin resistance at the level of adipocytes does not dictate resistance at the level of the ovaries. For example, ovarian tissue in women with PCO may be less insulin-resistant than adipose tissue or muscle, or may not be insulin-resistant at all. Lending support to this argument is the observation that insulin receptors on ovaries of premenopausal women do not appear to be regulated in the same fashion as insulin receptors present on other cell types and, unlike other tissues, are not downregulated by elevated serum insulin levels [44].

Moreover, several potential mechanisms exist by which a woman could be resistant to insulin's effects on glucose transport, yet remain sensitive to insulin's stimulation of ovarian androgenic pathways. For example, insulin could stimulate ovarian androgen production directly via activation of hybrid insulin receptors [45] or activation of an alternate signal transduction system such as inositolglycan second messengers [46]. Alternatively, insulin could act indirectly by promoting stimulation of ovarian androgen production by IGF-I. IGF-I is a potent stimulator of LH-induced androgen synthesis by ovarian interstitial cells [47,48], which may in part be due to an induction of LH receptors on these cells by IGF-I [49]. Insulin could accomplish this either by cross-reacting with and activating the ovarian IGF-I receptor [50], or by reducing intrafollicular levels of IGF-binding protein 1 (IGFBP-1) and thereby increasing intrafollicular concentrations of free IGF-I [51—54].

Insulin and SHBG

Recently, it has become apparent that insulin influences the clinical androgenic state not only by directly affecting the metabolism of ovarian androgens, but also indirectly by regulating circulating levels of the steroid-binding protein, SHBG. SHBG binds testosterone with high affinity, and it is commonly held that it is the unbound fraction of testosterone but not the SHBG-bound fraction, that is bioavailable to tissues. Regulation of circulating SHBG by insulin would constitute an important additional mechanism by which insulin could promote hyperandrogenism. By reducing circulating SHBG, insulin would increase the delivery of testosterone to tissues because more testosterone would be unbound and bioavailable.

As noted earlier, suppression of insulin with diazoxide in obese women with PCO led not only to a reduction in total testosterone but to a rise in SHBG levels as well. Although one might presume initially that the rise in SHBG was related to the fall in testosterone, several lines of evidence suggested that insulin itself might reduce

SHBG levels in women with PCO. For example, studies have demonstrated an inverse correlation between serum insulin and SHBG in women [55,56]. Insulin suppresses SHBG production by cultured HepG2 cells [57]. Furthermore, when women with PCO are matched for levels of androgens and estrogens, those with higher insulin levels have lower SHBG levels [58–60].

To determine whether insulin can directly influence SHBG metabolism in vivo, the effect of insulin suppression by diazoxide on serum SHBG levels was recently examined under conditions where serum androgen and estrogen levels remained unchanged [23]. Ovarian steroidogenesis in six obese women with PCO was suppressed for 2 months by the administration of a long-acting GnRH agonist. Despite substantial reductions in both serum androgens and estrogens (the mean serum testosterone level fell by 82%), serum SHBG levels did not change. In contrast, when diazoxide was then administered for 10 days to inhibit insulin release, while concurrently continuing GnRH treatment, serum SHBG concentrations rose significantly from a mean value of 17.8 ± 2.6 nmol/l to 23.5 ± 2.0 nmol/l ($p < 0.003$). Because ovarian steroidogenesis was suppressed in these women, diazoxide treatment did not alter serum androgen or estrogen levels. Diazoxide does not affect SHBG production by cultured HepG2 cells (Stephen R. Plymate, personal communication, 1990), nor does it alter serum SHBG levels of nonobese healthy women with normal levels of circulating insulin [40]. Thus, these observations suggest that the rise in serum SHBG levels following the administration of diazoxide was due to suppression of insulin release, and that hyperinsulinemia can reduce serum SHBG levels in obese women with PCO independently of any effect on serum sex steroids.

Studies from other investigators confirm an independent effect of insulin to lower serum SHBG levels in women with PCO [61,62]. Recent in vivo studies also suggest that insulin regulates SHBG not only in women with PCO but in normal men and women as well [63,64]. The results of these studies suggest that regulation of SHBG metabolism by insulin may be a generalized physiologic phenomenon, and that SHBG may serve as a biological marker for hyperinsulinemic insulin resistance in humans [65].

Insulin and pituitary secretion of LH

PCO is characterized by abnormalities in LH secretion by the pituitary. Some studies have found that LH pulse frequency is increased in PCO [66–69], while other studies have found no difference in LH pulse frequency between PCO women and eumenorrheic women [58,70,71]. In general, however, LH pulse amplitude appears to be increased in women with PCO compared to healthy age- and weight-matched control women [69].

An issue that has not been addressed adequately is whether hyperinsulinemia might also influence the androgenic state of women with PCO by affecting pituitary gonadotropin secretion. Insulin receptors have been identified in the human pituitary [72]. Insulin has been shown to modulate anterior pituitary function [73], and insulin has been shown to specifically augment pituitary release of gonadotropins in vitro [74]. Hence, a potential mechanism whereby insulin could enhance ovarian androgen production would be stimulation of LH release by the pituitary. Theoretically, insulin-induced increases in LH pulse frequency and/or amplitude would result in enhanced ovarian androgen production. Clinical studies assessing this possibility are presently in progress in our laboratory.

Insulin and follicular development

Finally, insulin may participate in the pathogenesis of PCO not only by altering the androgen milieu, but by directly affecting ovarian follicular development as well. Insulin can act as a mitogenic factor, it can stimulate tissue production of other growth factors such as IGF-I and IGF-II [75], and, occasionally, it can potentiate the effects of growth factors [76]. In any one of these ways, insulin could stimulate ovarian folliculogenesis and, ultimately, the development of multiple ovarian cysts.

As outlined recently in an excellent review by Nobels and Dewailly [77], there is indeed evidence to suggest that insulin stimulates folliculogenesis. Clinical studies have shown that at the time of puberty girls become increasingly insulin-resistant and hyperinsulinemic [78,79]. At the same time, if the ovaries of adolescent girls are studied by ultrasonography, multicystic ovaries are frequently present [80]. In many of these girls, the multicystic ovaries resolve spontaneously [81]. Nonetheless, it seems reasonable to assume that in some of these girls the multicystic ovaries persist, and the girls go on to clinically develop PCO. It would be instructive to ascertain whether insulin resistance regresses in the girls who demonstrate resolution of the multicystic ovaries, whereas perhaps insulin resistance persists or worsens in those girls who progress to PCO.

The idea that insulin acts to promote folliculogenesis is further supported by the recent preliminary findings of Dellai and colleagues [82]. These investigators studied three groups of women: 1) women with PCO (defined as polycystic ovaries and hyperandrogenism); 2) women with multifollicular ovaries (MFO) and normal androgen levels; and 3) normal ovulatory women. The MFO women manifested hyperinsulinemic insulin resistance compared to the normal women. Moreover, circulating insulin levels correlated with ovarian volume in both PCO and MFO women. Based on these findings, the authors suggested that elevated insulin levels may contribute to multiple folliculogenesis in women with MFO. Our hypothesis would suggest that the MFO women lacked the putative PCO gene. Hence, these women were not susceptible to insulin's action to promote ovarian hyperandrogenism, but were not exempt from insulin's stimulation of folliculogenesis.

Therapeutic implications

The association of insulin with PCO has important clinical therapeutic implications.

It predicts that women with PCO could be treated effectively through weight loss, accomplished either through diet or weight reduction surgery. In fact, studies such as those conducted by Pasquali et al. [83,84] and others [85,86] have well established that substantial weight loss can result in improved fertility in women with PCO. It is even possible that substantial weight loss would not be required to improve reproductive function, and that dietary modification designed to decrease overall insulinemia might suffice. For example, by ingesting more complex carbohydrates in smaller amounts rather than intermittent large binges of food.

A recent report by Kiddy and colleagues [87] lends credence to the idea that dietary therapy constitutes a viable therapeutic option for anovulation. This group studied 13 women with refractory PCO, who were put on a 1,000 calorie diet for 7 months. The women lost more than 5% of weight, with an average weight loss of 11%. To put the weight loss into perspective, this might translate into a reduction in weight from 200 to 180 lbs in a typical woman with PCO. With this modest degree of weight loss, serum insulin levels fell. Not only did serum insulin fall, but, as one might now predict, serum SHBG rose and free testosterone fell as well. Moreover, 11 of the 13 women exhibited improved reproductive function, with five women conceiving spontaneously. The findings of this study constitute strong evidence that dietary therapy is overlooked as a viable treatment option for women with infertility due to PCO.

Finally, it is also possible that medications which reduce circulating insulin levels, such as metformin [88] or some calcium-channel blockers [89–91], might prove to be effective therapies for PCO. This idea is supported by the recent preliminary report by Velazquez and co-workers [92] that treatment of 26 women with PCO with metformin for 8 weeks resulted in a significant fall in serum total testosterone and rise in SHBG concentrations. Some women in this study also experienced resumption of menses and improved fertility during metformin treatment.

Summary

Experimental evidence suggests that hyperinsulinemia can produce hyperandrogenism in women with PCO via two distinct and independent mechanisms: 1) by increasing circulating ovarian androgens, and 2) by directly reducing serum SHBG levels. The net result of these actions is to lower circulating free testosterone levels. It appears likely that an inherent (probably genetically determined) ovarian defect must be present in women with PCO, which makes the ovary susceptible to insulin's stimulation of androgen production.

With this in mind, the strong association between obesity and PCO is not surprising. Obesity is the most common cause of insulin resistance. When a woman with the genetic predisposition to PCO gains weight, the acquired obesity exacerbates any pre-existing insulin resistance and causes heightened hyperinsulinemia. Once a requisite degree of hyperinsulinemia has been attained, it can act to promote hyperandrogenism. In turn, the hyperandrogenism may then act to induce anovulation.

Limited evidence suggests that hyperinsulinemia may also promote ovarian androgen production by influencing pituitary release of gonadotropins. This possibility, however, has not been critically evaluated. Finally, insulin, acting as a growth factor, may promote follicular development. Hence, hyperinsulinemia, through its growth-promoting actions, might contribute to the emergence of multiple ovarian follicles independently of its effects on circulating androgens.

The clinical implication of these findings is that therapy for women with PCO might consist of weight loss, dietary modification, or medications aimed at ameliorating hyperinsulinemic insulin resistance. Such measures could be instituted as primary treatment for infertility, or as therapy in preparation for other ovulation induction strategies. Finally, these treatment modalities might be especially germane in the clinical management of adolescent females before potentially irrevocable alterations in ovarian function have taken place.

Acknowledgements

Studies from the Medical College of Virginia were performed with the invaluable assistance of Drs John Clore and William Blackard, past/present endocrine fellows, and General Clinical Research Center staff. They were supported by NIH Grants DK-18903 and RR-00065, and grants from the American Diabetes Association and the Thomas F. and Kate Miller Jeffress Memorial Trust.

References

1. Yen SSC. Clin Endocrinol (Oxford) 1980;12:177–208.
2. Franks S. Clin Endocrinol (Oxford) 1989;31:87–120.
3. Nestler JE, Strauss JF III. Endocrinol Metab Clin North Am 1991;20:807–823.
4. Nestler JE, Clore JN, Blackard WG. Am J Obstet Gynecol 1989;161:1095–1097.
5. Pasquali R, Casimirri F. Clin Endocrinol (Oxford) 1993;39:1–16.
6. Rosenbaum D, Haber RS, Dunaif A. Am J Physiol 1993;264:E197–E202.
7. Ciaraldi TP, el Roeiy A, Madar Z, Reichart D, Olefsky JM, Yen SSC. J Clin Endocrinol Metab 1992; 75:577–583.
8. Dahlgren E, Janson PO, Johansson S, Mattson L-Å, Lindstedt G, Crona N, Knutsson F, Lundberg P-A, Odén A. Fertil Steril 1992;57:505–513.
9. Dunaif A, Segal KR, Shelley DR, Green G, Dobrjansky A, Licholai T. Diabetes 1992;41:1257–1266.
10. Kim H, Kadowaki H, Sakura H, Odawara M, Momomura K, Takahashi Y, Miyazaki Y, Ohtani T, Akanuma Y, Yazaki Y. Diabetologia 1992;35:261–266.
11. Dunaif A, Green G, Futterweit W, Dobrjansky A. J Clin Endocrinol Metab 1990;70:699–704.
12. Dunaif A, Segal KR, Futterweit W, Dobrjansky A. Diabetes 1989;38:1165–1174.
13. Dunaif A, Graf M, Mandeli J, Laumas V, Dobrjansky A. J Clin Endocrinol Metab 1987;65:499–507.
14. Geffner ME, Kaplan SA, Bersch N, Golde DW, Landaw EM, Chang RZ. Fertil Steril 1986;45:327–333.
15. Chang RJ, Nakamura RM, Judd HL, Kaplan SA. J Clin Endocrinol Metab 1983;57:356–359.
16. Shoupe D, Kumar DD, Lobo RA. Am J Obstet Gynecol 1983;147:588–592.
17. Burghen GA, Givens JR, Kitabchi AE. J Clin Endocrinol Metab 1980;50:113–116.

18. Pasquali R, Casimirri F, Venturoli S, Paradisi R, Mattioli L, Capelli M, Melchionda N, Labo G. Acta Endocrinol (Copenhagen) 1983;104:110–116.
19. Stuart CA, Peters EJ, Prince MJ, Richards G, Cavallo A, Meyer WJ III. Metabolism 1986;35:197–205.
20. Carmina E, Ditkoff EC, Malizia G, Vijod AG, Janni A, Lobo RA. Am J Obstet Gynecol 1992;167:1819–1824.
21. Imperato-McGinley J, Peterson RE, Sturla E, Dawood Y, Bar RS. Am J Med 1978;65:389–395.
22. Nagamani M, Minh TV, Kelver ME. Am J Obstet Gynecol 1986;154:384–389.
23. Nestler JE, Powers LP, Matt DW, Steingold KA, Plymate SR, Rittmaster RS, Clore JN, Blackard WG. J Clin Endocrinol Metab 1991;72:83–89.
24. Dunaif A, Green G, Phelps RG, Lebwohl M, Futterweit W, Lewy L. J Clin Endocrinol Metab 1991;73:590–595.
25. Richards GE, Cavallo A, Meyer WJ III, Prince MJ, Peters EJ, Stuart CA, Smith ER. J Pediatr 1985;107:893–897.
26. Moller DE, Flier JS. N Engl J Med 1988;319:1526–1529.
27. Yoshimasa Y, Seino S, Whittaker J, Kakehi T, Kosaki A, Kuzuy H, Imura H, Bell GI, Steiner DF. Science 1988;240:784–787.
28. Poretsky L, Smith D, Seibel M, Pazianos A, Moses AC, Flier JS. J Clin Endocrinol Metab 1984;59:809–811.
29. Jarrett JC II, Ballejo G, Tsibris JCM, Spellacy WN. J Clin Endocrinol Metab 1985;60:460–463.
30. Poretsky L, Grigorescu F, Seibel M, Moses AC, Flier JS. J Clin Endocrinol Metab 1985;61:728–734.
31. Barbieri RL, Makris A, Randall RW, Daniels G, Kristner RW, Ryan KJ. J Clin Endocrinol Metab 1986;62:904–910.
32. Nestler JE, Clore JN, Strauss JF III, Blackard WG. J Clin Endocrinol Metab 1987;64:180–184.
33. Stuart CA, Prince NJ, Peters EJ, Meyer WJ. Obstet Gynecol 1987;69:921–925.
34. Micic D, Popovic V, Nesovic M, Sumarac M, Dragasevic M, Kendereski A, Markovic D, Djordjevic P, Manojlovic D, Micic J. J Steroid Biochem 1988;31:995–999.
35. Dunaif A, Graf M. J Clin Invest 1989;83:23–29.
36. Smith S, Ravnikar VA, Barbieri RL. Fertil Steril 1987;48:72–77.
37. Rowe JW, Young JB, Minaker KL et al. Diabetes 1981;30:219.
38. DeClue TJ, Shah SC, Marchese M, Malone JI. J Clin Endocrinol Metab 1991;72:1308–1311.
39. Nestler JE, Barlascini CO, Matt DW, Steingold KA, Plymate SR, Clore JN, Blackard WG. J Clin Endocrinol Metab 1989;68:1027–1032.
40. Nestler JE, Singh R, Matt DW, Clore JN, Blackard WG. Am J Obstet Gynecol 1990;163:1243–1246.
41. Givens JR. Endocrinol Metab Clin North Am 1988;17:771–784.
42. Simpson JL. In: Dunaif A, Givens JR, Haseltine FP, Merriam GR (eds) Polycystic Ovary Syndrome. Cambridge, MA: Blackwell Scientific Publications, 1992;59–69.
43. Nestler JE, Clore JN, Blackard WG. In: Dunaif A, Givens JR, Haseltine FP, Merriam GR (eds) Polycystic Ovary Syndrome. Cambridge, MA: Blackwell Scientific Publications, 1992;265–278.
44. Poretsky L, Bhargava G, Saketas M, Dunaif A. Metabolism 1990;39:161–166.
45. Poretsky L. Endocr Rev 1991;12:3–13.
46. Nestler JE, Romero G, Huang LC, Zhang C, Larner J. Endocrinology 1991;129:2951–2956.
47. Cara JF, Rosenfeld RL. Endocrinology 1988;123:733–739.
48. Adashi EY, Resnick CE, Hernandez ER, Hurwitz A, Roberts CT, LeRoith D, Rosenfeld R. In: Dunaif A, Givens JR, Haseltine FP, Merriam GR (eds) Polycystic Ovary Syndrome. Boston: Blackwell Scientific, 1992;213–222.
49. Cara JF, Fan J, Azzarello J, Rosenfield RL. J Clin Invest 1990;86:560–565.
50. Nissley SP, Rechler MM. Clin Endocrinol Metab 1984;13:43–67.
51. Pekonen F, Laatikainen T, Buyalos R, Rutanen EM. Fertil Steril 1989;51:972–975.
52. Conway GS, Jacobs HS, Holly JM, Wass JA. Clin Endocrinol (Oxford) 1990;33:593–603.
53. Cataldo NA, Giudice LC. J Clin Endocrinol Metab 1992;74:695–697.

54. Homburg R, Pariente C, Lunenfeld B, Jacobs HS. Hum Reprod 1992;7:1379–1383.
55. Haffner SM, Katz MS, Stern MP, Dunn F. Metabolism 1988;37:683–688.
56. Peiris AN, Sothmann MS, Aiman EJ et al. Fertil Steril 1989;52:69.
57. Plymate SR, Matej LA, Jones RE, Friedl KE. J Clin Endocrinol Metab 1988;67:460–464.
58. Dunaif A, Mandeli J, Fluhr H, Dobrjansky A. J Clin Endocrinol Metab 1988;66:131–139.
59. Kiddy DS, Sharp PS, White DM et al. Clin Endocrinol (Oxford) 1990;32:213.
60. Plymate SR, Fariss BL, Bassett ML, Matej L. J Clin Endocrinol Metab 1981;52:1246–1248.
61. Franks S, Kiddy DS, Hamilton Fairley D, Bush A, Sharp PS, Reed MJ. J Steroid Biochem Mol Biol 1991;39:835–838.
62. Buyalos RP, Geffner ME, Watanabe RM, Bergman RN, Gornbein JA, Judd HL. Fertil Steril 1993;60:626–633.
63. Preziosi P, Barrett-Connor E, Papoz L, Roger M, Saint-Paul M, Nahoul K, Simon D. J Clin Endocrinol Metab 1993;76:283–287.
64. Peiris AN, Stagner JI, Plymate SR, Vogel RL, Heck M, Samols E. J Clin Endocrinol Metab 1993;76:279–282.
65. Nestler JE. J Clin Endocrinol Metab 1993;76:273–274.
66. Burger CW, Korsen T, van Kessel H, van Dop PA, Caron FJM, Schoemaker J. J Clin Endocrinol Metab 1985;61:1126–1132.
67. Waldstreicher J, Santoro NF, Hall JE, Filicori M, Crowley WF Jr. J Clin Endocrinol Metab 1988;66:165–172.
68. Imse V, Holzapfel G, Hinney B, Kuhn W, Wuttke W. J Clin Endocrinol Metab 1992;74:1053–1061.
69. Berga SL, Guzick DS, Winters SJ. J Clin Endocrinol Metab 1993;77:895–901.
70. Couzinet B, Brailly S, Thomas G, Schaison G, Thalabard JC. Fertil Steril 1989;52:42–50.
71. Kazer RR, Kessel B, Yen SSC. J Clin Endocrinol Metab 1987;65:233–236.
72. Unger JW, Livingston JN, Moss AM. Prog Neurobiol 1991;36:343–362.
73. Yamashita S, Melmed S. Diabetes 1986;35:440–447.
74. Adashi EY, Hsueh AJW, Yen SSC. Endocrinology 1981;108:1441–1449.
75. Giudice LC. Endocr Rev 1992;13:641–669.
76. Poretsky L, Glover B, Laumas V, Kalin M, Dunaif A. Endocrinology 1988;122:581–585.
77. Nobels F, Dewailly D. Fertil Steril 1992;58:655–666.
78. Laron Z, Aurbach-Klipper Y, Flasterstein B, Litwin A, Dickerman Z, Heding LG. Clin Endocrinol (Oxford) 1988;29:625–632.
79. Amiel SA, Caprio S, Sherwin RS, Plewe G, Haymond MW, Tamborlane WV. J Clin Endocrinol Metab 1991;72:277–282.
80. Venturoli S, Porcu E, Fabbri R, Paradisi R, Ruggeri S, Bolelli G, Orsini LF, Gabbi D, Flamigni C. Horm Res 1986;24:269–279.
81. Venturoli S, Porcu E, Fabbri R, Magrini O, Paradisi R, Pallotti G, Gammi L, Flamigni C. Fertil Steril 1987;48:78–85.
82. Dellai P, Cognigni G, Michelacci L, Arnone R, Falbo A, Filicori M. Program and Abstracts of the 75th Annual Meeting of The Endocrine Society 1993;(Abstract 651):213.
83. Pasquali R, Antenucci D, Casmirri F, Venturoli S, Paradisi R, Fabbri R, Balestra V, Melchionda N, Barbara L. J Clin Endocrinol Metab 1989;68:173–179.
84. Pasquali R, Fabbri R, Venturoli S, Paradisi R, Antenucci D, Melchionda N. Am J Obstet Gynecol 1986;154:139–144.
85. Bates GW, Whitworth NS. Fertil Steril 1982;38:406–410.
86. Harlass FE, Plymate SR, Fariss BL, Belts RP. Fertil Steril 1984;42:649–652.
87. Kiddy DS, Hamilton Fairley D, Bush A, Short F, Anyaoku V, Reed MJ, Franks S. Clin Endocrinol (Oxford) 1992;36:105–111.
88. DeFronzo RA, Barzilai N, Simonson DC. J Clin Endocrinol Metab 1991;73:1294–1301.
89. Beer NA, Jakubowicz DJ, Beer RM, Arocha IR, Nestler JE. J Clin Endocrinol Metab 1993;76:178–183.
90. Beer NA, Jakubowicz DJ, Beer RM, Nestler JE. J Clin Endocrinol Metab 1993;76:1464–1469.

91. Byyny RL, LoVerde M, Lloyd S, Mitchell W, Draznin B. Am J Hypertens 1992;5:459–464.
92. Velazquez EM, Mendoza S, Glueck CJ, Hamer T, Sosa F. Clin Res 1993;41(3):694A (abstract).

Hypergonadotropic amenorrhea

Robert W. Rebar and Marcelle I. Cedars
University of Cincinnati, Department of Obstetrics and Gynecology, 231 Bethesda Avenue, Cincinnati, OH 45267-0526, USA

Abstract. Hypergonadotropic amenorrhea in young women is due to many causes and occurs with a higher frequency than previously believed. Careful evaluation is warranted to eliminate any potentially serious associated autoimmune disorder. Estrogen replacement therapy is indicated because of the increased risk of osteoporosis. Spontaneous pregnancy may occur in affected women but is rare and almost always occurs while affected individuals are taking exogenous estrogen. To date, efforts at ovulation induction have been largely unsuccessful in increasing the likelihood of pregnancy. Thus, women desirous of achieving pregnancy are best served by IVF-ET with donor oocytes.

Introduction

We have argued that use of the term "premature ovarian failure" to describe young women under the age of 40 years with hypergonadotropic amenorrhea and at least intermittent hypoestrogenism is inappropriate inasmuch as elevated concentrations of serum follicle-stimulating hormone (FSH) do not always indicate the existence of permanent and irreversible ovarian failure [1,2]. In addition, it is clear that this clinical picture can be due to any of several causes. As a consequence, we continue to advocate use of the term "hypergonadotropic amenorrhea" until a specific etiology can be established in individual patients.

The supposition that amenorrheic women with elevated FSH levels had permanent ovarian failure is based on the studies of Goldenberg and colleagues [3], who reported that amenorrheic individuals with FSH levels greater than 40 mIU/ml of the 2nd IRP-hMG (International Reference Preparation-human Menopausal Gonadotropin) invariably had no oocytes present on ovarian biopsy. This reference preparation is no longer used or available, and values greater than 30 mIU/ml are probably more indicative of ovarian failure in most laboratories today.

Clinical features

Based on publication of several large series of women with presumptive premature ovarian failure, as summarized by Rebar and colleagues [4], and with the addition of another recent large series [1], it is now possible to enumerate the clinical features of affected individuals.

In just over 75% of women evaluated, intermittent symptoms of estrogen deficiency — most commonly hot flushes and/or dyspareunia — are present. Such symptoms occur far more commonly in those with secondary amenorrhea [1]. Conversely, failure to develop mature secondary sex characteristics and chromosomal abnormalities are far more common in women with primary amenorrhea, with over half the patients with primary amenorrhea having obvious karyotypic abnormalities. Women with primary amenorrhea tend to have deletions of all or a part of one X chromosome, while those with secondary amenorrhea more commonly have an additional X chromosome.

Abnormalities suggesting an autoimmune process have been present in about 20% of affected women [1,5]. The combined frequency of clinical and latent manifestations of autoimmune dysfunction, including autoantibodies to steroid-secreting cells, has been found to be as high as 50% in some series [5,6]. Most commonly affected is thyroid function, but Addison disease and hypoparathyroidism are potentially the most serious disorders.

Hypergonadotropic amenorrhea is being seen with increasing frequency in individuals treated for any of a variety of malignancies with chemotherapy, especially alkylating agents, and/or radiation therapy. It is now clear that the amenorrhea may or may not be permanent [7].

A number of studies have now documented that women with hypergonadotropic amenorrhea are at increased risk of developing osteoporosis [1,8]. In one recent study 43% of nonobese patients with hypergonadotropic amenorrhea were below the vertebral fracture threshold and 25% were below the hip fracture threshold at the time of presentation [8].

Withdrawal bleeding in response to exogenous progestin appears to be quite common in women with hypergonadotropic amenorrhea. In one large series just under 50% of the women tested had withdrawal bleeding, and over 20% of those with primary amenorrhea even had some bleeding [1]. Interestingly, there was no correlation between the response to progestin and the likelihood of subsequent spontaneous ovulation. Presumably, withdrawal bleeding occurs because estrogen is intermittently secreted by the ovaries of some women with this disorder.

Characteristically, many of the women with secondary hypergonadotropic amenorrhea have pregnancies prior to diagnosis. Evidence of ovulation following diagnosis has been detected in about one-fourth of women with secondary amenorrhea, and approximately 8% have conceived spontaneously [1]. Women typically do not resume regular cyclic menses after diagnosis, suggesting that ovulation, if and when it occurs, is sporadic.

A number of investigators have attempted to induce ovulation in young women with hypergonadotropic amenorrhea. One prospective double-blind, placebo-controlled, crossover trial compared the effectiveness of estrogen alone and estrogen with an added gonadotropin-releasing hormone agonist to determine if gonadotropin suppression improves ovarian follicle function or ovulation rates in patients with karyotypically normal spontaneous premature ovarian failure [9]. Evidence of follicular function was found in 11 of 23 women and four women (17%) ovulated.

However, the gonadotropin agonist did not significantly enhance recovery of follicular function or ovulation. In a smaller, prospective crossover study, the effectiveness of a GnRH analog alone or together with menopausal gonadotropins was compared in 8 women [10]. Two women in each group ovulated but none conceived. Thus, the effectiveness of neither therapy, given the natural history of the disorder, could be established. These findings are consistent with earlier series reporting attempts at ovulation induction [1,2,4]. No therapy more effective than chance has been identified.

The potential usefulness of high-dose glucocorticoids to suppress immune activity has not been examined critically. Blumenfeld and colleagues [11] have reported that pregnancies were achieved in eight of 15 patients with evidence of autoimmune dysfunction treated with high doses of fluocortolone and menopausal gonadotropins. The study was uncontrolled, however, and is in contrast to another uncontrolled, nonrandomized study finding that two of 11 women conceived in response to high-dose prednisone alone but the other nine had absolutely no response [12]. It would seem that high-dose steroids may well also be no more effective than chance alone in inducing ovulation in affected women.

For reasons that are unclear, almost all of the spontaneous pregnancies that have been reported in women with hypergonadotropic amenorrhea have occurred while the women were taking exogenous estrogen [1,2]. Several of the reported pregnancies have even occurred in women ingesting combination oral contraceptive preparations! Although it has been postulated that estrogens are "effective" because they suppress gonadotropin secretion, there is no conclusive evidence that this is the case.

Ovarian biopsies from women with hypergonadotropic amenorrhea have typically revealed apparently viable oocytes in perhaps half the specimens [1,4]. Because spontaneous pregnancies have subsequently occurred in some women with no oocytes on biopsy [4], ovarian biopsy cannot be recommended. Aiman and Smentek [13] have estimated that follicles are sought in specimens representing 0.15% of a 2 × 3 × 4 cm ovary. Thus, the absence of follicles in biopsies from some women who conceive subsequently should not be unexpected.

Classification

The observations outlined thus far document forcefully argue that there are many causes for hypergonadotropic amenorrhea (Table 1). In a sense the classification suggested may be artificial as many, if not all, of the possible causes may be due to alterations in DNA base pairs. Evidence supporting these causes of hypergonadotropic amenorrhea has been reviewed previously [1,4]. A few comments, however, regarding the association between autoimmune dysfunction and hypergonadotropic amenorrhea are warranted.

It is clear that a wide variety of autoimmune disorders — both endocrine and nonendocrine — frequently occur in association with hypergonadotropic amenorrhea. Supporting an autoimmune etiology are some cases of hypergonadotropic amenorrhea

Table 1. A tentative classification of hypergonadotropic amenorrhea in young women

I. Genetic alterations
   A. Structural alterations in or absence of an X chromosome
   B. Trisomy X with or without mosaicism
   C. Reduced number of germ cells
   D. Accelerated atresia of germ cells (?)
   E. In association with myotonia dystrophica
   F. Enzymatic defects
      1. 17α-Hydroxylase deficiency
      2. Galactosemia

II. Immune dysfunction
   A. In association with other autoimmune disorders
   B. Isolated
   C. Congenital thymic aplasia

III. Physical insults
   A. Chemotherapeutic (especially alkylating) agents
   B. Ionizing radiation
   C. Viral infection
   D. Surgical extirpation

IV. Defective gonadotropin secretion or action (?)
   A. Secretion of biologically inactive gonadotropin
   B. α or β subunit defects
   C. Gonadotropin receptor or postreceptor defects

V. Gonadotropin-secreting pituitary tumors (extremely rare)

VI. Idiopathic

in which lymphocytic infiltrates have been observed in the ovary [4]. Characteristically, such infiltrates are composed of lymphocytes and plasma cells surrounding and infiltrating any remaining developing follicles. It is tempting to suggest that an antigen-specific suppressor cell defect, perhaps to an ovarian cell surface antigen such as the FSH receptor, might allow a "forbidden" clone of helper T cells to stimulate production of antibodies to the ovarian antigen by sensitized B lymphocytes. These antibodies to ovarian antigens might lead to cytotoxicity directly by fixation of complement or indirectly by activation of "killer" (K) cells. Similar mechanisms have been proposed for autoimmune thyroiditis [14]. In this regard, alterations in the T cell population have been reported in patients with premature ovarian failure, although it appears that estrogen deficiency is the cause for the changes in the lymphocyte subsets because the changes are reversed when exogenous estrogen is administered [15].

    Determining precisely which patients with early ovarian "failure" might have autoimmune etiologies is important because such patients might be treated to prevent accelerated loss of the remaining oocytes. Supporting this possibility are individual case reports of women who ovulated following treatment with high-dose glucocorticoids or plasmapheresis [2,5]. No controlled trials have confirmed the efficacy of such therapy. Moreover, even if autoantibodies to ovarian antigens are present, the antibodies may not be the cause of the ovarian failure. Similarly, cell-mediated autoimmunity may arise only after the process initiating destruction of oocytes has been initiated [5].

Evaluation of affected women

How thorough the laboratory evaluation of women with hypergonadotropic amenorrhea should be is subject to debate. In addition to clinical evaluation, measurement of circulating LH, FSH and estradiol concentrations on more than one occasion may help to determine if any functional oocytes remain. If the estradiol concentration is greater than 50 pg/ml or if the LH level is greater than the FSH (in terms of mIU/ml) in any sample, then it is likely that some viable oocytes still remain. Irregular uterine bleeding, indicative of continuing estrogen production, also may indicate the presence of viable oocytes. However, subsequent ovulation can occur even if none of these criteria is fulfilled. For example, we have observed a spontaneous pregnancy in a young woman with hypoestrogenic, hypergonadotropic amenorrhea treated with chemotherapy and radiation therapy for a childhood malignancy and who required estrogen in her late teenage years to effect development of secondary sex characteristics (unpublished). It is clear that intermittent estrogen deficiency, menstruation and occasional ovulation can occur in the same individual [1].

Simple laboratory tests should be performed to rule out thyroid disease, hypoparathyroidism, hypoadrenalism, diabetes mellitus and other evidence of autoimmune dysfunction. Any value of screening for antibodies to steroid-secreting cell antibodies remains to be established. How extensive testing for autoimmune disorders should be is unclear.

It would seem reasonable to perform chromosomal studies in women under age 30 at the time of diagnosis to identify those with gonadal dysgenesis of any kind and in those with female children to identify any transmittable disorder. If a Y chromosome is present, gonadal removal is warranted because of the increased risk of malignancy.

Evaluation of bone density appears warranted in women with hypergonadotropic amenorrhea because of the increased incidence of osteopenia [1,8]. Periodic assessment of bone density may be warranted after institution of therapy to assess its efficacy.

Because a gonadotropin-secreting pituitary neoplasm is a potential cause of hypergonadotropic amenorrhea, evaluation of the sella turcica is believed to be indicated by some clinicians. No cases of such tumors are reported in young women in the Western world. Such cases, therefore, if they exist, must be extremely rare. Because any such neoplasm would no doubt be a macroadenoma, a lateral coned down radiograph of the sella turcica should be adequate.

Therapy

Exogenous estrogen replacement is the mainstay of therapy regardless of the desire for pregnancy. Estrogen will prevent any accelerated loss of bone. Moreover, as previously noted, almost all spontaneous pregnancies have occurred during exogenous estrogen therapy. In spite of the administration of exogenous estrogen, the possibility of spontaneous pregnancy is quite low, certainly less than 10% in our series, even though perhaps 25% of women will ovulate at least occasionally while taking estrogen [1]. Because of the possibility of pregnancy, we advise affected women taking estrogen to contact their physician if they develop any signs or symptoms of pregnancy or do not withdraw to periodic progestin. We do not routinely advise additional contraception if pregnancy is not desired but do discuss this possibility in detail.

Because of the poor responses to ovulation induction, we do not encourage this approach in couples attempting to achieve a pregnancy. Because spontaneous remission is always a possibility, attempts to induce ovulation should be limited to controlled trials designed to determine safety and effectiveness. We encourage the use of donor oocytes for women desiring pregnancy.

Oocyte donation

Oocyte donation has now become an integral part of the assisted reproductive technologies. According to the National IVF Registry of the United States in 1990, 67 separate clinics reported performing in vitro fertilization and embryo transfer (IVF-ET) with donated oocytes [16]. There were 498 patients who received 547 donor transfers. A clinical pregnancy resulted in 160 (29%) of the donor transfers. At the time of the report, 122 (22%) live deliveries had resulted, including 36 sets of twins, three sets of triplets, and one set of quadruplets.

Our own use of oocytes from anonymous donors, transferred to women with presumptive premature ovarian failure, while more modest in number than the national statistics, provides additional revealing information about this enigmatic disorder and the likelihood of pregnancy in affected patients. Between 9/88 and 12/93, 29 patients participated in 38 cycles resulting in embryo transfer at the University of Cincinnati. These patients ranged in age from 28 to 45 years, with a mean of 35.7 years, at the time of IVF-ET. At diagnosis of hypergonadotropic amenorrhea the mean age of these patients was 28.8 years, with a range of 13 to 40. Fifteen patients had idiopathic hypergonadotropic amenorrhea, five had various forms of gonadal dysgenesis, four had their ovaries removed previously for various reasons, three had evidence of an autoimmune disturbance, and one each had previous chemotherapy and radiation therapy for a malignancy.

There were a total of 26 pregnancies which occurred in 22 of the patients. Two of the pregnancies occurred spontaneously following IVF-ET cycles. In one of these two women, a previously transferred embryo resulted in a clinical pregnancy which ended in spontaneous abortion. Excluding frozen embryo transfers in subsequent cycles, 16 clinical pregnancies occurred during the 38 IVF-ET cycles (42.1%). There were 19 conceptions during the first IVF-ET cycle (50%), seven of which resulted from transfer of embryos frozen during this initial cycle. There were five twin and one triplet pregnancy. Three pregnancies ended in spontaneous abortion, and one was an ectopic pregnancy. Interestingly, six of the seven patients over 40 years of age at the time of IVF-ET conceived, and all delivered viable children. In total, 21 of these 29 women (72.4%) with hypergonadotropic amenorrhea desiring children either have delivered viable infants or have ongoing pregnancies. Together, these data indicate that pregnancies can be achieved in these patients, regardless of age or diagnosis, at a very high success rate. Approaches involving ovulation induction must be compared with these high success rates.

To achieve these pregnancies, we have utilized a hormone replacement regimen in the patients consisting of transdermal estradiol-17β and intramuscular progesterone similar to that used by others and reportedly associated with the highest pregnancy rates of any regimen aimed at preparing the endometrium to receive an embryo [17]. Certainly our data are in agreement with this conclusion.

References

1. Rebar RW, Connolly HV. Fertil Steril 1990;53:804–810.
2. Rebar RW, Cedars MI. Endocrinol Metab Clin North Am 1992;21:173–191.
3. Goldenberg RL, Grodin JM, Rodbard D, Ross GT. Am J Obstet Gynecol 1973;116:1003–1012.
4. Rebar RW, Erickson GF, Coulam CB. In: Gondos B, Riddick D (eds) Pathology of Infertility. New York: Thieme Medical Publishers, Inc., 1987;123–141.
5. LaBarbera AR, Miller MM, Ober C, Rebar RW. Am J Reprod Immunol Microbiol 1988;16:115–122.
6. Betterle C, Rossi A, Dalla Pria S, Artifoni A, Pedini B, Gavasso S, Caretto A. Clin Endocrinol 1993;39:35–43.
7. Damewood MD, Grochow LB. Fertil Steril 1986;45:443–459.
8. Bagur AC, Mautalen CA. Calcif Tissue Int 1992;51:4–7.
9. Nelson LM, Kimzey LM, White BJ, Merriam GR. Fertil Steril 1992;57:50–55.
10. Rosen GF, Stone SC, Yee B. Fertil Steril 1992;57:448–449.
11. Blumenfeld Z, Halachmi S, Peretz BA, Shmuel Z, Golan D, Makler A, Brandes JM. Fertil Steril 1993;59:750–755.
12. Corenblum B, Rowe T, Taylor PJ. Fertil Steril 1993;59:988–991.
13. Aiman J, Smentek C. Obstet Gynecol 1985;66:9–14.
14. Volpé R. In: Volpé R (ed) Autoimmunity and Endocrine Disease. New York: Marcel Dekker, 1985;109–285.
15. Ho PC, Tang GWK, Lawton JWM. Hum Reprod 1993;8:714–716.
16. In vitro fertilization/embryo transfer in the United States: 1990 results from the National IVF-ET Registry. Fertil Steril 1992;57:15–22.
17. Benshushan A, Schenker JG. J Assist Reprod Genet 1993;10:105–111.

Ovulation induction with gonadotropins

Purified FSH: characteristics and applications

C. Flamigni, S. Venturoli*, L. Dal Prato and E. Porcu

Institute of Reproductive Physiology and Pathology, University of Bologna, Bologna, Italy

Introduction

The first steps towards the clinical use of gonadotropins were taken in 1926 when Zondek and Smith (cited in [1]) independently discovered that gonadal functions were controlled by the pituitary gland.

Subsequently, intensive research in the area of the extraction and purification of gonadotropins from human sources was simultaneously carried out in Italy, England, Scotland, Switzerland and Sweden. Gemzell et al. [2] reported the first successful induction of ovulation using human pituitary gonadotropins in 1958 and the first pregnancy in 1960. At the same time, Bettendorf [3] succeeded in extracting a potent gonadotropic agent from human pituitaries, and Donini [4] obtained a similar hormone from the urine of postmenopausal women.

The first pregnancy following administration of a human gonadotropin preparation derived from the urine of postmenopausal women (HMG) was obtained by Lunenfeld et al. in 1962 [5] in a patient with hypothalamic amenorrhea. Over the ensuing 30 years HMG has been proven to be effective; its use has become even more widespread due to the introduction of assisted conception techniques for the treatment of many different aspects of human subfertility.

HMG preparations have both LH and FSH activity; however, it is the FSH which is critical for stimulating folliculogenesis.

In 1978 Brown [6], using a pituitary FSH preparation, demonstrated that only a modest increase in circulating FSH levels (about 10—30%) is required in order to initiate follicular growth. In fact, the importance of LH in the follicular phase and its role in the stimulation of the follicle is uncertain, although — according to the "two-cells" theory — a critical sequence of hormones (FSH; FSH+estradiol; FSH+LH+estradiol) seems to be essential for the maturation and proliferation of granulosa cells as well as for the expression of their maximal steroid biosynthetic activity before and after ovulation.

The theory that both gonadotropins are required for complete stimulation of follicle maturation (two cells—two gonadotropins theory) dates back over 50 years.

---

*Address for correspondence: Prof Stefano Venturoli, Clinica Ostetrica e Ginecologica, Via Massarenti 13, I-40138 Bologna, Italy. Fax: +39-51-349774.

Fevold [7] was the first to demonstrate, in 1941, that treatment with FSH increased ovarian growth and follicle development in immature, hypophysectomized rats without stimulating the release of estrogens. Since then, contrasting results have been obtained in rats, monkeys and women in different experimental conditions. As a consequence, we must assess not only the importance of LH in the follicular phase together with its role in the stimulation of the follicle, but also the optimal amount of LH and the ratio of FSH:LH existing in the stimulating drugs.

In the early 80s, Serono provided researchers with a preparation of urinary FSH with minor LH activity (Pergonal FSH — later marketed as Metrodin — 75 IU FSH:<1 IU LH), still not pharmaceutically pure (less than 3% of the total protein content being FSH). The first pregnancy obtained with Metrodin was reported by Flamigni et al. [8] in a woman with polycystic ovary syndrome (PCOS). Originally Metrodin was used to treat women with this disorder. More recently, Metrodin has also been used, in combination with GnRH agonists, for the stimulation of multiple follicular development in patients undergoing assisted conception techniques. The first pregnancy obtained using this combination regimen was reported by Shaw et al. [9].

A number of prospective randomized studies have subsequently demonstrated that Metrodin is as effective as HMG when combined with a GnRH agonist in a long pituitary desensitization protocol. It may be concluded that in the current protocols which utilize pituitary desensitization, there is sufficient residual bioactive LH to support normal follicular development and ovarian steroidogenesis following stimulation with exogenous FSH. Only in the event that a patient is diagnosed as having hypogonadotropic hypogonadism may there be the need for exogenous LH [10].

An increasing number of reports suggest that the excessively high levels of LH during follicular development may be associated with reduced fecundity. Consequently it is possible that a preparation containing only FSH may be preferred for the vast majority of women who require gonadotropin therapy.

Metrodin has recently been further purified by employing additional procedures, such as immunoextraction using monoclonal antibodies and reverse-phase HPLC (Metrodin HP). These steps have resulted in the clinical availability of highly purified urinary FSH — with a specific activity of more than 9,000 IU FSH/mg protein — at least 60 times purer than Metrodin. This preparation can be administered s.c. The residual LH content is less than 0.1 IU per 1,000 IU FSH. Over 95% of the protein content in a 75 IU ampoule of Metrodin HP is FSH.

The following topics should be analyzed and discussed as far as the clinical application of purified FSH is concerned:
— Safety and efficacy of purified FSH used to induce ovulation in patients with PCOS;
— Safety and efficacy of purified FSH used to induce follicular growth and ovulation and optimal FSH:LH ratio in different clinical conditions.
— Safety and efficacy of "highly purified" FSH (HP FSH) used to induce multiple follicular growth in patients undergoing in vitro fertilization.

In the treatment of infertility due to lack of ovulation in patients with PCOS, clomiphene citrate is the drug of choice. In many cases, however, this treatment does not lead to pregnancy: this may be explained by ovulation failures, luteal phase defects, LUF syndrome and antiestrogenic effects on cervical mucosa. In clomiphene-resistant patients HMG has been used but many patients appear to have highly sensitive ovaries and a significant risk of superovulation and hyperstimulation may follow.

The causes of the frequent complications and failures encountered with different treatments may be due to the high levels of LH and the low levels of FSH, which are responsible for the arrest of aromatization and follicular growth and the altered steroid pattern, which is prevalently androgenic. The ovaries are characterized by the presence of an elevated number of follicles in different stages of development and atresia, and are markedly sensitive to stimulation. It has been suggested that treatment with HMG containing additional LH, may increase the risk of hyperstimulation; therefore the use of pure FSH has been advocated for the treatment of PCOS.

In 1977 Ray et al. [11] obtained ovulation in 14 out of 18 cycles and achieved two pregnancies using an FSH preparation obtained from human pituitary extracts. Two years later we obtained a pregnancy using an FSH preparation extracted from postmenopausal urine [8].

We treated two groups of anovulatory women suffering from PCOS in an open trial [12]. The first group consisted of 21 women who received FSH and the second group consisted of 22 women who received HMG. No statistical differences in ovulation rate were found (95.2% vs. 100%); pregnancy rate was 38.1% and 50%, respectively, and a similar abortion rate (9.5% vs. 13.6%) was also observed. No multiple pregnancies occurred. Serum E_2 levels and the number of maturing follicles prior to HCG injections were higher with FSH than with HMG. Ovarian hyperstimulations were more frequent after FSH (40%) than after HMG (22.2%) but cases of severe hyperstimulation were not observed. These data do not confirm an effective advantage in the use of purified FSH as far as induction of ovulation for PCOS is concerned. In a different study [13] we compared the effects of administration of FSH and HMG on the hormonal balance of five patients suffering from PCOS (Fig. 1).

FSH levels increased during both treatments and adequate follicular development was also obtained without substantial differences, but FSH stimulation induced a more rapid maturation and a higher estradiol response, perhaps related to its "head-start". The plasma levels of LH were always high under basal conditions; LH dropped with a clear-cut profile in both types of treatment. A spontaneous LH peak was observed in both types of treatment in four of the five patients but did not occur in the same subjects. Prolactin (PRL) and 17αOH progesterone (17αOH P) showed an increase in both treatments, particularly in the active phase, but no differences were seen. Progesterone (P) did not show any variation up to the LH peak. Plasma levels of testosterone (T), 5αDHT, and Δ_4 androstenedione (A) showed similar profiles in both kinds of treatments with wide daily fluctuations; only A increased more significantly after FSH. A marked turnover of follicles with diameters not exceeding 10 mm and multiple follicles were also found upon human chorionic gonadotropin administration in both treatments.

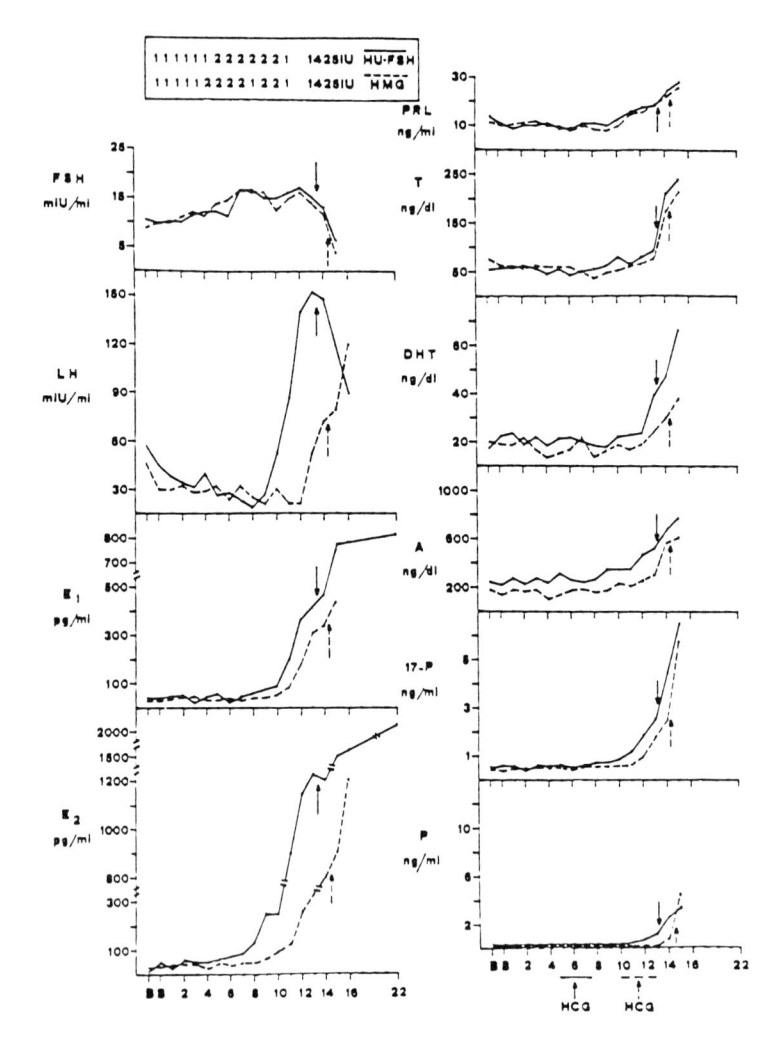

Fig. 1. Comparison between human urinary follicle-stimulating hormone (HU-FSH) and human menopausal gonadotropin treatment in the same patient suffering from PCOS. From Venturoli et al. [13].

Similar results have been described by Larsen et al. [14], Abdel Gadir et al. [15] and Homburg et al. [16].

Contrary to these findings, other authors have reported different kinds of advantages following treatment with FSH in PCOS [17–19].

Furthermore, several different protocols of administration of FSH have been proposed by a large number of authors.

Good results have been reported by Bouvat et al. [20] with a low-dose protocol, (only in part similar to Seibel [21] low-dose protocol). Pulsatile administration of FSH (i.v. or s.c.) has been carried out with and without pretreatment with GnRH analogs, with contrasting results.

Nakamura et al. [22] reported good clinical results, but a very high rate of hyperstimulation (23.5% per cycle); McFaul et al. [24] observed that pulsatile FSH required a greater total dose over a longer period of time to achieve ovulation; it also produced fewer follicles, lower maximum E_2 serum levels and the lowest incidence of hyperstimulation.

Pretreatment with an analog of GnRH has been attempted by a number of authors, however, with a few exceptions, results have been discouraging [16,22] because of either an impaired ovarian response or a high rate of hyperstimulation. A randomized, comparative trial of leuprolide plus FSH vs. FSH alone revealed that the pregnancy rate was significantly higher when leuprolide was not given (16.7% vs. 4.6%) even though the number of follicles on the day of HCG administration was higher in the leuprolide-treated group: in fact the number of patients treated with the analog who had midluteal serum progesterone levels >5 ng/ml was particularly low.

At present, it seems quite difficult to draw a general conclusion concerning the induction of ovulation with FSH in PCOS. Part of the conflict among data reported in the literature may arise from the varying criteria, from one study to another, concerning patient selection and the method used to classify the pathological condition.

The most common unclarified points concern:
— the actual meaning of "clomiphene resistance" (Failure to ovulate? Failure to menstruate? Failure to conceive? Failure after how many cycles? With what hormonal profile?).
— The failure of GnRH therapy, which should be included.
— The obese patients and those with "HAIR-AN" syndrome who should be separately evaluated and reported.
— The influence of intra- and extraovarian factors, such as androgen levels, number of follicles, metabolic clearance rates of the various hormones including FSH.
— The optimal therapy protocol which is still lacking.

In 1971 Berger and Taymor [23] demonstrated that treatment of patients with hypogonadotropic amenorrhea having only pituitary FSH did not result in follicular estradiol secretion; they concluded that LH was essential for induction of ovulation. It was thought that, since the substrate for aromatase (mainly androstenedione) is produced in the theca cells under the influence of FSH, both LH and FSH should be essential for estradiol biosynthesis [25,26].

Recently, the need for LH has been questioned. Jones et al. [27] have suggested that in normal women exogenous LH is not required for adequate folliculogenesis.

In 1986 Venturoli et al. [28] treated five normally menstruating women either with FSH or with HMG in an attempt to induce the development of multiple follicles (Fig. 2).

All cycles were ovulatory; the follicular phase was short and the luteal phase was normal after both treatments. No substantial differences were seen in regard to plasma values of FSH, LH, E_2 and P. FSH, E_2 and P increased to supraphysiologic levels and LH fluctuated within the normal range. A large number of growing follicles were observed in both treatments and at HCG administration time, multiple preovulatory

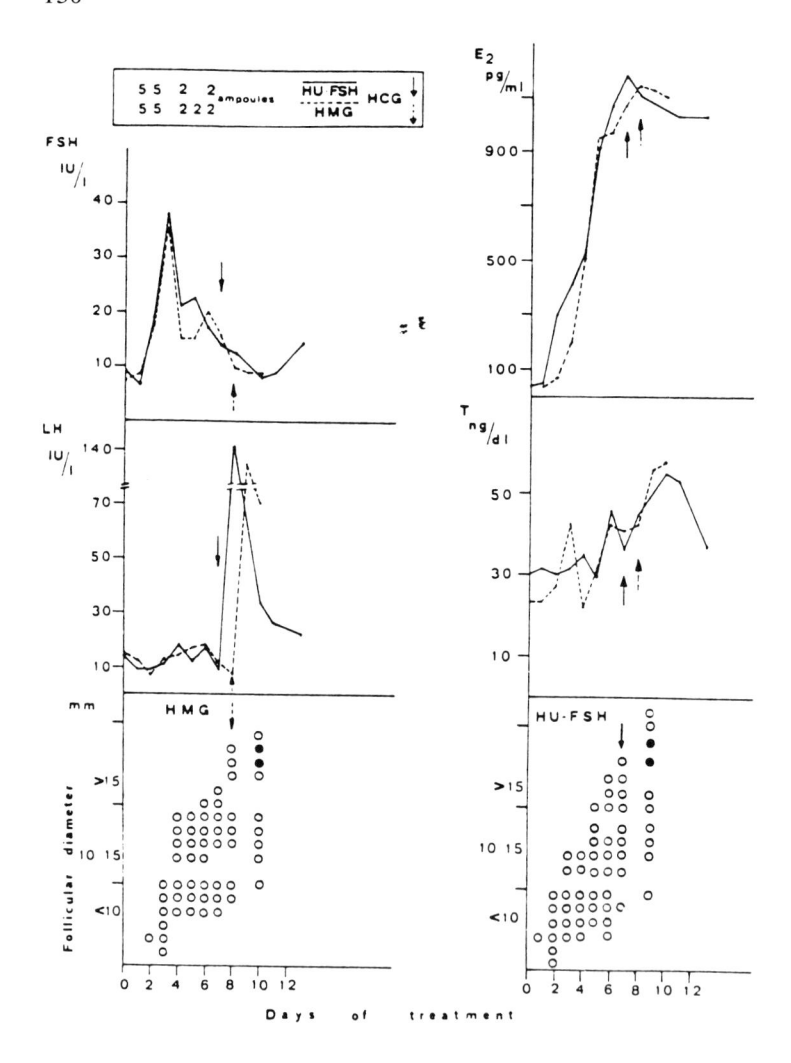

Fig. 2. Comparison between HU-FSH and HMG treatment in the same normal subject. ○: follicle; ●: corpus luteum. From Venturoli et al., 1986 [28].

follicles (>15 mm) were imaged without any difference between the two types of treatment. Pharmacological doses of FSH alone are apparently able to induce the growth of preovulatory follicles when the initiation of stimulation is timed early. Besides this, exogenous LH does not seem to interfere with follicular maturation and ovarian steroidogenesis when normal endogenous LH values are present.

Moreover, a second line of research employing both GnRH antagonists in monkeys [29,30] and GnRH agonists in humans [31,32] to virtually eliminate the pituitary gonadotropin production indicates that LH may be essential for normal steroidogenesis, but follicular growth may well proceed in the virtual absence of LH support.

A third very interesting line of study on this topic is the research started by Couzinet [25] who treated 10 patients with hypogonadotropic hypogonadism (Kallmann syndrome or hypophysectomy) with either purified FSH or HMG with a fixed dose of 225 IU/day for 10 days. Although follicle development could be induced by purified FSH alone, estradiol concentration was excessively low for the number of follicles, and the ovulation rate was lower than after HMG administration. The results highlight the predominant role of FSH in inducing E_2 production and its ability to induce ovulation when negligible amounts of LH (secreted or administered in the incompletely purified FSH preparations) are present.

Similar results have been obtained by Shoham et al. [33] with recombinant FSH in two women with hypogonadotropic hypogonadism; the treatment was sufficient to induce follicular growth but ineffective in increasing the synthesis of E_2. These results further support the notion that follicular development is predominantly dependent on FSH and that steroidogenesis is mainly supported by the synergistic action of FSH and LH.

Recently, we have evaluated the effects of administering FSH to patients with hypogonadotropic hypogonadism [34]. The absence of secretion of gonadotropin was confirmed evaluating circadian variation of LH and FSH levels. Increasing doses of purified FSH led to an increase of both number and diameter of ovarian follicles, but estrogens remained very low for many days and only a slight increment was observed after a prolonged stimulation. Similarly androgens, and in particular androstenedione, remained at their initial low levels — well below the normal range — throughout the entire stimulation period.

More recently, we have administered FSH and HMG in subsequent cycles in order to induce superovulation in patients suffering from hypogonadotropic hypogonadism and who are undergoing in vitro fertilization.

In patients treated with FSH, androgens and estrogens remained low; nevertheless the number of follicles detected, the number and quality of oocytes retrieved, the number of fertilized and cleaved oocytes and the number of embryos were similar in both treatment protocols (Table 1).

We may conclude that in the majority of experiments carried out so far we must not ignore the fact that either negligible endogenous amounts of LH and/or minimal LH contamination of the FSH preparation might explain the follicular maturation with consequent steroidogenesis that has been generally observed.

Moreover, pharmacological doses of FSH may induce an aromatizing system with sufficient activity to enhance estrogen production, even in the absence of normal ovarian androgen levels.

The majority of the studies seem to confirm the enhancing role of LH in ovarian steroidogenesis; more importantly, the results underline the predominant role of FSH in inducing E_2 production and its ability to induce ovulation when negligible amounts of LH are present and when LH activity is sufficient to support follicular development and ovarian steroidogenesis (as is the case in the majority of women).

Clomiphene citrate, HMG and GnRH analog, alone and in different combinations, have been used in a multitude of protocols, with varying degrees of success, in

Table 1. Comparison between the results obtained after the administration of FSH and HMG for an in vitro fertilization program, in subjects suffering from hypogonadotropic hypogonadism

	HMG	FSH
No of cycles	4	4
O.P.U.	4	3
Transfers	4	3
Pregnancies	0	1
Miscarriages	–	1
E2 on HCG day (pg/ml)	770 ± 150	205 ± 85
No of follicles:		
Tot.	11.3 ± 3.5	11.8 ± 3.8
>18 mm	5.0 ± 0.9	4.7 ± 0.8
No of oocytes	8.0 ± 2.0	8.8 ± 1.8
No of insemin. oocytes	8.0 ± 2.0	8.5 ± 2.3
No of fertilized oocytes	4.6 ± 1.5	6.3 ± 2.8
No of cleaved embryos	4.3 ± 1.1	5.3 ± 1.5
No of transf. embryos	3.4 ± 0.6	3.5 ± 0.5

O.P.U.= oocyte pick up.

patients participating in in vitro fertilization programs. More recently, purified FSH (alone; in conjunction with HMG and/or clomifene; with or without GnRH analog therapy) has raised expectations for an improved protocol that would allow variations in the amount of LH administered.

Recently, a multicentric study was carried out in Europe to assess the safety and efficacy of the new highly purified FSH which was administered alone, subcutaneously, to stimulate multiple follicular development in women undergoing in vitro fertilization and embryo transfer. The results of this study are now available [35].

There were 139 women recruited from 10 participating centers. Of these, 135 underwent pituitary desensitization with a long GnRH agonist protocol: following determination of ovarian inactivity, FSH-HP stimulation was started. There were 122 patients considered to be fully eligible for efficacy analysis: 118 of these women received HCG to induce final follicular maturation. The mean of oocyte recovery was 8.4 ± 4.7; 108 patients had an average of 5.3 oocytes fertilized and 105 of them had an average of 2.8 embryos transferred. Twenty-eight patients had a clinical pregnancy and 18 delivered normally.

Plasma E_2 levels rose significantly from baseline values over a 7-day period reaching 6,173 pmol/l on day of HCG. On analyzing the mean plasma E_2 by day of stimulation, levels first increased significantly from baseline concentrations on stimulation day 3. Plasma FSH concentrations in all patients who received HCG had risen significantly above baseline levels by stimulation day 2 and continued to increase to a plateau value of around 14–16 mIU/ml from day 6 of treatment.

Independent of the type and route of GnRH administration the mean pre-stimulation E_2, inhibin and LH were not significantly different, confirming an equivalent degree of pituitary suppression and ovarian inactivity at the time gonadotropin stimulation was started. However, in each case the mean plasma LH concentration was below the minimum value reported in spontaneous cycles. Following stimulation with Metrodin HP a further suppression of endogenous LH was recorded in those patients treated with triptoreline or with buserelin spray (as a consequence of the negative feed-back effects of rising estradiol on basal LH release).

To conclude, Metrodin HP can be safely administered subcutaneously leading to multiple follicular development even when LH concentrations are suppressed following the administration of a GnRH analog.

Conclusions

Purified FSH can be successfully used in the treatment of PCOS anovulation, as well as in other types of anovulation and in the induction of superovulation in women with GnRH analog pituitary desensitisation undergoing assisted reproduction.

Even in women with hypogonadotropic hypogonadism, purified FSH was found to be successful. Further investigations are needed to identify the most appropriate therapeutic protocols, according to the various clinical requirements. In addition, the recent availability of purified FSH and LH will enable researchers to utilize a combined treatment and determine the best FSH/LH ratio in each clinical condition.

Summary

FSH is useful in various clinical conditions and in particular:
— It may be used successfully in treating anovulatory sterility caused by PCOS, even if the ideal administration protocol to be used is not entirely clear.
— It may be used successfully in many cases of chronic anovulation not caused by PCOS and even in cases of extremely low endogenous LH levels.
— It may be utilized successfully to induce multiple follicular growth in patients who must undergo assisted reproduction.

References

1. Lunenfeld B, Insler V, Glezerman M. Diagnosis and treatment of functional infertility. Berlin: Blackwell Wissenschaft, 1993.
2. Gemzell CA, Diczfalusy E, Tillinger G. J Clin Endocrinol Metab 1958;18:1333.
3. Bettendorf G, Breckwoldt M, Neal CH. In: Rosemberg E (ed) Gonadotropins. Los Altos: Geron-X Inc., 1968;453–458.
4. Donini P, Puzzuoli D, Alessio ID, Lunenfeld B, Eshkol A, Parlow AF. Acta Endocrinol (Copenh) 1966;52:169–185.
5. Lunenfeld B, Sulimovici S, Rabau E, Eshkol A. Comptes rendus de la Societé Française de Gynecologie 1962;5:30.
6. Brown JB. Aust NZ J Obstet Gynaecol 1978;18:47–54.
7. Fevold HL. Endocrinology 1941;28:33–36.

8. Flamigni C, Venturoli S, Paradisi R. Induction of ovulation with human urinary FSH. 10th Congreso Mundial de Fertilidad et Esterilidad, Madrid 1980;abstract 358.
9. Shaw RW, Ndukwe G, Imoedemhe DA, Bernard AG, Burford G. Lancet 1985;ii:506.
10. Shoham Z, Balen A, Patel A, Jacobs HS. Fertil Steril 1991;56:1048−1053.
11. Raj SG, Berger MJ, Grimes EM, Taymor ML. Fertil Steril 1977;28:1280.
12. Venturoli S, Paradisi R, Fabbri R, Porcu E, Orsini LF, Flamigni C. Int J Fertil 1987;32:66−70.
13. Venturoli S, Paradisi R, Fabbri R, Magrini O, Porcu E, Flamigni C. Obstet Gynecol 1984;63:6−11.
14. Larsen T, Larsen JF, Schiøler V, Bostofte E, Felding C. Fertil Steril 1990;53:426−431.
15. Abdel-Gadir A, Mowafi RS, Alnaser HM, Alrashid AH, Alonezi OM, Shaw RW. Clin Endocrinol (Oxford) 1990;33:585−592.
16. Homburg R, Eshel A, Kilborn J, Adams J, Jacobs HS. Hum Reprod 1990;5:32−35.
17. Polan ML, Daniele A, Russell JB, DeCherney AH. J Clin Endocrinol Metab 1986;63:1284.
18. Anderson RE, Cragun JM, Chang RJ, Stanczyk FZ, Lobo RA. Fertil Steril 1989;52:216−220.
19. Garcea N, Campo S, Panetta V, Venneri M, Siccardi P, Dargenio R, de Tomasi F. Am J Obstet Gynecol 1985;151:635.
20. Buvat J, Buvat-Herbaut M, Marcolin G et al. Fertil Steril 1989;52:553−559.
21. Seibel MM, Kamrava MM, McArdle C, Taymor ML. Int J Fertil 1984;29:39.
22. Nakamura Y, Yamada H, Yoshida K, Manno T, Ubujata Y, Suzuki M, Yoshimura Y. Horm Res 1990;33(suppl 2):43−48.
23. Berger MJ, Taymor ML. Am J Obstet Gynecol 1971;11:708−710.
24. McFaul PB, Traub AL, Thompson W. Fertil Steril 1990;53:792−797.
25. Hsueh AJ, Adashi EY, Jones PB, Welsh TH Jr. Endocr Rev 1984;5:76−127.
26. Couzinet B, Lestart N, Brailly S, Forest M, Schaison G. Fertil Steril 1988;66:552−556.
27. Jones GS, Acosta A, Garcia JE, Bernardus RE, Rosenwaks Z. Fertil Steril 1985;43:696−702.
28. Venturoli S, Orsini LF, Paradisi R, Fabbri R, Porcu E, Magrini O, Flamigni C. Fertil Steril 1986;45:30−35.
29. Zelinski-Wooten MB, Hutchinson JS, Hess DL, Wolf DP, Stouffer RL. The American Fertility Society/The Canadian Fertilty and Andrology Society. 1993 Annual Meeting Program Supplement, S61.
30. Karnitis VJ, Townson DH, Friedman CI, Danforth DR. The American Fertility Society/The Canadian Fertility and Andrology Society. 1993 Annual Meeting Program Supplement, S5.
31. Bentick B, Show RW, Iffland CA, Burford G, Bernard A. Fertil Steril 1988;50:79−84.
32. Edelstein MC, Brzynsky RG, Jones GS, Simonetti S, Muasher SJ Fertil Stertil 1990;53:103−106.
33. Shoham Z, Mannaerts B, Insler V, Coelingh-Bennink H. Fertil Steril 1993;59:738−742.
34. Porcu E, Sganga E, Dal Prato L, Giacomucci E, Longhi M, Ramilli E, Rocchi G, Burgio K, Venturoli S. Induzione della maturazione follicolare multipla con FSH, in assenza di steroidogenesi in un' adolescente con ipogonadismo ipogonadotropo. LXVI Congresso Nazionale della Società Italiana di Ginecologia e Ostetricia. Sorrento, 23−27 Ottobre 1989.
35. Howles CM, Loumaye E, Giroud D, Luyet G. Multiple follicular development and ovarian steroidogenesis following subcutaneous administration of a highly pirified urinary FSH preparation (Metrodin HP) in pituitary desensitised women undergoing IVF/ET: results of a multicentre European phase III study. Hum Reprod (in press).

Induction of ovulation with gonadotrophins: hMG versus purified FSH

David T. Baird[1] and Colin M. Howles[2]

[1]*Department of Obstetrics and Gynaecology, Centre for Reproductive Biology, University of Edinburgh, 37 Chalmers Street, Edinburgh EH3 9EW, UK;* [2]*Ares-Services SA., 15 bis Chemin des Mines, CH-1202 Geneva, Switzerland*

Abstract. Menopausal gonadotrophin (hMG), which for the last 20 years has been the basis of preparation to induce ovulation in anovulatory women, contains equal amounts of FSH and LH as measured by in vivo bioassay. Recently, purified FSH which contains <1% LH has been prepared by immunochromatography and compared to hMG for induction of ovulation. In women devoid of gonadotrophins (hypogonadotrophic hypogonadism WHO type I) both FSH and hMG stimulate follicular development but the LH in hMG is required for normal secretion of oestrogen. In anovulatory women who have some endogenous LH and FSH (WHO type II e.g., PCOD) there is no difference between FSH and hMG in any of the clinical parameters of efficacy i.e., incidence of ovulatory cycles, monovulation, hyperstimulation, pregnancy or miscarriage. In the majority of anovulatory women minimal amounts of endogenous LH are sufficient to maintain normal oestrogen synthesis when follicular development is induced by FSH alone.

Introduction

The first successful use of gonadotrophins to induce ovulation in anovulatory women was by Carl Gemzell and colleagues in Sweden in 1958 [1]. Follicular development was stimulated by injection of an extract obtained from human pituitary glands (hPG) containing both FSH and LH. Very shortly afterwards, Brown and colleagues initiated widespread collection of pituitary glands in Australia and provided gonadotrophins for ovulation induction through a National Pituitary Agency [2]. Although it was reported in preliminary studies that preparations containing different amounts of FSH and LH had different biological activity, there was no systematic study of the optimum ratio of gonadotrophins to induce follicular development [3,4].

Because the supply of pituitary glands from cadavers was limited, when the technique of extracting gonadotrophins from menopausal urine was perfected, most physicians turned to using these preparations of hMG [5]. It was fortunate because it has subsequently turned out that there is a risk of transmitting the virus which causes the fatal Creutzfeldt-Jakob disease following treatment with pituitary extracts [6].

Gonadotrophins are extracted from urine using immunochromatography and hMG contain both FSH and LH in equal amounts. It has been very difficult to standardise the amount of LH and both commercial preparations (Humegon and Pergonal) contain

Table 1. Commercial preparations of gonadotrophins prepared from urine of menopausal women (hMG)

	FSH:LH	Company
Humegon	1:1	Organon
Pergonal	1:1	Serono
hMG 3:1	3:1	Organon
Metrodin	>60:1	Serono
HP Metrodin	>60:1	Serono

detectable amounts of hCG. In recent years, additional preparations containing different ratios of FSH and LH (as determined by in vivo bioassay) have become available (Table 1).

These purified preparations have some theoretical advantage over the crude urinary extracts i.e., they contain much less nonactive protein and they permit variation in relative amounts of gonadotrophins. Moreover, they provided powerful experimental tools with which to investigate the physiological requirements for follicular development. But do they really offer any real therapeutic advantage? In this paper we shall consider the evidence as to whether purified gonadotrophins (Metrodin or HP Metrodin) are more effective at inducing ovulation in anovulatory women. We shall confine ourselves to their use in hypogonadotrophic women and in women with anovulatory infertility in association with polycystic ovarian disease (PCOD). Use of gonadotrophins for stimulation of multiple follicular development in association with assisted conception is considered elsewhere in this symposium, as are gonadotrophins prepared by recombinant techniques.

Pharmacokinetics of urinary gonadotrophins

Gonadotrophins which are extracted from menopausal urine contain a species of FSH which is heavily glycosylated and has a relative acidic electrophoretic charge and, hence, a long terminal half-life of about 9–16 h [7]. The rate of clearance from the bloodstream is even longer after intramuscular injection and therapeutic levels may persist for up to 3 days [8]. As expected, the pharmacokinetics of FSH in both commercial preparations of hMG are identical and similar to those in the highly purified forms [9,10]. Less predictable is the fact that recombinant FSH has a similar half-life to native urinary FSH.

LH is cleared from the circulation much more quickly than FSH with a half-life of about 2 h. After intramuscular injection in normal women, there is a modest rise in concentration of LH to a maximum of 15% at 2 h, but thereafter, there is no significant difference in the concentration of LH in plasma of women treated with hMG or FSH [11]. As expected, in women treated with both preparations there is a sustained rise in the concentration of FSH while the basal concentration of LH (collected at least 18 h after the previous day's injection) declines progressively as follicle development is stimulated (see later). In summary, the pharmacokinetics of

FSH in both hMG and purified FSH are identical while the LH in hMG is cleared much more rapidly.

In order to simulate the physiological secretion more accurately and to maintain the levels of FSH and LH throughout the 24 h, hMG and FSH have been given by frequent pulses via a portable infusion pump programmed to deliver a bolus subcutaneously or intravenously at intervals of 60–120 min [12–15]. There are no comprehensive data on the pattern of concentration of FSH and LH achieved following this treatment, although in a single woman there was a constant level of FSH and pulsatile pattern of LH, as one might expect [15]. Based on single daily samples of blood collected just prior to the pulse, there is no difference in the concentration of FSH or LH between women given hMG or FSH [13].

In summary, because of the long half-life of FSH there appears to be no significant difference in the pharmacodynamics whether the preparation is delivered as a single daily intramuscular injection or by frequent pulsatile subcutaneous injections.

Induction of ovulation in women with hypogonadotrophic hypogonadism (WHO type I)

When women with anovulatory infertility due to an absence or severe depletion of gonadotrophins are treated with hMG, over 90% of cycles are ovulatory and the pregnancy rate per cycle is about 25% [16,17]. However, each woman appears to have a separate threshold level of FSH which will stimulate follicular development and it is very difficult to reach this level without stimulating the development of multiple follicles. For this reason even with careful monitoring, the incidence of multiple births is almost 25%. The therapeutic objective of selecting a single follicle for ovulation as in the spontaneous cycle has not been achieved in part because of the limitations of the existing preparations of hMG. In many women with hypogonadotrophic hypogonadism e.g., Kallmann syndrome, weight-related amenorrhoea, in whom the defect is hypothalamic, it is possible to induce ovulation with GnRH [18]. It is necessary to administer the GnRH in a series of pulses at intervals of 60–120 min in order to simulate the physiological pattern of secretion of GnRH from the hypothalamus [19]. Normal feedback of ovarian hormones at the level of the anterior pituitary remains intact, and hence, a single ovulation usually occurs. The cumulative pregnancy rate is very high if the women are selected appropriately.

There are, however, some women with absent or malfunctioning pituitary glands e.g., following hypophysectomy, who still require gonadotrophins. There is now convincing evidence that both FSH and LH are required to induce normal ovarian function in women who are totally devoid of gonadotrophins. Couzinet et al. showed that although follicular development could be induced in such amenorrhoeic women with purified FSH, the addition of some LH in the form of hMG was required for normal secretion of oestrogen [20]. Similar results have recently been reported in women with Kallmann syndrome using recombinant FSH which is totally devoid of

LH [21]. These results, therefore, confirm in women the two-gonadotrophin–two-cell hypothesis for action of gonadotrophins on the follicle i.e., while FSH acts to induce growth and differentiation of granulosa cells, LH stimulates the theca cells to produce androgens which are used as precursors for the synthesis of oestrogen [22]. We do not know whether the low levels of oestrogen produced during treatment with purified FSH are due to minimal levels of endogenous LH or synthesised from androgen precursors of adrenal origin. It seems unlikely, however, that the concentration of oestrogen would be adequate to induce development of the endometrium to a degree sufficient to support implantation. Thus, although there is no direct evidence, it is assumed that pure FSH alone would not be a suitable treatment for infertile women with hypogonadotrophic hypogonadism.

In order to prevent the stimulation of multiple follicles and to reduce the risk of multiple births, various regimens of treatment with hMG have been tried. We have suggested previously that it may be necessary to use several different preparations of FSH with different half-lives, in combination with varying amounts of LH in order to reproduce more closely the changes which occur in the normal ovarian cycle [23]. As recombinant pure FSH and LH become available, it will be possible to investigate these therapeutic options.

Treatment of polycystic ovarian syndrome (WHO type II)

While the cause of anovulation and treatment of women lacking gonadotrophins is obvious, it is less clear why the majority of women with evidence of some ovarian activity fail to ovulate [24]. In many, persistent anovulation is associated with polycystic ovarian disease (PCOD) which is characterised by a disturbance in the regular pattern of menses and polycystic ovaries accompanied in many cases with hirsutism, obesity and insulin resistance [25]. The majority of women with PCOD will ovulate when given antioestrogens such as clomiphene or tamoxifen. The reason why some fail to respond to antioestrogens is not known but these women require treatment with gonadotrophins.

Characteristically, women with PCOD have relatively high levels of LH due to high amplitude pulses of LH which occur at a frequency of 60–120 min. There is some evidence that this high level of LH impairs normal follicular development perhaps by stimulating excessive production of androgens by hypertrophied theca cells. While this cannot be the sole explanation for PCO which persists even if the raised levels of LH are suppressed with progestogens or GnRH agonists, raised levels of LH in the follicular phase are associated with premature luteinisation of the follicle (as indicated by raised concentration of progesterone) and a relatively high incidence of miscarriage [26]. It may be that in addition to increased secretion of progesterone, LH induces premature reactivation of the oocyte from the dictyate stage of the first meiotic division and, hence, fertilisation of an "ageing" oocyte occurs [27].

Because women with PCOD are very sensitive to gonadotrophins, the risk of hyperstimulation and multiple births is increased. A number of authors have recommended starting with a very low daily dose of hMG (usually 37.5 U) and only increasing gradually after a period of 7–10 days [28–30]. Because the level of endogenous LH is already raised, it seems logical to treat women with purified FSH rather than the mixture found in hMG [31–34]. Moreover, following a single bolus injection of hMG the concentration of LH might be high enough to induce premature luteinisation of the follicle. Theoretically, there could be some advantage in giving the hMG by continuous or pulsatile administration rather than by single daily injections.

What is the evidence that any of these theoretical concepts offer any real clinical benefit? Unfortunately, there are very few randomised control trials of FSH versus hMG and none in which the power has been sufficient to demonstrate whether there are significant differences in pregnancy rate. The pharmacokinetics of FSH and LH after intramuscular or subcutaneous injection do not suggest that there is any significant difference in the therapeutic levels of gonadotrophins achieved by either route.

Comparison of FSH and hMG

Treatment with gonadotrophins is usually restricted to those women with anovulatory infertility who are unresponsive to clomiphene or other antioestrogens. As such, the published studies are unrepresentative of a general population of women with PCOD because many of the more fertile women may have already become pregnant by treatment with simpler methods e.g., clomiphene. As mentioned above, as PCOD is characterised by excessive secretion of LH, it would seem logical to select a gonadotrophin preparation with relatively little LH. An alternative approach has been to render women with PCOD relatively hypogonadotrophic by pretreatment with analogues of GnRH [35,36]. In this way it was hoped that the results of treatment with gonadotrophins in women with PCOD could be as successful as treatment of women with hypogonadotrophic hypogonadism. Unfortunately, the evidence so far suggests that neither of these assumptions is correct.

Pharmacodynamic studies have revealed that there is little if any difference in the concentrations of FSH or LH found after the administration of purified FSH or hMG to women with PCOD [11,37]. In both the level of FSH is elevated throughout the course of treatment. The concentration of LH is slightly higher (15% for a few hours after the injection) but in both groups of women there is a significant and progressive decrease in the concentration of LH in the days after commencement of treatment. This decrease has been reported in normal women receiving FSH or hMG by pulsatile subcutaneous or by intramuscular injection [13]. The decrease coincides with stimulation of follicular development and presumably is due to suppression of endogenous LH by oestradiol or some other hormone(s) e.g., gonadotrophin surge attenuating factor (GnSAF) secreted by the developing antral follicles.

Clinical results of FSH and hMG in PCOD

There are numerous reports of the induction of follicular development and ovulation in women with PCOD with either FSH or hMG [31–34]. Women with PCOD are notoriously sensitive to hMG and the incidence of multiple ovulation and hyperstimulation is disturbingly high. Moreover, the pregnancy rate per treatment cycle is usually reported to be much lower than that following similar treatment in women with hypogonadotrophic hypogonadism. Is there any evidence that the results can be improved by using purified FSH?

There are very few randomised trials comparing the two preparations in the same group of patients. In a randomised crossover study involving 12 women with PCOD, Larsen et al. were unable to find any difference in the dose of FSH and hMG necessary to induce preovulatory follicles [37]. There were no differences in the concentration of pituitary or ovarian hormones during treatment. Moreover, the increase in ovarian volume, as a prediction of potential hyperstimulation, was similar in the two treatments. The number of pregnancies (one in each group) was too few to determine clinical efficacy. A similar conclusion was reached by Homburg et al., who compared FSH with hMG in a small number of women treated with hMG or FSH (Table 2) [36].

Whether or not the women were downregulated with GnRH agonist prior to gonadotrophins, there was no difference between the groups in pregnancy rate, ovulatory cycles or hyperstimulation between the women treated with hMG or FSH (Table 3).

It is of interest that the incidence of hyperstimulation was significantly higher in the group treated with GnRH agonists, presumably because it was possible to give greater doses of FSH or hMG for longer in this group.

Both these studies have confirmed the high incidence of hyperstimulation which occurs when women with PCOD are treated with gonadotrophins. The stimulation of many follicles associated with this potentially serious complication could lead to a high incidence of multiple pregnancies if ovulation was induced with hCG. In an attempt to reduce the risk of multiple follicular development, there have been several reports of low-dose gonadotrophin treatment [28–30]. Following the principles established by Brown and Gemzell that each woman has her own "threshold" of FSH

Table 2. FSH versus hMG in PCOD

	With GnRH analogue		Without GnRH analogue	
	hMG	FSH	hMG	FSH
Patients	14	11	11	10
Cycles	30	27	42	23
Ovulation	17 (56%)	15 (56%)	34 (81%)	17 (74%)
Pregnancies (% cycle)	2	3	3	3
Hyperstimulation	10 (33%)	9 (33%)	3 (7%)	2 (9%)

From Homburg et al., 1990 [36].

Table 3. GnRH analogue and treatment with FSH or hMG

	GnRH analogue	FSH/hMG alone	Significance
No. cycles	57	65	
Mean ampoules/cycle	27.7	16.5	$p < 0.001$
Mean duration treatment (days)	18.2	13.8	$p < 0.004$
% Hyperstimulation	33	8	$p < 0.007$

From Homburg et al., 1990 [36].

[2,16], this treatment starts with a low dose (usually ½ ampoule — 37.5 IU) per day for a period of at least 10 days. If there has been no response as indicated by a rise in serum oestradiol level and/or an increase in the growth of one or two follicles, the dose is increased by no more than 30% until the threshold dose is found. Using this technique in 100 women with PCOD, it has been possible to achieve ovulation in 72% of cycles in which 73% were uniovular [29]. Although the cumulative pregnancy rate was 55% at 6 months and there were only two multiple births, the pregnancy rate per cycle started was only 11% and only 26 of 45 pregnancies resulted in a viable birth. The rate of early pregnancy loss (32%) was disappointingly high.

In a small series these same authors reported a comparison of urine FSH and hMG in 30 women with PCOD [38]. The women were randomly allocated to low-dose treatment with either hMG or FSH after consent for randomisation had been obtained. The overall results of the total of 75 cycles of treatment given (35 and 40 to FSH and hMG, respectively) were similar to the large series quoted above. There was no difference in the ovulation rate or incidence of single follicular development of pregnancy rate between the two groups. The authors concluded that in women with PCOD the amount of LH in hMG is insignificant compared to the amount of endogenous LH.

Summary and Conclusions

In the last 30 years, gonadotrophins have been used successfully in the treatment of women with anovulatory infertility. Although extracts of human pituitary glands with different relative amounts of FSH and LH were used initially, in the last 20 years preparations of urinary gonadotrophins (hMG) have contained a fixed ratio of FSH to LH. There is substantial evidence that the active ingredient of hMG in stimulating follicular development is FSH. In women who are totally devoid of gonadotrophins, LH is required for the production of normal amounts of oestradiol confirming the "two-gonadotrophin–two-cell" hypothesis for follicular development and steroid synthesis.

In normal women or women with PCOD, there is no evidence that there is a significant difference in the clinical efficacy of hMG and purified FSH. The pharmacodynamic profiles of the two preparations are identical with regard to FSH and show biologically insignificant difference of LH. Current evidence suggests that recombinant FSH is similar to FSH extracted from menopausal urine. Further experience will be required to determine whether there is any clinical advantage in preparations which contain different relative amounts of FSH and LH and of different half-lives. The problem of multiple pregnancies due to lack of our ability to stimulate the development of a single ovulatory follicle remains.

References

1. Gemzell CA, Diczfalusy E, Tillinger G. J Clin Endocrinol Metab 1958;18:1333–1348.
2. Brown JB, Evans JH, Adey FD, Taft HP, Townsend SL. In: Baird DT, Strong JA (eds) Control of Gonadal Steroid Secretion. Baltimore: Williams and Wilkins & Co., 1970;210–225.
3. Bertran PV, Coleman JR, Crooke AC, McNaughton MC, Mills IH. J Endocrinol 1972;53:231–248.
4. Berger MJ, Taymor ML, Karam K, Nudemgerg F. Fertil Steril 1972;23:783–790.
5. Lunenfeld B, Insler V. Bailliere's Clin Obstet Gynaecol 1990;4:473–489.
6. Healy DL, Evans J. Br Med J 1993;307:517–518.
7. Baird DT. In: Howles CM (ed) Gonadotrophins, Gonadotrophin-releasing Hormone Analogues and Growth Factors in Infertility: Future Perspectives. Medifax International, 1992;43–55.
8. Dicsfalusy E, Harlin J. Hum Reprod 1988;3:21–27.
9. Mannaerts B, Coelingh Bennink H. In: Shaw RW (ed) The Control and Stimulation of Follicular Growth. Carnforth, UK: Parthenon Publishing, 1993;75–86.
10. Chappel S, Kelton C, Nugent N. In: Genazzani AR, Petraglia F (eds) Hormones in Gynaecological Endocrinology. Carnforth, UK: Parthenon Publishing, 1992;179–184.
11. Anderson RE, Cragon JM, Chang, RJ, Stanczyk FZ, Lobo RA. Fertil Steril 52;216–220.
12. Messinis IE, Templeton AA, Baird DT. J Clin Endocrinol Metab 1985;61:1076–1080.
13. Messinis IE, Templeton AA, Baird DT. Hum Reprod 1986;1:223–226.
14. Nakamura Y, Yoshimura Y, Tanabe K, Iizuka R. Fertil Steril 1986;46:46–54.
15. Polson DW, Mason HD, Saldahna MBY, Franks S. Clin Endocrinol 1987;26:205–212.
16. Gemzell CA. Rec Prog Horm Res 1965;21:179–198.
17. Brown JB. In: Insler V, Lunenfeld B (eds) Infertility: Male and Female. Edinburgh, London, Melbourne, New York: Churchill Livingstone, 1986;359–396.
18. Leyendecker G, Wildt L. J Reprod Fertil 1983;69:397–409.
19. Filicori M, Falmigni C, Meriggiola MC, Ferrari P, Michelacci L, Campaniello E, Valdiserri A, Cognigni G. J Clin Endocrinol Metab 1991;72:965–972.
20. Couzinet B, Lestrat N, Brailly S, Forest M, Schaison G. J Clin Endocrinol Metab 1988;66:552–556.
21. Schoot DC, Coelingh Bennink HJT, Maanaerts BMJL, Lamberts SWJ, Bouchard P, Fauser BCJM. J Clin Endocrinol Metab 1992;74:1471–1473.
22. Greep RO, vanDyke HB, Chow BF. Endocrinology 1942;30:635–649.
23. Baird DT. In: Adashi EY, Leung PCK (eds) The Ovary. New York: Raven Press, 1993;529–544.
24. Baird DT. In: DeGroot LJ (ed) Endocrinology, 2nd edn. Philadelphia: WB Saunders 1989;1950–1968.
25. Yen SSC. Clin Endocrinol 1980;12:177–208.
26. Regan L, Owen EJ, Jacobs HS. Lancet 1990;336:1141–1144.
27. Howles CM, Macamee MC, Edwards RG, Goswamy R, Steptoe PC. Lancet 1986;ii:521–528.
28. Kamrava MM, Seibel MM, Berger MJ, Thompson I, Taymor ML. Fertil Steril 1982;37:520–523.
29. Hamilton-Fairley D, Kiddy D, Watson H, Sagle M, Franks S. Hum Reprod 1991;6:1095–1099.
30. Shoham Z, Patel A, Jacobs HS. Fertil Steril 1991;55:1051–1056.
31. Schoemaker J, Wentz AC, Jones GS, Dubin HH, Karan C. Obstet Gynecol 1978;51:270–277.
32. Venturuli S, Paradisi R, Fabbri R, Margini O, Porcu E, Flamigni C. Obstet Gynecol 1984;63:6–11.
33. Seibel MM, McArdle C, Smith D, Taymor ML. Fertil Steril 1985;43:703–708.

34. Buvat J, Buvat-Herbaut M, Marcolin G, Dehaene JL, Verbecq P, Renouard O. Fertil Steril 1989;52: 553–559.
35. Fleming R, Haxton MJ, Hamilton MPR, McCune GS, Black WP, Macnaughton MC, Coutts JRT. Br J Obstet Gynaecol 1985;92:369–373.
36. Homburg R, Eshel A, Kilburn J, Adams J, Jacobs HS. Hum Reprod 1990;5:32–35.
37. Larsen T, Larsen JF, Schioler V, Bostofe E, Fielding C. Fertil Steril 1990;53:426–431.
38. Sagle MA, Hamilton-Fairley D, Kiddy DS, Franks S. Fertil Steril 1991;55:55–60.

Low-dose gonadotropin regimens for induction of ovulation

S. Franks, D.W. Polson, M. Sagle, D. Hamilton-Fairley and D.M. White

Department of Obstetrics and Gynaecology, Imperial College of Science Technology and Medicine (University of London), St Mary's Hospital Medical School, Norfolk Place, London W2 1PG, UK

Abstract. Low-dose gonadotropin therapy in women with polycystic ovary syndrome is associated with a high rate of unifollicular ovulation and a correspondingly low (7%) rate of multiple pregnancy. The outcome of treatment is influenced by age, obesity and persistently raised concentrations of luteinising hormone (LH). The most successful results have been obtained in women of normal weight who are under the age of 36 and whose serum concentration of LH normalises in the late follicular phase.

Introduction

In women with polycystic ovary syndrome (PCOS), induction of ovulation by conventional doses of exogenous gonadotropins is associated with a number of problems. These include lower rates of ovulation and pregnancy than in hypogonadotropic women, multiple follicle development (and an associated increase in the risk of hyperstimulation syndrome and of multiple pregnancy) and a higher rate of miscarriage compared with gonadotropin-deficient patients. There is an increasing awareness of the adverse medical and sociological implications of multiple gestation and it should be the aim of an induction of ovulation programme to achieve unifollicular ovulation. It was for this reason that we have adopted a low-dose regimen for induction of ovulation with gonadotropins in women with PCOS.

The "threshold concept"

The threshold concept was highlighted by Brown et al. [1,2] in reports of results of a large series of women who received human pituitary gonadotropin (HPG). He observed that by making small, stepwise increments in the dose of FSH of about 30% at 5 day intervals, it was possible to define a "threshold" dose at which a significant rise is estrogen excretion was detectable and beyond which multiple folliculogenesis was more likely. Although the results of his programme showed a multiple pregnancy rate of 26 and a 3% rate of hyperstimulation [1], we felt that the idea of small increments of FSH was, in principle, correct. The failure to achieve a high proportion of uniovulatory cycles may have been related to various factors, including the relatively high initial dose of HPG and the interval of only 5 days before changing dose.

The low-dose gonadotropin regimen

Subsequently Kamrava et al. [3] reported successful induction of ovulation in two patients with PCOS following the administration of FSH at a fixed daily dose of only one ampule (75 IU). A protocol was, therefore, devised for the treatment of clomiphene-resistant women with PCOS, in which purified urinary FSH (Metrodin) was given, subcutaneously, at a starting dose of 75 IU/day to be followed by small (30–50%) stepwise increments if necessary. Initial results in 10 patients demonstrated a 78% rate of unifollicular ovulation [4]. Subsequent studies showed that similar results could be obtained with hMG [5] and by daily, intramuscular injection [6,7]. The regimen has since been modified as follows.

Gonadotropin treatment (hMG or FSH) is started at a dose of 52.5 IU (0.7 ampule) by daily intramuscular injection following the onset of spontaneous or progestogen-induced menses. Ultrasound and endocrine assessment is performed initially at three to 4-day intervals and, in the preovulatory phase, on alternate days (or daily, if indicated). Decisions about changes in treatment are usually made on the basis of ultrasound scanning with retrospective analysis of LH and estradiol measurements when necessary. The initial dose of hMG is maintained for up to 14 days in the first cycle and the dose is increased to 75 IU, only if no follicle >10 mm is observed by that stage. Further increments of 37.5 IU (half ampule) are made, if necessary, at weekly intervals, to a maximum of 225 IU/day. If a dominant follicle emerges, that dose of hMG (the "threshold" dose) is continued until the follicle has reached a diameter of at least 18 mm.

Ovulation is triggered by a single, intramuscular dose of hCG, 5,000 IU, and hMG is stopped. HCG is given routinely because, although some patients will have a spontaneous LH surge, it is not possible to predict this with any reliability. Treatment is discontinued if there are more than three follicles of 15 mm (or more) in diameter, to minimize the risk of hyperstimulation and/or multiple pregnancy. Serum progesterone is measured 5 to 8 days after hCG.

If further cycles of treatment are necessary, hMG is reintroduced at a dose below the previous threshold (and no more than 75 IU/day). In the second and subsequent cycles, the first increment in dose is usually made after 7 days, rather than 14 days. In women who develop multiple follicles, either a smaller starting dose (i.e., 37.5 IU) is given or the dose is increased by only 25 IU.

Results of treatment with low-dose gonadotropins

The results of treatment of 134 women (505 cycles of treatment) are summarized in Table 1 [8].

The threshold (mean maximum daily) dose for all cycles was 95.3 IU/day (range 52.5–225 IU). The threshold dose varied little from cycle to cycle but it was noted that a small variation (e.g., of 25–37.5 IU) might represent the difference between a single dominant follicle and hyperstimulation. This was the rationale for starting

Table 1. Results of low-dose gonadotropin treatment in 134 women with PCOS

No. of cycles	505
No. of ovulatory cycles	368 (73%)
No. of uniovulatory cycles	265 (72%)
No. of nonresponders	7 (5%)
Total no. of pregnancies	60
No. of women pregnant	57 (43%)
Delivered or ongoing	37 (28%)
Early pregnancy loss	18 (30%)
Multiple pregnancies (all twin)	4 (7%)
Mean threshold dose	95 IU
(range)	(52–225)
Mean total dose per cycle	18.5 ampules
(range)	(5-81)
Mean time to hCG	14.2 days
(range)	(range) (5–34)

subsequent cycles at subthreshold doses of gonadotropin (see above). The total dose of gonadotropin per cycle was 18.5 (5–81) IU and the mean interval from start of treatment to administration of hCG was only 14.2 days (range 5–34).

There were 60 pregnancies in 57 (43%) of women treated. Of the 60 pregnancies only four (7%) were multiple gestations (all twins). Two pregnancies were ectopic. There were 18 miscarriages before the 12-week gestation (30%), two 2nd-trimester abortions and one neonatal death following premature delivery at 28 weeks. The cumulative pregnancy rate, calculated for 100 consecutive patients [9] was 63% at 6 months (Fig. 1).

The conception rate of 10% per cycle and the relatively high frequency of early pregnancy loss are in keeping with the results of treatment with conventional gonadotropin dosage regimens. The obvious difference between these results and those of standard gonadotropin treatment is the low rate (7%) of multiple pregnancy and the absence of triplet and higher order pregnancies in this series. The multiple pregnancy rate is, indeed, somewhat better than the overall figures reported in hypogonadotropic women treated with pulsatile GnRH [10,11]. Importantly, there were no cases of severe hyperstimulation syndrome. However, despite the success of the low-dose regimen in avoiding the complications related to multiple folliculogenesis, this protocol is not associated with an improvement in fecundity or reduction in miscarriage rate compared with standard treatment regimens. The results of this and other studies were therefore examined to see whether it was possible to define factors, endocrine or otherwise, which might predict the outcome of treatment.

Factors influencing the outcome of low-dose gonadotropin treatment

The principle nonendocrine factors affecting the outcome of treatment with low-dose

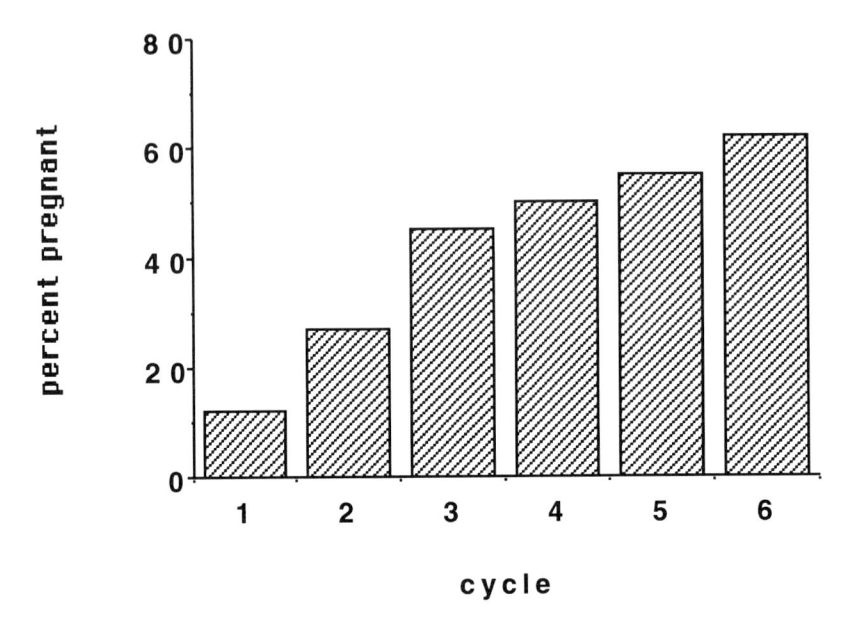

Fig. 1. Cumulative conception rate, calculated by life-table analysis, in 100 women treated with low-dose gonadotropin (excluding women who never ovulated and those with male factor infertility) (redrawn from [9]).

gonadotropin were other (tubal or male factor) causes of infertility and age. Women with tubal disease were not included in this study, nor were those whose partners who had an obviously abnormal semen analysis. Nevertheless, persistently negative postcoital tests were subsequently identified in 6% of cases, none of whom conceived. The adverse effect of age on fertility was illustrated by the finding of a 48% pregnancy rate in women of 35 or under, compared with only 15% (two of 13) aged 36 or above.

Obesity

Women whose BMI was greater than 28 kg/m^2 were excluded from treatment but the results of therapy in women who were moderately overweight (BMI 25.1–28.0 kg/m^2) were strikingly different from those in subjects whose BMI was within the normal range (Table 2) [12]. Overweight women required 50% more gonadotropin per day and twice as much per cycle in order to obtain a dominant follicle. Serum levels of FSH in the circulation were appropriately higher in the obese than in the lean women so that the increased dose requirement could not be explained simply on the basis of poor absorption or more rapid clearance of FSH in the overweight group. From these data, it would appear that the ovary is relatively resistant to FSH in obese women with PCOS.

The ovulation rate was lower in the obese group than in lean women – 57% compared with 77% – and there was a lower proportion of uniovulatory cycles (60

Table 2. Results of low-dose gonadotropin treatment in lean and obese women with polycystic ovary syndrome

	Lean (BMI 19–24.9)	Obese (BMI 25–28)
No. of women treated	75	25
No. of cycles:		
total	308	97
ovulatory	237 (77%)	55 (57%)[a]
uniovulatory	177 (75%)	33 (60%)[b]
Gonadotropin dose:		
total (ampules)	14.9 (9.1)	28.4 (11)[c]
maximum daily (IU)	85.1 (25.1)	126 (33.9)[c]
No. of women pregnant	29 (39%)	12 (48%)
No. of pregnancies	30	15
Miscarriages:		
total	8 (27%)	9 (60%)[b]
early	8 (27%)	7 (47%)[b]

Values are mean ± SD or n (%); [a] $p < 0.05$; [b] $p < 0.01$; [c] $p < 0.001$.
From Hamilton-Fairley et al. [12].

vs. 75%). Pregnancy rates were similar but 60% of pregnancies miscarried (nine of 15) in the obese group compared with 27% (eight of 30) in the lean group. This effect of BMI was independent of serum LH concentrations.

The adverse effect of obesity on outcome of pregnancy was not only observed in women with PCOS who had received induction of ovulation. Analysis of the large obstetric database from the North West Thames Health Regional Health Authority (UK) [12,13], using logistic regression, indicated that the risk of miscarriage rose with increasing BMI (Fig. 2). This relationship was maintained even after correcting for maternal age. The risk of miscarriage before first viable birth in women with a BMI of 25–27.9 was 26% higher than in the reference group (BMI 19–24.9).

Hypersecretion of LH

An adverse effect of raised serum LH concentrations on fertility and miscarriage has been described in women with PCOS who were undergoing induction of ovulation by pulsatile GnRH [14]. In particular, hypersecretion of LH in the midfollicular phase of ovulatory cycles was related to either a lower pregnancy rate or a greater risk of early miscarriage when compared with the outcome of cycles in which LH levels had normalised during treatment.

In women treated by low-dose gonadotropins, 53% had raised pretreatment concentrations of LH but, as in those treated with pulsatile GnRH, this abnormality proved to be a less important predictor of outcome than the level of LH in the midfollicular phase [9,14]. In approximately 25% of ovulatory cycles, LH concentrations remain higher than those in the normal follicular phase and this appears to have a marked adverse influence on outcome. Only one of 12 cycles resulted in a success-

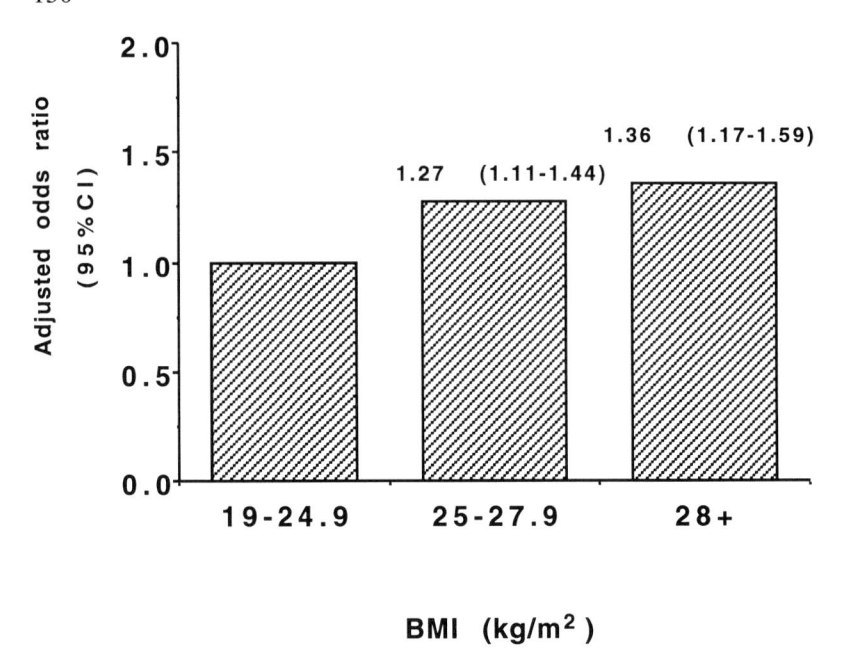

Fig. 2. Risk of one or more miscarriages before first viable birth in 13,128 consecutive primiparous women, related to maternal BMI. Adjusted odds ratio corrects for influence of maternal age. (Data from Northwest Thames Regional Health Authority [UK] obstetric data base) [12].

ful pregnancy compared with 54% of cycles in which the midfollicular LH was normal. It remains to be determined whether suppression of LH (e.g., by GnRH agonist analogues) during induction of ovulation would improve the chance of successful pregnancy.

Comparison of conventional and low-dose gonadotropin treatment

Two studies have made a direct comparison between standard and low-dose regimens [15,16]. In the publication by Buvat and colleagues, a much lower rate of multiple folliculogenesis and hyperstimulation and a *higher* pregnancy rate were noted following low-dose treatment [15]. In a more recent study, in a smaller number of patients, Shoham et al. reported similar findings [16]. Previously reported non-controlled studies had suggested that low-dose therapy may result in lower fecundity than conventional therapy [17] but the results from these direct, comparative studies suggest otherwise.

Recombinant human FSH

There has already been a short report of the use of human recombinant FSH for successful induction of ovulation in a woman with PCOS [18]. White and colleagues, in the proceedings of this meeting [19], presented data in 17 women with PCOS who were treated with low-dose recombinant FSH (Org 32489, Organon, Oss, The Netherlands). Eight of these women have conceived within three cycles of treatment.

References

1. Brown JB, Evans JH, Adey FD, Taft HP, Townsend L. J Obstet Gynaecol Br Commonw 1969;76: 289–306.
2. Brown JB. Aust NZ J Obstet Gynaecol 1978;18:47–54.
3. Kamrava MM, Seibel MM, Berger MJ, Thompson I and Taymor ML. Fertil Steril 1982;37:520–523.
4. Polson DW, Mason HD, Saldahna MB and Franks S. Clin Endocrinol 1987;26:205–212.
5. Sagle MA, Hamilton-Fairley D, Kiddy DS and Franks S. Fertil Steril 1991;55:56–60.
6. Polson DW, Mason HD, Kiddy DS, Winston RM, Margara R and Franks S. Br J Obstet Gynaecol 1989;96:746–748.
7. Quartero HW, Dixon JE, Westwood O, Hicks B and Chapman MG. Hum Reprod 1989;4:247–249.
8. Franks S, Hamilton-Fairley D. In: Adashi EY, Rock JA, Rosenwaks Z (eds) Reproductive Endocrinology, Surgery and Technology. New York: Raven (in press).
9. Hamilton-Fairley D, Kiddy D, Watson H, Sagle M and Franks S. Hum Reprod 1991;6:1095–1099.
10. Braat DDM, Ayalon D, Blunt SM et al. Gynecol Endocrinol 1989;3:35–44.
11. Homburg R, Eshel A, Armar NA et al. BMJ 1989;298:809–812.
12. Hamilton-Fairley D, Kiddy D, Watson H, Paterson C, Franks S. Br J Obstet Gynaecol 1992;99:128–131.
13. Maresh M, Dawson AM, Beard RW. Br J Obstet Gynaecol 1986;93:1239–1245.
14. Homburg R, Armar NA, Eshel A, Adams J, Jacobs HS. Br Med J 1988; 297:1024–1026.
15. Buvat J, Buvat HM, Marcolin G, Dehaene JL, Verbecq P, Renouard O. Fertil Steril 1989;52:553–559.
16. Shoham Z, Patel A, Jacobs HS. Fertil Steril 1991;55:1051–1056.
17. Hull MGR. In: Howles CM (ed) Gonadotrophins, Gonadotrophin-releasing Hormone Analogues and Growth Factors in Infertility: Future Perspectives. Hove (UK): Medi-Fax International, 1991;56–70.
18. Donderwinkel PF, Schoot DC, Coelingh BH, Fauser BC. Lancet 1992;340(8825).
19. White DM, Franks S. Efficacy of recombinant human FSH (rFSH) for induction of ovulation in women with polycystic ovary syndrome. Proceedings of Symposium "Induction of Ovulation: Basic Science and Clinical Advances", Palm Beach, Florida, USA, 20–22 January 1994.

Step-down follicle-stimulating hormone regimens in polycystic ovary syndrome

Bart C.J.M. Fauser*

Department of Obstetrics and Gynaecology, Dijkzigt Academic Hospital, and Erasmus University Medical School, Rotterdam, The Netherlands

Abstract. Multiple follicle development underlies the majority of complications (i.e., multiple pregnancies and ovarian hyperstimulation) following gonadotrophin induction of ovulation. During conventional (low-dose) step-up regimens follicle-stimulating hormone (FSH) serum levels are high in the late follicular phase. This condition contradicts normal physiological circumstances where FSH is elevated during the luteal-follicular transitions. High FSH later in the cycle interferes with selection of a dominant follicle (prevents remaining follicles from the recruited cohort going into atresia) and may therefore give rise to complications. Based on this conception a step-down dose regimen has been developed and tested for induction of ovulation. Data obtained so far have revealed evidence that follicles continue to grow although late follicular-phase serum FSH concentrations decrease significantly. Clinical outcome so far has suggested acceptable success and complication rates. Early monitoring of ovarian response may further improve treatment outcome.

A considerable proportion of patients that suffer from infertility and anovulation exhibit insufficient response to antioestrogen medication. Urinary gonadotrophins represent an effective second line treatment in this group of patients. However, chances of multiple follicle development and subsequent complications are substantial due to the fact that regulatory mechanisms operative under normal conditions are overruled by direct stimulation of the ovary.

Treatment outcome has improved substantially over the years, mainly because of improved treatment monitoring and the introduction of low-dose step-up dose regimens. Nevertheless, even today, gonadotrophin therapy should be considered an effective therapy with a high complication rate. In fact, many clinicians believe that frequent complications are inevitable in order to obtain good success rates. In as many as 50% of patients complications (chiefly multiple pregnancies, ovarian hyperstimulation and early pregnancy wastage) do occur, and it seems that (unintended) stimulation of multiple follicles to ongoing growth underlies most of these complications [1]. Besides the doses administered, numerous factors may affect outcome of gonadotrophin therapy, such as indication for treatment, patient diagnosis of underlying endocrine abnormalities, patient age and body weight, previous

---

Address for correspondence: Dijkzigt Academic Hospital, Dr Molewaterplein 40, 3015 GD Rotterdam, The Netherlands. Fax: +31-10-436-7306.

medication, use of gonadotrophin preparation (human urinary menopausal gonadotrophin (HMG) versus purified follicle-stimulating hormone (FSH)), adjuvant medication, monitoring of ovarian response, and luteal support (for review see [2]). This review addresses attempts by our group to diminish the magnitude of multiple follicle development during gonadotrophin induction of ovulation using a decremental ("step-down") dose regimen by reducing interference with the process of selection of the dominant follicle. Since this concept is based on considerations with regard to regulation of follicle development under normal conditions, this topic will also be discussed in greater detail.

History and present approach for gonadotrophin induction of ovulation

The clinical use of gonadotrophins became reality with the extraction of biologically active FSH and luteinizing hormone (LH) from urine of postmenopausal women [3]. Since its introduction in the early 60s many dose regimens have been tested, such as daily administration of fixed, incremental or decremental doses, and intermittent or single gonadotrophin injections [4–6]. It was concluded that the preferred dose regimen should be individualized with initial daily intramuscular doses of 1 or 2 ampoules (each consisting of 75 IU of LH and FSH activity based on in vivo bioassays) with dose increments of 1 ampoule/day every 3 days in case of insufficient response. The amount of gonadotrophins needed to elicit ovarian response was referred to as the "daily effective dose", which was followed by a "latent" (absent oestrogen production) and subsequently an "active phase" (from initial oestrogen rise until ovulation) [7]. These "step-up" dose regimens have since been applied by most clinicians. Combined data of individual studies reveal a pregnancy rate per cycle of 17–23%, multiple pregnancy rates of 23–28% and abortion rates of 17–28% [8,9]. The incidence of moderate and severe ovarian hyperstimulation may be up to 9% [10]. Results have improved over the years mainly because of improved monitoring of ovarian response by measurement of estrogen secretion and visualization of follicle growth by pelvic sonography (for review see [11]). A single dose of human chorionic gonadotrophin (hCG) is administered to induce ovulation. Timing of hCG is still controversial (when hCG is administered early oocyte maturation may be insufficient, but administration late in the follicular phase may enhance multiple follicle development and subsequent ovarian hyperstimulation). Some investigators also use repeated, low dose hCG injections after ovulation to support corpus luteum function.

In the mid 80s a new method of stimulation was introduced by Seibel and colleagues referred to as "low-dose, step-up" dose regimens [12]. The initial dose was low (½ to 1 ampoule/day) with no dose adjustment for 1–2 weeks. Thereafter doses could be increased with ½ ampoule/day at weekly intervals, if needed. This empirical method was based on data generated by Brown and colleagues [13] introducing the concept of the "FSH threshold". It was hypothesized that the ovarian requirement for FSH operates in a very narrow range. If FSH concentrations are below the threshold follicle development does not occur. Only a minor increase of FSH administered resulting in serum levels just above the threshold would induce normal follicle growth, whereas a further increase would cause excessive stimulation. Recently — with the use of intravenous gonadotrophin infusion and rapid FSH serum measurements — the concept of an FSH threshold requirement for follicle growth has been further substantiated [14,15]. During recent years various groups have reported their results regarding low-dose step-up regimens [16,17], and indeed, in general, complication rates appear to be reduced. A cumulative conception rate of over 50%, with minimal multiple pregnancies and no cases of severe hyperstimulation was reported by a single centre [17]. Combined results of 6 different studies using low-dose, step-up regimens [9] indicate an overall pregnancy rate of 15% per cycle, with 11% multiple pregnancies and 39% miscarriage rate.

Pathophysiology of ovarian function

Regulation of normal follicle development

A better understanding of regulation of ovarian function under normal conditions may help to improve treatment outcome following exogenous gonadotrophins. Once growth of a primordial follicle is initiated it takes several month to develop into a preovulatory follicle [18]. Initiation of growth takes place continuously (approximately 1,000 follicles enter the growing pool each month) and its regulation is at present unknown. If follicles reach a certain stage of development at a size of approximately 2–5 mm they undergo atresia unless FSH levels are elevated [18]. Only if the "FSH threshold" is surpassed — which under normal conditions takes place around the luteal-follicular transition [19] due to reduced oestrogen secretion by the corpus luteum [20] — a restricted number of follicles will gain gonadotrophin dependence and continue their development [21] (for review see [22–24]). The longer FSH serum concentrations are above the threshold (i.e., the wider the "FSH window") the more follicles will continue their development. This is the goal of controlled ovarian hyperstimulation for in vitro fertilization, where the aim is to override the selection process by extended pharmacological FSH levels to allow maturation of many oocytes. During the normal menstrual cycle early follicular phase FSH levels control follicle development [25], and serum concentrations start to decrease in the early/mid-follicular phase [26] — presumably due to gonadal feedback activity — ensuring a small "FSH window" (number of days where FSH levels are above the threshold). Consequently, a restricted number of follicles is recruited and selection of a single dominant follicle will take place in the early to midfollicular phase. Under normal conditions from cycle day 6 and a diameter of 10 mm onwards a dominant follicle can be visualized by transvaginal sonography [27] and only thereafter a substantial elevation in serum oestrogen levels can be observed [26]. The selected follicle continues its growth despite decremental serum FSH levels presumably due to local (auto- or paracrine) upregulation [28,29]. Remaining follicles from the recruited cohort undergo atresia due to insufficient stimulation by FSH [21,22].

Table 1. Key physiological considerations related to normal follicle development

* Perimenstrual elevation of serum FSH rescues follicles from atresia (referred to as "follicle recruitment")

* Decrease in serum FSH during the follicular phase is essential for development of a single dominant follicle and atresia of remaining follicles from the recruited cohort

* The dominant follicle continues to grow despite decreasing serum FSH due to local (auto- or paracrine) upregulation

For references see text.

Various aspects of recruitment and dominant follicle selection have been substantiated in vivo in the monkey model and a proportion of these observations have also been confirmed in the human (see also Table 1). These studies have convincingly demonstrated that:
1. A rise in serum FSH provoked by removal of the corpus luteum or the dominant follicle does induce new follicle recruitment irrespective of the phase of the menstrual cycle [30–32]. For human studies see [33–35].
2. Follicle development is arrested following a premature decrease in FSH in the early follicular phase [36].
3. Atresia has been initiated in nondominant follicles in the late follicular phase and consequently these follicles can no longer be stimulated [37] (in the human a progressive abolition of the ability of HMG to stimulate follicle growth as ovulation approaches has also been reported [38].
4. Interference with the gonadotrophin suppressing actions of oestrogens results in continued recruitment and maturation of secondary follicles in the presence of a dominant follicle [21] (i.e., decreasing serum FSH levels are essential for monofollicle development).
5. Follicles can continue to mature with decremental FSH stimulation after initial stimulation by elevated FSH [39]. See next section for studies in the human.
6. Decremental gonadotrophin stimulation better synchronizes follicular rupture and reduces susceptibility to delayed ovulation [40].

Polycystic ovary syndrome and the significance of patient selection for gonadotrophin induction of ovulation

Most patients that exhibit insufficient response following antioestrogen medication suffer from the polycystic ovary syndrome (PCOS) and the majority of these patients will need exogenous gonadotrophins to induce ovulation. Since it is known that these patients are very "sensitive" to exogenous gonadotrophins and that complication rates during treatment are high, ovarian abnormalities in these patients should be discussed in greater detail. If we attempt to incorporate physiological principles in our treatment strategies there is a distinct need to gain knowledge concerning what is different from normal in these ovaries.

Underlying mechanisms of anovulation in PCOS patients are largely unknown, but in the majority of patients elevated serum androgen or LH levels are believed to be important for initiation and maintenance of polycystic transformation of ovaries. Mainly based on studies in the early 60s measuring steroid levels in follicle fluid or using cultures of human ovarian cells or tissue it was generally believed that in patients with PCOS induction of granulosa cell aromatase activity was absent. Low intrafollicular oestrogen levels would provoke follicle development arrest and subsequent atresia. However, it can be inferred from several more recent human in vitro [41,42] as well as in vivo [26,43] studies that a substantial rise in oestrogens occurs only after dominant follicle selection has taken place. Therefore it came as no surprise that sonography studies revealed that in polycystic ovaries follicle development is arrested at a stage where dominant follicle formation takes place under normal conditions [44]. Moreover, analysis of steroid and inhibin levels in individual follicles also showed that the endocrine profile is not different from normal nondominant follicles [45]. The above-mentioned morphologic as well as clinical observations are all in favour of the concept of normal early follicle growth and disturbed dominant follicle selection in PCOS (for review see [46]). Normal serum FSH levels are observed in these patients suggesting that the FSH threshold for ongoing follicle stimulation is elevated due to intraovarian abnormalities.

Gonadotrophin step-down regimens for induction of ovulation

Keeping regulatory mechanisms underlying normal follicle development in mind it should be considered that the empirical approach of low-dose step-up regimens ignores various of its aspects (see Fig. 1). It should also be emphasized that the relatively long half-life of FSH of approximately 30–40 h [47,48] following intramuscular administration brings about steady-state levels of serum FSH concentrations that are reached only after 5 to 7 days of gonadotrophin administration in equal amounts. Hence, FSH accumulates in serum and reaches maximum levels in the late follicular phase, completely opposing normal circumstances. Mechanisms ensuring monofollicular development [21] are overruled and follicles are rescued from atresia. Moreover, during the course of elevated FSH levels additional follicles will be recruited and undergo further maturation [40]. Indeed, differences in magnitude of ovarian stimulation following a similar dose of gonadotrophins for in vitro fertilization were found to be dependent on the magnitude of late follicular phase FSH accumulation [49]. Low-dose step-up regimens may partly overcome these shortcomings since the FSH threshold will be surpassed to a minor extent and the FSH window may not be as wide. However, it is not yet clear what can be gained from an extended period of time before the FSH threshold is reached (can the ovary be sensitized?) and maximum FSH levels will still be obtained in the late follicular phase. Indeed, "overstimulated cycles" have been reported even after low-dose gonadotrophin administration [50].

Surely, physiological circumstances should not be mimicked during gonadotrophin

- Enhanced sensitivity of the dominant follicle for FSH

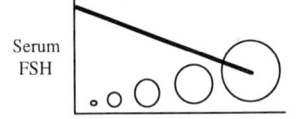

follicular phase of normal menstrual cycle

- Accumulation of serum FSH levels with similar doses of gonadotropins

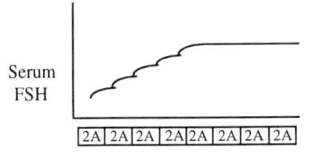

daily im. injections (2 Amp HMG/FSH)

- Wide FSH window plus FSH accumulation elicits continuous recruitment and interferes with selection

follicle development

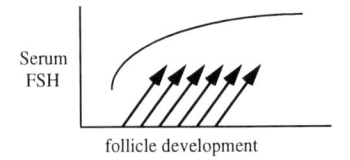

Fig. 1. Step-up regimens for gonadotrophin induction of ovulation not taken into account.

induction of ovulation according to step-down dose regimens since (mainly PCOS) patients involved suffer from ovarian dysfunction. Again, the majority of these patients may indeed have intraovarian abnormalities. It should therefore be kept in mind that ovaries from these patients may respond differently as compared to normal, and therefore doses administered should be adjusted on the basis of estimates of individual ovarian response. For that reason patient selection and adequate monitoring of ovarian response is extremely important, and better understanding of ovarian abnormalities (and related differences in FSH threshold) in these patients should further improve treatment outcome. Incidentally, results applying high initial doses followed by decremental steps have been reported [51,52]. One prospective study reported comparison between a fixed dose (150 IU/day purified FSH) and a step-down (225 IU/day for 2 days followed by 75 IU/day) regimen in 23 PCOS patients [53]. Obtained data suggested similar ovulation rates with lower amounts of exogenous FSH and less medium-sized follicles in the step-down group. Testing the decremental dose regimen for gonadotrophin induction of ovulation, our group initially addressed the following issues; a) a rapid rise in serum FSH levels above the threshold would not be harmful if followed by a subsequent decline (resulting in a narrow FSH window); b) the dominant follicle would continue to grow although gonadotrophin doses (and FSH serum levels) were decreased; and c) whether we could find evidence of diminished interference with the selection process (i.e., less multiple follicle development). We elected GnRH agonist adjuvant medication, mainly to exclude potential interference between exogenous and late follicular phase changes in endogenous gonadotrophin secretion. We compared initial doses of 225 IU/day HMG for 2 days followed by 150 IU/day (fixed) with a further decrease to 75 IU/day (step-down) in a prospective randomized study [54]. The timing of decremental doses was based upon a follicle exceeding a size of 9 mm diameter as observed by transvaginal sonography (this equals dominant follicle selection in the normal menstrual cycle [27]). Although a major individual variability in FSH serum levels as well as ovarian response was found, evidence of a decline in functional medium-sized follicles could be generated. In addition, we learned that the initial dose chosen was too high, resulting in extended FSH elevations throughout most of the follicular phase even if FSH doses were diminished. In subsequent studies as well as in clinical practice we then elected initial doses of 150 IU/day followed by decremental steps to 1½ ampoules followed by 1 ampoule/day (Fig. 2). Using this dose regimen for the first time proof could be obtained in the human of ongoing growth of the dominant follicle although late follicular-phase serum FSH concentrations were decreasing significantly [55]. In a proportion of patients treated according to a step-down dose regimen monofollicular growth could be obtained indistinguishable from normal circumstances [56], indicating that — at least in a proportion of patients — ongoing follicle development is normal once growth was stimulated by a transient elevation of serum FSH. It seems reasonable to suggest that to some extent physiological mechanisms are still operative in these patients. However, overall ovarian response is heterogeneous. This variable response is not related to differences in FSH serum levels and therefore represents variable FSH threshold levels (Schoot

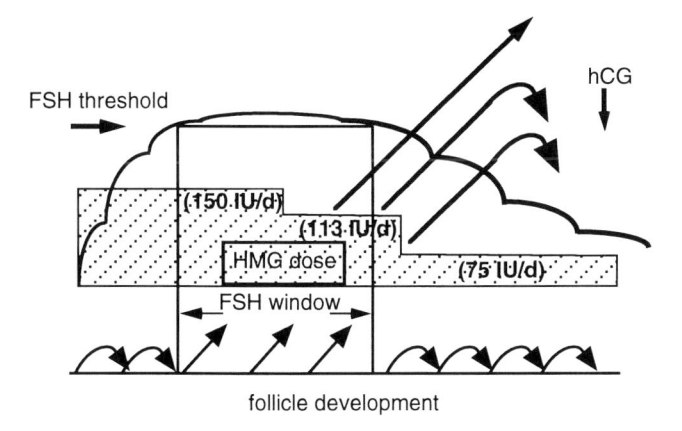

Fig. 2. Schematic representation of stimulation of follicle growth following exogenous gonadotrophins. Once the FSH threshold is surpassed (due to the administration of 150 IU/day of HMG/ pFSH) follicles will continue to grow. When an ovarian response is observed daily doses will be reduced by ½ ampoule eliciting decreasing FSH serum concentrations. Interference with selection of the dominant follicle may be reduced by decremental FSH levels which may give rise to less complications.

Table 2. Potentials for improvement of gonadotropin step down regimens for induction of ovulation

* Improved patient diagnosis
  (adjustment of initial dose based on differences in FSH threshold)
* Improved monitoring ovarian response during treatment
  (reduction of initial dose based on sonography and estrogen secretion)

et al., unpublished observations) in keeping with recent observations indicating that ovarian sensitivity in PCOS is different from normal [57]. Our preliminary, overall clinical results obtained so far were reported recently [58]. With ovulation rates of 84%, pregnancy rates of 18% per ovulatory cycle, cumulative pregnancy rates of 51% and a 6% rate of multiple pregnancy, as well as absent severe hyperstimulation, this approach seems promising. However, there is room for further improvement of clinical outcome by including early monitoring of oestrogen secretion following initial (high dose) FSH stimulation (Schoot et al., unpublished observations) (see also Table 2). Based on a prospective, multicentre, comparative study presented recently [59] it was concluded that a step-down dose regimen suffered from similar stimulation of multiple follicle growth and reduced efficacy because of low pregnancy rates. This conclusion seems premature for various reasons: 1) PCOS patients were not included in this study; 2) the step-down regimen included a high initial dose (225 IU/day) and a fixed regimen (after 3 days decrease to 75 IU/day); 3) timing of hCG was rather early at 16 mm of the largest follicle (making the extended elevation of serum FSH levels due to the high initial dose even more prominent); and 4) ovulation rates themselves were similar. We feel that for the step-down regimen a strategy should first be worked out which deals with doses administered (which takes individual response differences into consideration) and on the other hand is realistic for "routine" use in clinical practice. Only thereafter should a prospective comparative study test whether clinical outcome is indeed improved.

Acknowledgements

The author would like to emphasize that performing clinical studies in a complex academic organization is a major team effort involving various disciplines. The author is grateful to Drs Peter Donderwinkel, Dick Schoot, Thierry van Dessel and Evert van Santbrink for performing the induction of ovulation studies as well as to the staff of the outpatient clinic and clinical research unit for their much-appreciated help. In addition, the author would like to thank Prof F. de Jong (endocrine laboratory), Drs Hop (Department of Epidemiology and Biostatistics) and Dr H.J.T. Coelingh Bennink (Organon Int BV) for their support of these studies. Financial support was provided by the "Stichting Voortplantingsgeneeskunde Rotterdam".

References

1. Blankstein J, Shalev J, Saadon T, Kukia EE, Rabinovici J, Pariente C, Lunenfeld B, Serr DM, Mashiach S. Fertil Steril 1987;47:597—602.
2. Fauser BCJM. In: Bouchard P, Cataldy C, Pavlou S (eds) GnRH Analogues, Gonadotropins and Gonadal Peptides. Park Ridge, UK: Parthenon Publishing, 1993 (in press).
3. Lunenfeld B, Insler V. Baillieres Clin Obstet Gynaecol 1990;4:473—489.
4. Thompson CR, Hansen LM. Fertil Steril 1970;21:844—853.
5. Rabau E, David A, Serr DM, Mashiach S, Lunenfeld B. Am J Obstet Gynecol 1967;98:92—98.
6. Taymor ML, Sturgis SH, Goldstein DP, Lieberman B. Fertil Steril 1967;18:181—190.
7. Insler V. Int J Fertil 1988;33:85—97.
8. Schwartz M, Jewelewicz R. Fertil Steril 1981;35:3—12.
9. Hull MG. In: Howles CM (ed) Gonadotrophins, GnRH Analogues and Growth Factors in Infertility: Future Perspectives. Oxford, UK: Alden Press, 1991;56—61.
10. Schenker JB, Weinstein D. Fertil Steril 1978;30:255—262.
11. Schoot DC, Fauser BCJM. Exp Clin Endocrinol 1992;11:303—306.
12. Seibel MM, Kamrava MM, McArdle C, Taymor ML. Int J Fertil 1985;29:39—43.
13. Brown JB. Aust N Z J Obstet Gynaecol 1978;18:47—54.
14. Van Weissenbruch MM, Schoemaker HC, Drexhage HA, Schoemaker J. Hum Reprod 1993;8:813—821.
15. Scheele F, Hompes PG, van der Meer M, Schoute E, Schoemaker J. Fertil Steril 1993;60:620—625.
16. Buvat J, Buvat-Herbaut M, Marcolin G, Dehaene JL, Verbecq P, Renouard O. Fertil Steril 1989; 52:553—559.
17. Hamilton-Fairley D, Kiddy D, Watson H, Sagle M, Franks S. Hum Reprod 1991;6:1095—1099.
18. Gougeon A. In: Adashi EY, Leung PCK (eds) The Ovary. New York: Raven Press, 1993;21—39.
19. Hall JE, Schoenfeld DA, Martin KA, Crowley WF. J Clin Endocrinol Metab 1992;74:600—607.
20. Le Nestour E, Marraoui J, Lahlou N, Roger M, de Ziegler D, Bouchard P. J Clin Endocrinol Metab 1993;77:439—442.
21. Zeleznik AJ, Hutchison JS, Schuler HM. Endocrinology 1985;117:991—999.
22. Hodgen GD. Fertil Steril 1982;38:281—300.
23. Goodman AL, Hodgen GD. Recent Prog Horm Res 1983;39:1—73.
24. Baird DT. J Steroid Biochem 1987;27:15—23.
25. Messinis IE, Templeton AA. Hum Reprod 1990;5:153—156.
26. Fauser BCJM, Pache TD, Schoot DC. In: Hsueh AJ, Schomberg DW (eds) Ovarian Cell Interactions: Genes to Physiology. Serono Int Symposia Series. New York: Raven Press, 1993 (in press).
27. Pache TD, Wladimiroff JW, De Jong FH, Hop WC, Fauser BC. Fertil Steril 1990;54:638—642.
28. Hsueh AJ, Adashi EY, Jones PB, Welsh THJ. Endocr Rev 1984;5:76—127.
29. Hillier SG. Sem Reprod Endocrinol 1991;9:332—340.
30. Goodman LA, Hodgen GD. Endocrinology 1979;104:1304—1309.
31. Goodman AL, Nixon WE, Hodgen GD. Endocrinology 1979;105:69—73.
32. DiZerega GS, Nixon WE, Hodgen GD. J Clin Endocrinol Metab 1980;50:1046—1048.
33. Nilsson L, Wikland M, Hamberger L. Fertil Steril 1982;37:30—34.
34. Araki S, Chikazawa K, Akabori A, Ijima K, Tamada T. Endocrinol Jpn 1983;30:55—70.
35. Baird DT, Backstrom T, McNeilly AS, Smith SK, Wathen CG. J Reprod Fertil 1984;70:615—624.
36. Zeleznik AJ. Endocrinology 1981;109:352—355.
37. DiZerega GS, Hodgen GD. J Clin Endocrinol Metab 1980;50:819—825.
38. Gougeon A, Testart J. Fertil Steril 1990;54:848—852.
39. Zeleznik AJ, Kubik CJ. Endocrinology 1986;119:2025—2032.
40. Abbasi R, Kenigsberg D, Danforth D, Falk RJ, Hodgen GD. Fertil Steril 1987;47:1019—1024.
41. Erickson GF, Hsueh AJW, Quigley ME, Rebar RW, Yen SSC. J Clin Endocrinol Metab 1979;49: 514—519.

42. Hillier SG, van der Boogaard AMJ, Reichert LE, van Hall EV. J Clin Endocrinol Metab 1980; 50:640—647.
43. Baird DT, Fraser IS. Clin Endocrinol (Oxford) 1975;4:259—266.
44. Pache TD, Wladimiroff JW, Hop WC, Fauser BC. Radiology 1992;183:421—423.
45. Pache TD, Hop WC, De Jong FH, Leerentveld RA, van Geldorp H, Van de Kamp TM, Gooren LJ, Fauser BC. Clin Endocrinol (Oxford) 1992;36:565—571.
46. Fauser BCJM, Pache TD. In: Schoemaker J (ed) Ovarian Endocrinopathies. Park Ridge, UK: Parthenon Publishing, 1993 (in press).
47. Mizunuma H, Takagi T, Honjyo S, Ibuki Y, Igarashi M. Fertil Steril 1990;55:440—445.
48. Mannaerts B, Shoham Z, Schoot D, Bouchard P, Harlin J, Fauser BC, Jacobs H, Rombout F, Coelingh Bennink H. Fertil Steril 1993;59:108—114.
49. Ben-Rafael Z, Strauss JF, Mastroianni LJ, Flickinger GL. Fertil Steril 1986;46:586—592.
50. Herman A, Ron-El R, Golan A, Soffer Y, Bukovsky I, Caspi E. Hum Reprod 1993;8:30—34.
51. Glasier AF, Baird DT, Hillier SG. J Steroid Biochem 1989;32:167—170.
52. Baird DT. In: Adashi EY, Leung PCK (eds) The Ovary. New York: Raven Press, 1993;529—544.
53. Mizunuma H, Takagi T, Yamada K, Ibuki Y, Igarashi M. Fertil Steril 1991;55:1195—1197.
54. Schoot DC, Pache TD, Hop WC, De Jong FH, Fauser BC. Fertil Steril 1992;57:1117—1120.
55. Fauser BC, Schoot DC, van Dessel T. Serum hormone levels during gonadotropin induction of ovulation in a decremental dose regimen in PCOS. 75th Annual Meeting Endocrine Society, Las Vegas 1993;75 (Abs 100).
56. Schoot DC, Hop WC, Pache TD, De Jong FH, Fauser BC. Acta Endocrinol (Copenhagen) 1993;129:- 126—129.
57. Caruso A, Fortini A, Fulghesu AM, Pistilli E, Cucinelli F, Lanzone A, Mancuso S. Fertil Steril 1993; 59:115—120.
58. Fauser BC, Donderwinkel P, Schoot DC. Baillieres Clin Obstet Gynaecol 1993;7:309—330.
59. Steinkampf MP, Banks KS. Step-down versus conventional FSH treatment in patients with WHO group II amenorrhea: Results of a US Multicenter clinical trial. Ann Meeting American Fertility Society, 1993, Montreal, Canada 1993;S21—S22 (Abs 0-044).

Use of FSH threshold administration in polycystic ovarian disease

J. Schoemaker, M.M. van Weissenbruch and M. van der Meer

Department of Obstetrics and Gynecology, Division of Reproductive Endocrinology and Fertility, Free University Hospital, P.O. Box 7057, 1007 MB Amsterdam, The Netherlands

Abstract. Experiments in which the FSH threshold is determined and in which the FSH level is manipulated in relation to this threshold level are herewith described. In these experiments we have found that monofollicular growth can be induced by manipulating the FSH level to just above the threshold level. Only minor further elevations will predictably induce multifollicular growth.

Also, the use of GnRH analogues in low-dose step-up protocols alters the FSH pharmacodynamics and blocks the feedback on the endogenous component of the FSH concentration. As such they have an important effect on the manipulation of the FSH level in relation to the FSH threshold. If they are used in ovulation induction, which according to the authors is not advisable, then the dose should not be increased by more than a quarter of an ampule at a time. GnRH analogues do not change the threshold level as such.

A model has been developed for follicular selection, in which each follicle has its own threshold for continued FSH dependent growth.

The principle of the FSH threshold concept has been explained in the previous chapters by Zeleznik and Franks. So far, in the clinical practice of ovulation induction, the principle has been applied to the FSH dose. It is clear, however, that follicles in the ovary do not respond to FSH doses but to FSH levels.

Until recently no quantitative data were available in the literature on the FSH threshold levels under different physiological and pathological conditions. Even at this moment we know little about the exact FSH dependency of large preovulatory Graafian follicles, e.g., just before the LH surge. Yong et al. pointed out that steroidogenesis at this time is greatly enhanced by LH rather than by FSH [1]. Therefore the need for FSH of these follicles may well be close to nothing.

In an analysis of FSH levels measured during ovulation induction with different types of gonadotropin preparations, in patients with clomiphene resistant polycystic ovarian syndrome (PCOS), van Weissenbruch and co-workers [2] found that FSH levels, at which follicular growth did not occur and those at which growth did occur, showed a considerable overlap between 6.3 and 10.4 IU/l. This means that the actual threshold levels varied to a great extent in this group of patients. Also in this study, as in Brown's original threshold paper [3], it was shown that the intraindividual variation was much greater than the intraindividual cycle to cycle variability. This finding contrasted with van Weissenbruch's findings in patients with hypothalamic amenorrhea and in those with normal cycles whose pituitaries had been desensitized with long-term GnRH infusion. In these patients the FSH threshold level was found to be stable at approximately 7.8 IU/l [4].

Our group applied the concept of the FSH threshold level in a prospective study in clomiphene resistant PCOS patients, developing a technique whereby the FSH level through intravenous administration and daily rapid FSH determinations was manipulated to just above the FSH threshold level. During a first induction cycle where we initially aimed to bring the FSH level at 1 IU/l above the prestimulation value for 10 days, and subsequently increased the level by 1 IU/l every 7 days, the threshold was determined. In subsequent cycles the FSH level was manipulated just above this threshold level. Van der Meer's data confirm that only minor changes in FSH level, translating in as little a difference of ¼ ampule/day or 19 IU/day, may determine whether mono- or multifollicular growth will occur. Of the 13 first cycles in which the threshold was established, seven patients ovulated and were monofollicular. Of the 21 subsequent cycles, in each of which the threshold information of the first cycle was used, 19 patients ovulated and 15 were monofollicular. It thus seems that monofollicular growth can be attained by a technique of ovulation induction in which the FSH threshold concept is rigorously applied.

Next, an experiment was performed in three patients who had shown a stable threshold level for three cycles, whose cycles all had shown monofollicular growth. When in the fourth cycle the FSH level was increased to 1 IU/l above the threshold found in the previous cycles, multifollicular growth was induced in all three patients.

These findings brought us to a new model concerning the threshold concept, which has now evolved from a threshold dose for the individual patient, through a threshold level in the individual patient to a threshold level for each individual follicle. We call this model the Cornet model.

The Cornet model

By the end of the luteal phase of a menstrual cycle, the ovaries of a woman contain a cohort of follicles, all between 2 and 5 mm in diameter [5], and all, to a certain extent, but all differently, sensitive to FSH. The FSH threshold of the most sensitive follicle in either of her two ovaries is the FSH threshold for this woman. Every follicle of this cohort has its own sensitivity and therefore its own threshold, although it may be so that the less sensitive follicles are more numerous and may have the same threshold level.

This leads to a cone-shaped model of the cohort at the beginning of each new cycle. We therefore like to call this the Cornet Model. In the lower apex of the cone the most sensitive follicle is situated, i.e., the one with the lowest threshold level.

When the FSH concentration increases to a certain level, e.g., 1 IU/l above the threshold level, a number of follicles will start to grow. It is not known whether this number is stable from cycle to cycle and from patient to patient. In other words, the density of follicles in the cohort is not known and neither do we know whether there is any variation in this.

In patients with PCOS, according to van Weissenbruch et al. [2], the threshold varies from patient to patient and therefore so does the sensitivity of the most sensitive follicle. Whether the density of the cohort is different in PCOS ovaries compared to normal ovaries, is also unknown. The size and density of the cohort most probably varies from patient to patient.

In women with normal menstrual cycles the sensitivity of the growing follicles in the ovary increases with their further development [6]. This means that, if the actual FSH level is kept constant, more follicles will drop their threshold level under the actual level, therefore becoming stimulated to further growth and development. This is the mechanism behind the open gate as described in the model David Baird introduced in 1987 [7].

This can only last for a few days because, probably by an intraovarian regulatory mechanism, the sensitivity of the follicles that have not yet been selected now rapidly decreases so that they can no longer be stimulated, not even with large doses of hMG [8–10]. This is not to say that all follicles that have been selected will indeed continue to grow and ovulate. The rate of decrease of FSH concentration will now determine whether this will happen. When the FSH level decreases faster than the increase in the sensitivity of an individual follicle, the level will drop below the threshold of that particular follicle, and it will become atretic due to insufficient FSH stimulation. Several follicles, that initially have been stimulated, will be lost in such a way.

To test whether indeed the decrease in FSH levels was of importance, once monofollicular growth had already been obtained by a low-dose step-up regimen, Scheele, from our group, compared two groups of patients treated with low-dose step-up stimulation without (15 patients for 39 cycles) and with (13 patients for 33 cycles) GnRH-a cotreatment. He found that despite equal stimulation regimens, the number of follicles >13 mm and those from 11–13 mm were significantly higher in the analogue treated group [11]. In examining the FSH levels he detected that this was probably due to profoundly altered pharmacodynamics of FSH under cotreatment with GnRH-a. The increase of the FSH level per ampule of FSH appeared to be twice as high under GnRH-a suppression compared to without suppression. Therefore, it is likely that under analogues the chance that, with each step of dose increase, the FSH level rises to high above the FSH threshold level and thus leads to multifollicular growth is greater than without analogues.

Therefore, if the low-dose step-up stimulation is applied under GnRH-a suppression, the weekly increments should be of ¼ ampules rather than of ½ ampules.

As, in this experiment, due to the altered pharmacodynamics of FSH, it did not become clear whether a lack of negative feedback on FSH also played a role in the development of multifollicular growth, van der Meer designed an experiment in which the FSH levels were again increased by 1 IU/l/week. This eliminated the effect of altered pharmacodynamics of FSH.

Patients were treated with a regular low-dose step-up regimen in the first cycle and were then randomised to receive a low-dose step-up regimen again, without or with cotreatment of an analogue. It appeared that, in contrast to the analogue-cotreated patients, the FSH level of the patients who did not receive the GnRH analogue decreased significantly during the 6 days before the largest follicle reached a diameter of 18 mm. In the same experiment, van der Meer was able to demonstrate that the GnRH analogue did not change the threshold level of the most sensitive follicle.

References

1. Yong EL, Baird DT, Yates R, Reichert LEJ, Hillier SG. J Clin Endocrinol Metab 1992;74:842–849.
2. van Weissenbruch MM, Schoemaker HC, Drexhage HA, Schoemaker J. Hum Reprod 1993;6:813–821.
3. Brown JB. Aust N Z J Obstet Gynaecol 1978;18:47–54.
4. van Weissenbruch MM. Gonadotrophins for induction of ovulation. Thesis. Vrije Universiteit, Amsterdam, The Netherlands, 1989.
5. Gougeon A. In: Adashi EY, Leung PCK (eds) The Ovary. New York: Raven Press, 1993;21–39.
6. Zeleznik AJ, Kubik CJ. Endocrinology 1986;119:2025–2032.
7. Baird DT. J Steroid Biochem 1987;27:15–23.
8. diZerega GS, Hodgen GD. J Clin Endocrinol Metab 1980;50:819.
9. van Hooff MH, Alberda AT, Huisman GJ, Zeilmaker GH, Leerentveld RA. Hum Reprod 1993;8:369–373.
10. Gougeon A, Testart J. Fertil Steril 1990;54:848–852.
11. Scheele F, Hompes PG, van der Meer M, Schoute E, Schoemaker J. Fertil Steril 1993;60:620–625.

Endometrial receptivity in controlled ovarian hyperstimulation (COH): the hormonal factor

Dominique de Ziegler and Renato Fanchin

Hôpital A. Béclère, Department of Obstetrics and Gynecology, 92141 Clamart, France

Introduction

Controlled ovarian hyperstimulation (COH), which was conceived to enhance the efficacy of in vitro fertilization (IVF), has been feared to simultaneously hamper endometrial receptivity. The first mechanism put forth to explain the seemingly suboptimal endometrial receptivity of COH is the excessively elevated levels of plasma estradiol (E_2) [1,2], an interpretation that has subsequently been challenged [3]. Another factor, the premature elevation of plasma progesterone (P), has also been singled out by some [4–6] as capable of encumbering endometrial receptivity. But this has been similarly challenged [7,8]. In spite of this complexity the interest for studying endometrial receptivity in COH has remained high because embryo implantation rates remain distressingly low and clearly represent the single steps limiting IVF outcome the most.

One area of IVF that has been particularly successful, IVF with oocyte donation conducted in women deprived of ovarian function (IVF-OD), has provided an unexpected model to study the hormonal control of endometrial receptivity [9–12]. Originally considered as a nearly heroic procedure, IVF-OD conducted in women deprived of ovarian function and receiving E_2 and P substitution was recognized to have excellent pregnancy rates [13–18]. Research on the hormonal control of endometrial receptivity conducted in E_2 and P substitution cycles has led to a finer perception of the interval of endometrial receptivity or window of implantation [15]. Further, studies conducted after modifying E_2 and P substitution cycles have permitted researchers to delineate the impact of changes in hormonal levels [11,12,19] or that of fertility drugs such as clomiphene citrate [20] on endometrial morphology.

We will describe how investigations using the E_2 and P replacement cycle model led the authors to challenge the prevailing concepts on the role of plasma E_2 to P ratio and single out an unsuspected sensitivity of the endometrium to P [19]. The present paper will also analyze our current views on how ovarian hormones affect endometrial morphology and receptivity in actual COH cycles and discuss the practical implications.

A new experimental model: E_2 and P replacement cycles

At first glance, egg donation was perceived as an almost heroic endeavor because of the seemingly complex tasks it involved [13,14]. Indeed, to succeed, egg donation required that oocyte maturation in the donor be synchronized with endometrial transformations induced in the recipient with exogenous hormones. Yet, it has rapidly become apparent that egg donation was universally rewarded by excellent pregnancy rates, that by and large exceeded results of corresponding regular IVF programs [21] that have validated egg donation hormonal replacement regimens as study model for elucidating the physiology and physiopathology of the hormonal control of endometrial receptivity.

Attempting to simplify the hormonal replacement regimens prescribed to egg donation recipients, numerous investigators have questioned whether it is necessary to reproduce the cyclical increase in E_2 levels that normally takes place just prior to ovulation in the menstrual cycle. In the menstrual cycle, it has been amply documented that the cyclical increase in E_2 exerts a facilitatory role on the neuroendocrinological mechanisms governing the preovulatory LH surge [22]. The classical reproductive endocrinology reference texts, however, usually remain silent about the possibility that the preovulatory increase in E_2 has any associated endometrial effects. The report by Craft et al. [23], which shows excellent pregnancy rates after egg donation recipients received constant dose of E_2, has seriously challenged the possibility that the endometrium benefits from specific endometrial priming brought by the preovulatory pattern of E_2 increase. Hence, looking at egg donation data it appears that sufficient estrogen priming (time and dose wise) is all that is needed as prerequisite for P to trigger proper endometrial receptivity.

Egg donation protocols have also enriched our understanding of the therapeutic dilemmas pertaining to P administration. Here, the situation differs slightly from that experienced with E_2 treatment because oral P administration has rightfully not been attempted for priming endometrial receptivity. Indeed, the extremely poor bioavailability of orally administered P [24] precludes the use oral P for egg donation. The remaining options for P administration in egg donation are the intramuscular (IM) and transvaginal routes.

A corollary to the excellent pregnancy rates observed after transferring embryos in women whose endometrium has been prepared solely with exogenous hormone is that ovarian factors other than E_2 and P are not strictly necessary for triggering prime endometrial receptivity. Hence it can be said that as far as endometrial priming is concerned, "less", i.e., E_2 and P only, not only suffices for triggering optimal endometrial receptivity, but may also benefit from avoiding potentially deleterious effects on the endometrium of other ovarian factors such as, for example, androgens.

The role of the E_2/P ratio

We and others have become interested in the role played by the plasma E_2/P ratio on endometrial receptivity because COH cycles have been associated with marked changes in this ratio. Specifically, we were interested whether decreases or increases in the E_2/P ratio could explain the suboptimal endometrial receptivity of COH cycles. Yet it appeared that a preliminary step to any meaningful analysis of E_2/P required that the role of one of the component of this ratio, luteal E_2, on endometrial morphology and receptivity be clarified.

It has long been established that sufficient priming of the endometrium by endogenous or exogenous E_2 is a specific requisite for proper endometrial action of P [34]. On the other hand, the physiological significance of E_2 produced by the corpus luteum concomitantly to P, i.e., luteal E_2, has remained a puzzling enigma. Hence, to understand the physiological significance of luteal E_2 has been viewed as an obligatory premise to analyzing the consequences on endometrial receptivity of alterations in E_2/P ratio encountered in COH cycles. Therefore, we have conceived an experimental paradigm based on the E_2 and P replacement cycle model to analyze the physiological role played by luteal E_2 [12]. For this, 24 women whose ovaries were absent or inactive as a result of POF, ovarian dysgenesis or prior surgery received transdermal E_2 and vaginal P. All women received 0.1 to 0.4 mg of E_2 per 24 h from day 1 to 14, according to a regimen designed to duplicate the menstrual cycle levels of plasma E_1 and E_2. This was achieved by wearing one or several transdermal therapeutic systems (Estraderm-TTS 100, Ciba Pharmaceuticals, Rueil, France) delivering approximately 0.1 mg $E_2/24$ h, each [10]. Micronized P (Utrogestan, Besins-Iscovesco, Pharmaceuticals, Paris, France) was administered vaginally from day 15 to 28 (300 mg/day) in all women. Between days 15 and 28 administration of E_2 varied between the two study groups. Women in group I received 0.3 to 0.1 mg of $E_2/24$ h in order to duplicate the E_2 production of the corpus luteum. On the other hand, women in group II removed all their transdermal systems on the morning of day 15 and received no E_2 from day 15 to 28. In groups I and II endometrial biopsies were obtained on days 20 and 24. Endometrial biopsies obtained on day 20 showed the characteristic findings described earlier [25], heralding an abundant development of subnuclear vacuoles in the glandular epithelium and no difference was observed between groups I and II. On day 24 endometrial specimens of groups I and II showed predecidualization of stromal cells around the spiral arteries and again no difference was noticed between women who received luteal E_2 (group I) and those who did not (group II). Therefore, our results indicate that luteal E_2 is not essential to the proper action of P on the E_2 primed endometrium, while it is a requisite cofactor to the inhibitory action of P on plasma gonadotropins.

As in COH cycles plasma E_2 is often found more profoundly elevated than plasma P, a fear exists that it is an increase rather than a decrease in the E_2/P ratio that might be deleterious to endometrial receptivity. In agreement with this long prevailing concept, Forman et al. [1] analyzed their IVF results in relation to pre-hCG levels of E_2. These authors have observed data corroborating the suspicion that exceedingly high levels of E_2 are deleterious, as pregnancy rates decreased when pre-hCG levels of E_2 exceeded the 90th percentile. Yet opinions about the possible detrimental effects of high E_2 levels are far from being unanimous. Indeed, there have been recent reports that failed to observe that very high levels of E_2 were detrimental to the outcome of IVF [3].

To clarify this much debated issue we further modified the E_2 and P replacement cycle model. The question that we wished to answer was whether extremely high levels of E_2 interfere with the endometrial action of P. To address this issue, six other women (group IV), also deprived of ovarian function, received physiological E_2 and P replacement as described for the participants of group I. In addition these women also received IM injections of 5 mg E_2-benzoate (E_2-B) every 12 h, from days 15 to 20. Blood samples were obtained twice a week as in groups I and II and an endometrial biopsy was obtained on day 20. Mean plasma E_2 levels reached nearly 3,000 pg/ml on day 20 in women of group IV, thus mocking the highest levels of E_2 encountered in COH cycles. Here again, contrary to our expectations, no difference was observed in the endometrial morphology of endometrial specimens obtained in women in groups III and I (controls).

Taken together, our results obtained by altering E_2 and P in the replacement cycle model indicated that even extreme alterations in plasma E_2/P ratio remained without effect on the endometrial action of P. It appears, therefore, that our data seriously challenge the frequently heeded concept that one should strive for maintaining an ideal plasma E_2/P ratio. If confirmed, our data fail to justify such practice on the basis of equilibrating the E_2/P ratio.

The glandular stromal dyssynchrony heralding a delay of the glands and an advance of the stroma that has been reported in some COH cycle may result from a mechanism closely related to dyssynchrony seen in by E_2-P cycles and not be related to the altered E_2/P ratios. Indeed, in COH cycles the duration of exposure of early luteal phase endometrial glands to P has been shortened by preventing the slight P rise that is seen in the menstrual cycle just prior to and during ovulation. This phenomenon has been particularly marked since gonadotropins have been routinely suppressed by an agonistic analog of gonadotropin-releasing hormone (GnRH-a). Hence, as in the E_2 and P cycles of IVF-OD, the delay in the secretory changes of endometrial glands seen in COH cycles may also result from a shortening of the exposure to P. Conversely, the advance seen in the secretory changes of the endometrial stroma on day 20 may result from plasma P levels surpassing those encountered during the early luteal phase of the menstrual cycle. We are currently conducting a clinical trial to determine precisely the P profile that follows the injection of hCG in COH cycles. As in E_2 and P cycles the closure of the window of endometrial receptivity (after day 19 or day 5) is contemporaneous with the development of secretory changes in the endometrial stroma, there are reasons to fear that the advancement of stromal changes in COH may impair receptivity by putting the endometrium out of synchrony with the transferred embryos. If proven valid, this hypothesis could lead to a timely use of anti-P compounds such as RU 486 to delay endometrial changes in COH cycles. Therefore, the practice of prescribing luteal support with P or hCG should not be abruptly relinquished solely on the basis of our experimental data.

Endometrial receptivity in IVF: the "third factor" hypothesis

Originally, the suboptimal implantation rates that appear to cripple the COH results have been blamed on the excessively high plasma E_2 levels and the resulting alterations in E_2/P ratio [1]. According to this concept it was proposed that plasma P had to be raised in proportion to the high E_2 levels in order to maintain the hypothetical magical value of the E_2/P ratio. Yet the concept that high E_2 levels resulting from COH are responsible of the suboptimal implantation rates of IVF has now been challenged by numerous recent observations [3].

Using the egg donation model to elucidate the physiopathology of endometrial receptivity in COH, we have failed to observe findings in support of the hypothesis that altered E_2/P ratios are at fault in the altered IVF implantation rates. On the contrary, we have observed that even maximal increases and decreases in E_2/P ratio failed to affect endometrial morphology. Our results, therefore, tend to disclaim the excessively high E_2 levels from their role of the designated scapegoats responsible for hampering IVF results. Thus, we must envision that P and hCG supplementation may affect endometrial receptivity through mechanisms having no morphological expression or that the reported improvements might have resulted from statistical flukes.

These observations have led us to formulate a new hypothesis to explain the suboptimal endometrial receptivity of IVF cycles. This new concept or "third factor" proposes that ovarian factors other than E_2 and P, yet also induced by the hMG driven ovarian hyperstimulation, are responsible for lowering endometrial receptivity in some IVF cases. First among the substances produced in excessive amounts in COH that are susceptible to hamper endometrial receptivity are the ovarian androgens. Supporting data in favor of our newly proposed concept is the observation that ovarian androgens, androstenedione (Δ^4) and testosterone (T), increase more in COH [26] than in the menstrual cycle [27]. Preliminary work from our group has confirmed that in COH, hMG treatment increases plasma androgens more than 2-fold, while hCG administration does not further elevate plasma Δ^4 and T above the levels achieved at the end of follicular maturation (Society for Gynecologic Investigation, 1994).

The above notwithstanding, COH may also result in the excessive production of nonsteroidal ovarian products that may also affect endometrial blood flow and receptivity. Be it the ovarian androgens or a yet to be defined peptide, the "third factor" affecting endometrial receptivity in COH is believed to either interfere with the action of E_2 on uterine vessels or to exert vascular and/or endometrial properties of its own.

Conclusion

Data from our work and that of others studying physiological replacement cycles originally designed to prime endometrial receptivity in recipients of IVF-OD support the abandonment of the deeply anchored belief that an ideal plasma E_2/P ratio is a requisite for endometrial receptivity. Indeed, imbalances in E_2/P have been universally designated as responsible for the suboptimal embryo implantation rates observed in various forms of assisted conception, including IVF. Yet none of our observations made after inducing maximal alterations in the plasma E_2/P ratio in the E_2 and P replacement cycle model has suggested that these hormonal changes affect the endometrial action of P. Therefore, we think that the detrimental role of non-physiological plasma E_2/P ratios on endometrial receptivity has been overemphasized and that its significance should now be seriously challenged.

Results obtained through studying the E_2 and P model suggest that endometrial glands and stroma respond differently to P. While endometrial glands seem to be influenced mainly by the duration of exposure to even minimal increments in plasma P levels, advancement in the secretory changes of the stroma appear to depend mostly on the actual levels of plasma P. It is suggested that the glandular-stromal dyssynchrony observed in the early luteal phase of E_2 and P and COH cycles may be mediated by a similar mechanism combining a shorting of the duration of exposure P and an increase in the levels of P. Levels of P are higher than normal in COH which may hasten secretory changes occurring in endometrial stroma which, in turn, may participate in lowering pregnancy rates in IVF by an early closing of the window of receptivity. An alternative mechanism that may account for pregnancy rates being lower in IVF than in IVF-OD is the possibility that the high doses of hMG used in COH trigger an overproduction of ovarian products (other than E_2 and P) resulting in elevated uterine artery resistance and suboptimal endometrial receptivity.

References

1. Forman R, Fries N, Testart J, Belaisch-Allart J, Hazout A, Frydman R. Fertil Steril 1988;49:118–122.
2. Mac Namee MC, Edwards RG, Howles CM. Human Reprod 1988;3:43–52.
3. Chenette PE, Sauer MV, Paulson RJ. Fertil Steril 1990;54:858–863.
4. Fanchin R, de Ziegler D, Taieb J, Hazout A, Frydman R. Fertil Steril 1993;59:1090–1094.
5. Silverberg KM, Burns WN, Olive DL, Riehl M, Schenken RS. J Clin Endocrinol Metab 1991;73: 797–803.
6. Schoolcraft W, Sinton E, Schlenker T, Huyinh D, Hamilton F, Meldrum DR. Fertil Steril 1991;55: 563–566.
7. Edelstein MC, Brzyski RG, Jones GS, Simonetti S, Muasher SJ. Fertil Steril 1990;53:103–105.
8. Hofmann GE, Bentzien F, Bergh PA, Garrisi GJ, Williams MC, Guzman I, Navot D. Fertil Steril 1993;60:675–679.
9. Navot D, Anderson TL, Droesch K, Scott RT, Kreiner D, Rosenwaks Z. J Clin Endocrinol Metab 1989;68:801–807.
10. de Ziegler D, Bessis R, Frydman R. Fertil Steril 1991;55:775–779.
11. Navot D, Bergh PA, Williams M, Garrisi GJ, Guzman I, Sandler B, Fox J, Schreiner-Engel P, Hofman GE, Grunfeld L. J Clin Endocrinol Metab 1991;72:408–414.
12. de Ziegler D, Bergeron C, Cornel, Médalie DA, Massai MR, Milgrom E, Frydman R, Bouchard P. J Clin Endocrinol Metab 1992;74:322–331.
13. Lutjen P, Traunson A, Leeton J, Findlay J, Wood C, Renow P. Nature 1984;307:174–175.
14. Navot D, Laufer N, Kopolovic J et al. N Engl J Med 1984;314:806–811.
15. Rosenwacks Z. Fertil Steril 1987;47: 895–909.

16. Frydman R, Letur-Könirsch H, de Ziegler D, Bydlowski D, Raoul-Duval A, Selva J. Fertil Steril 1990;53:666–672.
17. Edwards RG, Morcos S, Macnamee M, Balmaceda JP, Walters DE, Asch R. Lancet 1991;338:292–294.
18. Edwards RG. Human Reprod 1992;7:773–774.
19. de Ziegler D, Bouchard P. Curr Opin Obstet Gynecol 1993;5:378–388.
20. Massai MR, de Ziegler D, Lesobre V, Bergeron C, Frydman R, Bouchard P. Fertil Steril 1993; 59:1179–1186.
21. Sauer MV, Paulson RJ, Lobo RA. JAMA 1992;268:1275–1279.
22. Hoff JD, Quiegley ME, Yen SSC. J Clin Endocrinol Metab 1983;57:792–796.
23. Serhal PF, Craft IL. Fertil Steril 1987;48:265–269.
24. Nahoul K, Dhemin L, Jondet M, Roger M. Maturitas 1993;16:185–202.
25. Steingold KA, Matt DW, de Ziegler D, Sealey JE, Fratkin M, Reznikov S. J Clin Endocrinol Metab 1991;73:275–280.
26. Cedars MI, Surey E, Hamilton F, Lapolt P, Meldrum DR. Fertil Steril 1990;53:627.
27. Judd HL, Yen SSC. J Clin Endocrinol Metab 1973;36:475.

Recombinant gonadotropins: basic aspects

Structure-function studies of gonadotropins using site-directed mutagenesis and gene transfer: design of a long-acting gonadotropin agonist

I. Boime[1*], F. Fares[1], M. Furuhashi[1], P.D. LaPolt[2], K. Nishimori[2], T. Shikone[2], T. Sugahara[1] and A.J.W. Hsueh[2*]

[1]*Washington University School of Medicine, St. Louis, MO 63110;* [2]*Stanford University Medical School, Stanford, CA 94305-5317, USA*

Abstract. Follitropin (FSH) is a pituitary glycoprotein hormone that is essential for the development of ovarian follicles and testicular seminiferous tubules. FSH is used clinically to stimulate follicular maturation for in vitro fertilization and treatment of anovulatory women. One issue regarding the clinical use of FSH is its short half-life in the circulation. To address this point, we constructed a chimeric gene containing the sequence encoding the carboxy-terminal peptide (CTP) of the chorionic gonadotropin β subunit (CGβ) containing the four serine-linked oligosaccharides fused to the translated sequence of the human FSH β subunit (FSHβ). This region of CGβ is important for maintaining the prolonged plasma half-life of human CG dimer. The presence of CTP did not significantly affect assembly of FSHβ with the α subunit or secretion of the dimer. In vitro receptor binding and steroidogenic activity of dimer bearing the FSH-β-CTP chimera were the same as wild type FSH. However, the in vivo potency and the chimera was enhanced.

Since the α subunit is common to LH, FSH, hCG and TSH, the CTP was inserted in the subunit to increase the half-life of all four hormones (and derivatives thereof) with one change. When inserted near the amino terminus of the α subunit, the CTP sequence did not effect receptor binding or steroidogenesis of FSH or hCG in vitro. The in vivo activity of the hCG chimera was increased compared to wild type hCG. The results show the potential for the FSH and hCG chimeras as therapeutic agents. In addition, the presence of the CTP sequence may represent a general method for enhancing the in vivo longevity of different proteins.

Introduction

Follitropin (follicle-stimulating hormone; FSH) is a pituitary glycoprotein hormone essential for maintenance of ovarian follicle and testicular tubule development. FSH, together with luteinizing hormone (LH), thyroid-stimulating hormone and human chorionic gonadotropin (CG), constitute a family of glycoprotein hormones that are heterodimers containing two nonidentical subunits: α and β [1]. Within an animal

---

Address for correspondence: 1) I. Boime, Washington University School of Medicine, Department of Molecular Biology & Pharmacology, 660 S. Euclid Avenue, Box 8103, St. Louis, MO 63110. 2) A.J.W. Hsueh, Department of Obstetrics and Gynecology, Division of Reproductive Medicine, Stanford University Medical School, Stanford, CA 94305-5317, USA.

species the amino acid sequences of the α subunits are identical, and although the β subunits determine the biological specificity of the hormones, there is significant amino acid sequence similarity among them [1]. This is readily apparent for the LHβ and CGβ subunits as they share >80% sequence identity, which is presumably responsible for the similar biological activity of their dimers [2,3]. CGβ is distinguished among the β subunits because of the presence of a C-terminal extension with four O-linked oligosaccharides (Fig. 1). This extension is believed to play a role in maintaining the prolonged half-life of CG compared to the other hormones [3–6]. Recent studies using site-directed mutagenesis and gene transfer techniques indicated that the dimer containing CGβ devoid of the C-terminal peptide (CTP) was 3-fold less active than native CG in stimulating ovulation in rats [6]. Together with site-directed mutagenesis, these methods have been valuable tools for elucidating structure/function determinants of the glycoprotein hormone family [6–11]. Similar methodology provides a powerful approach for designing therapeutic analogs of these hormones. FSH is used clinically to stimulate development of ovarian follicles for in vitro fertilization [12,13], and to initiate follicular maturation in anovulatory women with chronic anovulatory syndrome [14] or luteal phase deficiency [15]. One major issue regarding the clinical use of FSH is its relatively short half-life in vivo [16,17]. To address this issue, the CTP of the CGβ subunit was fused to the human FSH β subunit coding sequence [18]. We reasoned that this FSH analog would have a prolonged half-life and enhanced bioactivity in vivo, as suggested from the experiments with CG lacking the CTP sequence. These constructs were transfected into Chinese hamster ovary (CHO) cells together with the wild type α subunit and stable clones were selected. Compared to wild type FSH, the addition of CTP sequences did not significantly affect assembly, secretion, or stimulation of steroidogenesis in vitro. However, the in vivo potency of the chimera was substantially increased. To assess the general nature of the approach, the CTP unit was also fused to the α subunit gene. Because the α subunit is common to the gene protein hormones, we reasoned that α-CTP subunit chimera would in one construct increase the in vivo stability of all hormone dimers. We tested hCG dimers containing an α chimera which had increased biopotency compared to wild type hCG. The data show the potential for this approach to generate long-acting FSH agonists.

CGβ O-linked Extension

```
              O                      O                   O                     O
              |                      |                   |                     |
-Ser Ser Ser Ser Lys Ala Pro Pro Pro Ser Leu Pro Ser Pro Ser Arg Leu Pro Gly Pro Ser
 118

Asp Thr Pro Ile Leu Pro Gln-COOH
              145
```

Fig. 1. The O-linked rich extension of hCGβ subunit. The O designates those serine residues containing oligosaccharides.

Methods

Construction of expression vector

An hFSHβ chimera bearing the CTP unit was created [19]. The chimera was transfected alone or with vector pM^2 containing the α subunit gene into CHO cells and was screened as described [19]. The nucleotide sequence encoding the CTP was inserted in frame with the human α subunit coding sequence using overlapping polymerase chain reaction [20]; the sequence was inserted at the carboxy end or between amino acids three and four of the subunit.

In vitro bioassay and radioligand receptor assay

FSH and chimeric proteins in conditioned medium obtained from cells incubated without serum were quantitated with an FSH immunoradiometric assay and a double-antibody radioimmunoassay (RIA) (Diagnostic Products, Los Angeles). The in vitro bioactivity was determined as described [8,21]. Stimulation of estrogen production by wild type FSH and the chimeras was compared after a 3-day culture period.

To measure bioactivity, immature female Sprague-Dawley rats were implanted with a 10-mm silastic capsule containing diethylstilbestrol. Rats were maintained in standard vivarium facilities with food and drinking water available ad libitum. Beginning the 4th day after estrogen treatment, rats received two equivalent intraperitoneal (i.p.) injections of wild type FSH or the chimeras at 24-h intervals. These hormones were quantitated by the radioreceptor assay and by radioimmunoassay with monoclonal antibody, and the determinations were in agreement within 15%. In the receptor assay, the amount of hormone required to achieve 50% binding was used to quantitate the derivatives. Animals were sacrificed by cervical dislocation 48 h after the initial injection, and ovaries were removed. The ovaries were decapsulated, weighed, and granulosa cells were isolated to determine levels of aromatase, a specific indicator of FSH bioactivity. Induction of aromatase activity was determined by the ability of isolated granulosa cells to convert androstenedione to estrogens in vitro. Granulosa cells isolated from ovaries described above were cultured (300,000 viable cells/well) in McCoy's 5A medium (GIBCO) containing 0.3 μmol/l androstenedione (Sigma) for 6 h at 37°C in a humidified atmosphere of 5% CO_2/95% air. After culture, the media were analyzed for estrogen content by RIA as described [22]. The viability of the cells were unaffected by addition of any of the conditioned media samples.

Results

Receptor binding and in vitro biological activity of chimeras

The CTP unit on FSHβ did not significantly interfere with assembly or secretion of the dimer [18]. Although the CTP is not critical for bioactivity of CG in vitro [6,23,24], the additional 29 amino acids on the heterologous subunit may affect signal transduction of the modified FSH protein. The chimera was quantitated in conditioned medium by using a monoclonal antibody-based RIA and receptor binding was assessed in a radioligand receptor assay by quantitating the displacement of ^{125}I-hFSH binding to rat testes membranes. Addition of the CTP unit to FSHβ did not affect receptor binding of the dimer [22]. Because FSH specifically induces aromatase in granulosa cells [25], in vitro signal transduction of the modified FSH dimers was assessed in the granulosa cell aromatase bioassay by measuring hormone-stimulated estrogen production [25]. The steroidogenic activity of FSH-CTP was comparable to that of wild type FSH. Thus, modification at the carboxyl end of FSHβ by adding the CTP sequence did not significantly affect in vitro receptor binding or signal transduction [22]. In addition, the chimera had no LH bioactivity as tested in a LH radioligand receptor assay (data not shown).

In vivo biopotency/half-life of chimeras

FSH treatment stimulates ovarian granulosa cell differentiation and increases follicle growth and antrum formation [25]. The in vivo biopotencies of wild type FSH and FSH-CTP were examined by determining ovarian weight augmentation and granulosa cell aromatase induction. The hormones were injected i.p. into immature estrogen-primed at 24-h intervals. Rats were killed 24 h after the second injection, and the ovaries were removed. Induction of granulosa cell aromatase activity was studied ex vivo by incubating granulosa cells with a saturating dose of the aromatase substrate androstenedione for 6 h. The ovarian weight increased significantly between animals treated with wild type FSH and FSH-CTP. In addition, estrogen production by granulosa cells from rats treated with the analog increased 3- to 5-fold over that seen in rats treated with wild type FSH.

Studies were performed to determine whether priming with a single i.p. injection of FSH-CTP could allow a high dose of CG given 48 h earlier to fail to induce ovulation, presumably due to the absence of sufficiently matured follicles. In contrast, priming with a single injection of FSH-CTP allowed CG to induce ovulation in a dose-dependent manner. Rats that received 3 or 10 IU FSH-CTP ovulated in response to CG with 20 ± 6 and 43 ± 5 oocytes/rat, respectively. Similarly, rats that received four 2.5-IU doses of wild type FSH 12 h apart also ovulated, with 35 ± 9 oocytes/rat. In addition, there was no significant difference in ovarian weight 18 h after CG treatment between unprimed animals (32 ± 4 mg; n = 4) and rats primed with a single injection (10 IU) of wild type FSH (35 ± 2) mg; n = 4). In contrast, there were marked increases in ovarian weight 18 h after CG treatment in rats primed with a single administration of 1, 3, or 10 IU FSH-CTP (47 ± 4, 76 ± 6 and 59 ± 6 mg, respectively; n = 4/group) and in females primed with four injections of 2.5 IU wild type FSH 12 h apart (105 ± 20 mg; n = 4).

Injection of CG to rats primed with a single subcutaneous dose of wild type FSH (10 IU) failed to induce ovulation in response to CG 48 h later, whereas CG effectively induced ovulation in rats primed with a single subcutaneous dose of either 3 or 10 IU FSH-CTP. Thus, there was no major difference in ovulatory potential between subcutaneous and i.p. administration.

Because the α subunit is common to the glycoprotein family, we reasoned that an α subunit CTP chimera would, in one construct, increase the in vivo stability of the entire glycoprotein hormone family. Moreover, since the α subunit sequence is dissimilar from the β subunits, the efficacy of this α-subunit derivative would test the general application of CTP-chimeras for increasing the biologic half-life of other bioactive proteins. Alpha-subunit CTP chimeras were constructed using overlapping PCR mutagenesis [20]. They were cotransfected with gene encoding the hCGβ subunit into CHO cells, stable clones were selected, and the in vitro biologic activity was tested (Fig. 2). CG dimers containing α subunit chimera with CTP at the carboxy end (αC) of the subunit had a much lower binding affinity for the human LH/hCG receptor. This is presumably due to the presence of determinants for receptor binding/signal transduction at the carboxy end of the α subunit [26–28]. The affinity of dimers composed of chimeric α subunit with the CTP inserted between amino acids three and four of the subunit (Cα) was comparable to wild type hCG. Preliminary data show that CαCG dimer stimulates testosterone in hypophysecto-

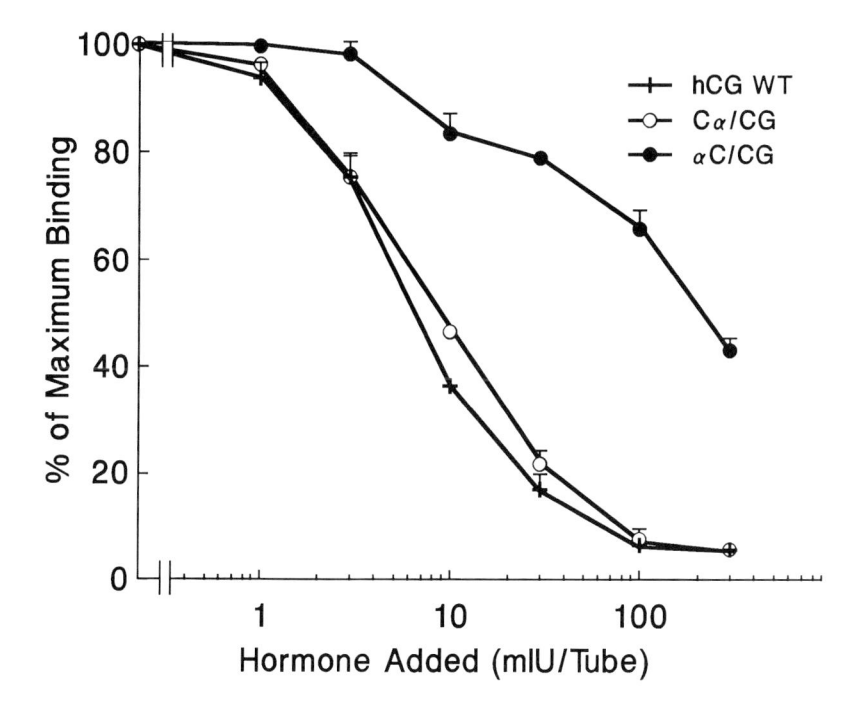

Fig. 2. Displacement of [^{125}I] hCG binding to human LH receptors by WT hCG and analogs. Human fetal kidney cells permanently expressing recombinant human LH receptors were incubated with [^{125}I] hCG in the absence or presence of varying concentrations of inhibited wild type or derivatives of hCG. Displacement curves are presented as the percentage of maximal binding at each dose of unlabeled hormone (mean ± SEM) of three replicate experiments.

mized rats with a potency greater than 3-fold compared to wild type hCG. These data further support the usefulness of using the CTP to increase the potency of bioactive glycoproteins.

Discussion

Here we describe the construction of several chimeric genes that contain the C-terminal peptide coding region of CGβ fused to FSHβ and the common α subunit. Compared to wild type FSH, the presence of the CTP did not interfere with combination to the α subunit or secretion of dimers. Similarly, in vitro receptor binding and steroidogenic activity of these chimeras were not significantly affected. The data are consistent with earlier studies, demonstrating that deletion of the CTP from CGβ does not affect secretion or in vitro receptor binding/signal transduction of CG dimer [6,23]. However, fusion of CTP to FSHβ clearly increases the in vivo serum half-life and biologic activity of the chimera.

Due to the relatively rapid clearance of native FSH in vivo, the commonly used therapeutic protocol requires frequent injection of the hormone. The chimera described here could be an effective long-acting agonist for clinical use. Moreover, CTP chimeras could be constructed for diverse proteins to enhance their in vivo biological half-life. The addition of the CTP could elicit immune reactions. However, several studies have demonstrated that the CTP region of CGβ is weakly immunogenic [29,30]. In addition, because the native CGβ which contains the CTP is normally secreted in both men and women, the immune system may not recognize the FSH chimera as a foreign protein.

Although the kidney is the main site of clearance for FSH [17], much less CG is cleared by this route [16,31]. It has been suggested that more negatively charged forms of human FSH (i.e., forms with increased sialic acid content) have longer half-lives, which may be related to a decreased glomerular filtration [32]. Thus, the presence of the CTP with it sialylated O-linked oligosaccharides may prolong the circulating half-life of the hormone secondary to a decrease in renal clearance. Alternatively, as proposed previously [6] the CTP sequences may affect the processing of asparagine-linked oligosaccharides, which in turn could influence extracellular levels.

Significantly, the CTP sequence can be shuttled to different proteins and still be an acceptor for O-linked oligosaccharides. This suggests a potential model system for elucidating the recognition sequences that determine why particular serine residues can accept O-linked oligosaccharide chains [33]. Since the CTP sequence terminates the carboxyl end of the CGβ subunit, and this sequence with the attached oligosaccharides apparently does not affect folding of CGβ, the CTP is a convenient sequence for site-directed mutagenesis. This is critical because if the O-linked glycosylation sites are in the interior of the subunit, amino acid replacements could lead to pronounced position effects.

These data establish a rationale for using these chimeras as long-acting gonadotropin analogs that can be used clinically where replacement therapy is indicated. Anovulatory women, or men with impaired testicular functions, would be candidates for such therapy.

Acknowledgements

This work was supported by NIH Contract #HD-92922, a Postdoctoral Fellowship from the Rockefeller Foundation (FF) and NRSA #HD-07252 (PSLP).

References

1. Pierce J, Parsons T. Annu Rev Biochem 1981;50:465–495.
2. Talmadge K, Vamvakopoulos N, Fiddes J. Nature (London) 1984;307:37–41.
3. Birken S, Canfield RE. J Biol Chem 1977;252:5386–5392.
4. Keutmann HT, Williams RM. J Biol Chem 1977;252:5393–5394.
5. Kessler MJ, Mise T, Ghai RD, Bahl OP. J Biol Chem 1979;254:7909–7914.
6. Matzuk MM, Hsueh AJW, LaPolt P, Tsafriri A, Keene JL, Boime I. Endocrinology 1990;126:376–383.
7. Matzuk MM, Spangler M, Camel M, Suganuma N, Boime I. J Cell Biol 1989;109:1429–1438.
8. Keene JL, Matzuk MM, Otani T, Fauser CJM, Galway B, Hsueh AJW, Boime I. J Biol Chem 1989;264:4769–4775.
9. Chen F, Wang Y, Puett D. J Biol Chem 1991;266:19357–19361.
10. Campbell R, Dean-Emig D, Moyle W. Proc Natl Acad Sci USA 1991;88:760–764.
11. Kaetzel D, Virgin J, Clay C, Nilson J. Mol Endocrinol 1989;3:1765–1771.
12. Jones GS, Acosta A, Garcia JE, Bernardus RE, Rosenwaks Z. Fertil Steril 1985;43:696–702.
13. Albert PJ, Schlafke J, Kaesemann H, Gille J. Arch Gynecol Obstet 1987;241:53–56.
14. Worley RJ. In: Garcia CR, Mastroianni L, Anelar RD, Dubin L (eds) Current Therapy of Infertility 3. Toronto: Decker, 1988;106–110.
15. Lightman A, Jones EE, Boyers SP. In: Cecherney AH, Polan ML, Lee RD, Boyers SP (eds) Decision Making in Infertility. Toronto: Decker, 1988;32–33.
16. Sowers JR, Pekary AE, Hershman JM, Kanter M, Distefano JJ. J Endocrinol 1979;80:83–89.
17. Amin HK, Hunter WM. J Endocrinol 1970;48:307–317.
18. Fares F, Suganuma N, Nishimori K, LaPolt P, Hsueh AJW, Boime I. Proc Natl Acad Sci 1992;89:4304–4308.
19. Matzuk MM, Krieger M, Corless CL, Boime I. Proc Natl Acad Sci USA 1987;84:6354–6358.
20. Ho SN, Hunt H, Horton R, Pullen J, Pease L. Gene 1989;77:51–59.
21. Jia X-C, Hsueh AJW. Endocrinology 1986;119:1570–1577.
22. Adashi EY, Hsueh AJW. J Biol Chem 1982;257:6077–6083.
23. El-Deiry S, Kaetzel D, Kennedy G, Nilson J, Puett D. Mol Endocrinol 1989;3:1523–1528.
24. Bousfield GR, Liu W-K, Ward D. Endocrinology 1989;124:379–387.
25. Hsueh AJW, Bicsak T, Jia X-C, Dahl K, Fauser B, Galway AB, Czekala N, Pavlou S, Papkoff H, Keene J, Boime I. Recent Prog Horm Res 1989;45:209–277.
26. Merz W, Dorner M. Biochem and Biophys Acta 1985;844:62–71.
27. Charlesworth M, McCormick O, Madden B, Ryan R. J Biol Chem 1987;262:13409–13416.
28. Bidari J, Troalen F, Bousfeld G, Gohoun C, Bellet D. Endocrinol 1989;124:923–929.
29. Birken S, Canfield R, Lauer R, Agosto G, Gabel M. Endocrinology 1980;106:1659–1664.
30. Matsuura S, Chen H-C. In: Liu D, Schechter A, Henrikson R, Candliffe P (eds) Chemical Synthesis and Sequencing of Peptides and Proteins. London: Elsevier, 1981;197–251.

31. Kalyan NK, Bahl OP. J Biol Chem 1983;258:67–74.
32. Wide L. Acta Endocrinol (Copenhagen) 1986;112:336–344.
33. Jentoft N. Trends Biochem 1986;14:272–275.

Control of gonadotropin-binding specificity

Robert K. Campbell
Ares Advanced Technology, 280 Pond Street, Randolph, MA 02368, USA

Abstract. Human chorionic gonadotropin (hCG) and follicle-stimulating hormone (FSH) are homologous heterodimeric trophic factors that act on the gonads. These proteins bind their respective receptors with high selectivity, exhibiting less than 0.01% cross-reactivity. The determinant for this binding specificity has been identified as a short linear sequence in the C-terminal region of the β subunit. Several lines of evidence suggest that this region acts as a conformational switch influencing the structure of the α subunit, rather than a direct binding contact with the receptor.

It has been 30 years since it was first reported that a glycoprotein hormone, luteinizing hormone (LH), could be dissociated by acid exposure into two subunits of similar size [1]. Subsequent analyses indicated that these subunits possessed different amino acid and carbohydrate content [2,3]. Hormone biological activity was lost following dissociation, but could be restored by recombining the subunits [4]. Studies with a second glycoprotein hormone, thyroid-stimulating hormone (TSH), demonstrated that it too was a heterodimer [5]. The dissociated subunits, designated α and β, could be recombined to reconstitute active TSH. When the β subunit of TSH was recombined with an α subunit from LH the resulting protein exhibited TSH activity. This suggested that the α subunit was common to all the glycoprotein hormones, whereas the β subunits were unique to each hormone and controlled binding specificity. Additional recombination studies demonstrated that α subunits could also be exchanged between placental and pituitary glycoprotein hormones [6], between glycoprotein hormones from different species [7,8], and even between different vertebrate classes [9]. In each case, the biological activity of the recombined heterodimers was related to the hormone from which the β subunit was derived. Amino acid sequencing of several glycoprotein hormones confirmed that within a species the α subunits were identical [10,11]. As a result of these various studies the role of the β subunit as the dominant determinant of receptor binding specificity was quickly established. However, the specific regions of the β subunit responsible for determining binding specificity were not readily apparent. Comparison of hormone amino acid sequences revealed numerous differences scattered throughout the proteins, precluding the localization of functional determinants.

A decade after the identification of the role of the β subunit in hormone-receptor binding, a powerful strategy for elucidating structural determinants of specificity in protein-protein interactions was devised by Smith-Gill and her colleagues at NIH. In this work, key amino acid residues in antibody epitopes on hen egg lysozyme (HEL) were identified by comparing antibody binding to HEL and several closely related lysozymes from other avian species [12,13]. These other proteins differed from HEL at only a few residue positions. This permitted fine localization of residues critical for antibody discrimination. In combination with the known crystallographic structure of HEL, the mapping data permitted the preparation of a model of the epitopes on the protein. The determination of structures for several HEL-antibody F_{ab} complexes by x-ray crystallography has shown that the predictions from the mapping studies were highly accurate [14].

Glycoprotein hormones with distinguishing characteristics, but that differ in sequence by only a few amino acid residues, have not been readily available. For example, despite the existence of highly selective antibodies that distinguish hCG from hLH, the sequence differences between hCG and hLH are too numerous and diffuse to permit ready interpretation of mapping studies of the native proteins. To apply the epitope mapping strategy to the gonadotropins it was necessary to obtain novel analogs that differ by only a few residues.

Mutagenesis of protein-encoding DNAs and subsequent characterization of the expressed protein analogs is a powerful strategy for modifying protein structure and evaluating the importance of specific amino acid residues to protein function. However, mutagenesis suffers from limitations and pitfalls. For example, mutations may introduce deleterious conformational changes in the protein. These may confound the interpretation of the sequence change. In addition, there are potential difficulties in accurately quantifying muteins in unpurified samples. The mutagenesis strategy most resistant to these risks is that of assembling chimeric constructs from homologous proteins. This can permit the study of a subset of residue differences, facilitating studies similar to those done with HEL.

Early applications of chimeric muteins were to localize the DNA binding domain in steroid hormone receptors [15] and to grossly localize determinants of receptor and antibody binding in α-interferon [16,17]. In these studies the muteins were characterized to determine which properties from the two parent molecules had been introduced or eliminated. By comparing the relative activities of chimeric analogs in different functional assays it is possible to conclusively detect changes in functional specificity (e.g., receptor or antibody binding) relative to the parent constructs, provided the doses used in the various assays can be normalized.

The initial application of chimeric mutagenesis to the glycoprotein hormones focused on identifying residues responsible for differences between hCG and hLH in secretion kinetics and antibody binding [18,19]. Coincident with these studies the chimera mapping strategy was also adapted to localize the β subunit sequences that determine receptor binding specificity. Since hCG and hLH bind similarly to LH receptors (from most species), hCG/hLH chimeras were not particularly suitable for identifying receptor binding determinants. For this purpose chimeras of hCG and hFSH were initially used. These two hormones have very little receptor cross-specificity [20]. The first hCG/hFSH chimeric β subunits [21] were designed to examine regions previously implicated as important for receptor binding, i.e., the large loop, hCG 38–57/hFSH 32–51 [22,23] and the determinant loop [24], hCG

93–100/hFSH 87–94. These regions differ markedly between the two hormones, suggesting that they might contribute to binding specificity. Subsequent hCG/hFSH chimeras investigated the carboxyl-termini of hFSH and hCG, regions that are also characterized by extensive heterogeneity between the hormones.

The results of these studies, which have been previously reported [21], support the notion that the various glycoprotein hormone β-subunits have highly homologous conformations. Even though the least conserved sequences in the proteins were selected for chimeric substitution, with the resulting introduction of numerous changes in side chain size, charge and hydrophobicity, nearly all of the mutant subunits retained binding sites for the other subunit and multiple monoclonal antibodies. Many of the mutant analogs also exhibited the ability to bind to FSH receptors and/or antibodies. These observations indicate that the transplanted sequences assume conformations similar to those in hFSH. Thus, not only can the intact subunits be exchanged between hormones to create novel analogs, but portions of their sequences can be exchanged (by mutagenesis).

A sequence from hFSHβ (residues 88–108) has been identified that acts as a determinant for near-exclusive FSH receptor binding specificity when transferred into hCGβ [21]. Substitution of this sequence for the carboxyl-terminus of hCG converts the hormone into a potent follitropin (equipotent to hFSH). This mutein retains only slight LH activity (about 0.01% the activity of hCG). The change in specificity occurs despite the retention of high sequence identity with hCGβ, i.e., the chimera is 86% identical to hCGβ (though it does lack the carboxyl-terminal peptide). In comparison, the β subunit from the naturally occurring hormone most closely related to hCG (i.e., hLH) is 85% identical to hCGβ (and also lacks the CTP). Unlike the hCG/hFSH chimera, hLH is functionally similar to hCG and exhibits strong LH receptor selectivity.

The change in binding specificity cannot be attributed to the removal of the hCGβ carboxyl-terminal peptide (CTP; residues 115–145) since certain chimeras lacking the CTP do not exhibit altered specificity [21]. Furthermore, addition of the hCGβ CTP to hFSHβ does not impair FSH receptor binding [25]. Thus, a small linear segment of the β subunit sequence is implicated as the dominant determinant of binding specificity. At present there is little evidence that any other β subunit regions contribute to binding specificity.

With regard to LH receptor binding, certain residues in the "determinant loop" (hCGβ residues 93–100) appear to be very important for binding and stimulation of LH receptors. All heterodimers containing analogs of hCGβ in which the 93–100 region was unchanged, bound and stimulated LH receptors, regardless of the changes beyond residue Cys100 in the β subunit [21]. Chimeras in which residues between 93–100 were disrupted exhibited diminished binding to LH receptors. Similar results have been observed by others using nonchimeric mutagenesis studies. Substitution of hCGβ Arg-94 with aspartic acid caused about a 10-fold change in LH-like activity, whereas substitution with lysine had little effect [26]. Replacement of hCGβ Asp-99 with arginine diminished hormone activity by at least two orders of magnitude, whereas substitutions with Asn or Glu had minor effects [27]. Deletion of the determinant loop (and all other carboxyl-terminal residues) prevented the β subunit from forming heterodimers with the α subunit [28]. Although residues in the determinant loop are not particularly well conserved across mammalian LH and CGβ subunits, many of these hormones exhibit strong species selectivity in LH receptor binding [29,30].

The strategy of using chimeric constructs to identify residues critical for receptor binding is strongly supported by the recent elucidation of the structure of growth hormone bound to the extracellular domain of its receptor [31]. This work demonstrated the extreme accuracy of predictions of hormone-receptor contact sites based on chimeric mutations required to convert prolactin into a high affinity ligand for the growth hormone receptor. With regard to other strategies for identifying binding determinants (using the growth hormone paradigm), mutagenesis studies employing negative endpoints (i.e., loss of binding activity) were less predictive of residues in the contact region. Some of these latter mutations may disrupt function by inducing disruptive, but nonlocalized conformational changes in the ligand. Antibody mapping studies were also predictive of hGH receptor binding regions [31].

Growth hormone and prolactin are monomeric ligands. Since the glyocoprotein hormones are multimeric proteins, it is not certain that acquisition of receptor binding activity in hCG/FSH muteins is necessarily mediated by direct involvement of the mutated residues in contacts with the receptor. In addition, in multimeric proteins disruptive mutations may be indicative of effects on subunit interactions, rather than direct involvement of the modified residues in receptor contacts. This is suggested by studies with tumor necrosis factors α and β [32,33]. Thus it is necessary to evaluate the conformational effects of the modifications on the protein in order to identify those that induce deleterious changes in quaternary structure. In the gonadotropin chimera studies, antibodies to hCG and FSH have been used to evaluate the extent of conformational effects. In nearly all instances the mutations affected only a subset of antibody binding activities [19,21].

As previously reported, several lines of evidence suggest that the β subunit region identified as a dominant FSH receptor binding determinant is near or in the contact region with the α subunit [21]. This includes the results of cross-linking studies with LH [34], epitope mapping of heterodimer-selective antibodies [19], and protection mapping studies [35]. In addition, peptides derived from this region of hCGβ or hFSHβ do not appear to interact with LH or FSH receptors [22,36]. A role for the β subunit influencing the conformation of α is suggested by observations that antibody binding to the α subunit differs between hormone heterodimers [37,38]. It is interesting to note that putative binding determinants in the hormones typically map to regions thought to lie in or near the subunit interface. In addition, epitopes for several antibodies that strongly inhibit hormone-receptor binding have been assigned to these sequences [19,21]. Although the effects of mutations on hormone functions are clear, it remains difficult to distinguish whether the mutated residues are in direct contact with the receptor or are located outside the receptor contact region. In the latter case the mutations may be acting to alter subunit conformation and subunit-subunit interactions.

In summary, recent studies using mutagenesis to study structure-activity relationships in the β subunits of glycoprotein hormones reveal these proteins to be tolerant of change and amenable to engineering. In combination with receptor and structural studies this is providing greater understanding of how gonadotropins act as well as an expanded range of possible interventions to modify gonadotropin properties and actions.

References

1. Li CH, and Starman B. Nature 1964;202:291–292.
2. Ward DN, Fujino M, Lamkin WM. Fed Proc 1966;25:348.
3. Papkoff H, Samy TSA. Biochim Biophys Acta 1967;147:175–177.
4. Papkoff H, Samy TSA. Proc Fed Amer Soc Exp Biol 1968;27:371.
5. Liao T-H, Pierce JG. J Biol Chem 1970;245:3275–3281.
6. Reichert LE Jr. Endocrinology 1971;90:1119–1122.
7. Reichert LE Jr, Midgley AR, Niswender GD, Ward DN. Endocrinology 1970;87:534–541.
8. Pierce JG, Bahl OP, Cornell JS, Swaminathan N. J Biol Chem 1971;246:2321–2324.
9. Licht P, Papkoff H, Farmer SW, Muller CH, Tsui HW, Crews, D. Recent Prog Horm Res 1977; 33:169–243.
10. Pierce JG, Liao T-H, Carlsen RB, Reimo T. J Biol Chem 1971;246:866–872.
11. Liu W-K, Nahm HS, Sweeny CM, Lamkin WM, Baker HN, Ward DN. J Biol Chem 1972;247: 4351–4364.
12. Smith-Gill SJ, Wilson AC, Potter M, Prager EM, Feldmann RJ, Mainhart CR. J Immunol 1982; 128:314–322.
13. Smith-Gill SJ, Lavoie TB, Mainhart CR. J Immunol 1984;133:384–393.
14. Davies DR, Sheriff S, Padlan EA. J Biol Chem 1988;263:10541–10544.
15. Green S, Chambon P. Nature 1987;325:75–78.
16. Shafferman A, Velan B, Cohen S, Leitner M, Grosfeld, H. J Biol Chem 1987;262:6227–6237.
17. Taylor-Papadimitriou J, Shearer M, Griffin D. J Immunol 1987;139:3375–3381.
18. Matzuk MM, Spangler MM, Camel M, Suganuma N, and Boime I. J Cell Biol 1989;109:1429–1438.
19. Moyle WR, Matzuk MM, Campbell RK, Cogliani E, Dean-Emig DM, Krichevsky A, Barnett RW, Boime I. J Biol Chem 1990;265:8511–8518.
20. Lee CY, Ryan RJ. Proc Natl Acad Sci USA 1972;69:3520–3523.
21. Campbell RK, Dean-Emig DM, Moyle WR. Proc Natl Acad Sci USA 1991;88:1760–1764.
22. Keutmann HT, Charlesworth MC, Mason KA, Ostrea T, Johnson L, Ryan RJ. Proc Natl Acad Sci USA 1987;84:2038–2042.
23. Schneyer AL, Sluss PM, Huston JS, Ridge RJ and Reichert LE, Jr. Biochemistry 1988;27:666–671.
24. Ward DN, Moore WT. In: Alexander NJ (ed) Animal Models for Research on Contraception and Fertility. New York: Harper & Row, 1979;151–164.
25. Fares FA, Suganuma N, Nishimori K, LaPolt PS, Hsueh AJW, Boime I. Proc Natl Acad Sci USA 1992;89:4304–4308.
26. Chen F, Puett D. Biochemistry 1991;30:10171–10175.
27. Chen F, Wang Y, Puett D. J Biol Chem 1991;266:19357–19361.
28. Chen F, Puett D. J Biol Chem 1991;266:6904–6908.
29. Davies TF, Walsh PC, Hodgen GD, Dufau ML, Catt KJ. J Clin Endocrinol Metab 1979;48:680–685.
30. Jia X-C, Oikawa M, Bo M, Tanaka T, Ny T, Boime I, Hsueh AJW. Mol Endocrinol 1991;5:759–768.
31. de Vos AM, Ultsch M, Kossiakoff AA. Science 1992;255:306–312.
32. Goh CR, Porter AG. Prot Eng 1991;4:385–389.
33. Eck MJ, Ultsch M, Rinderknecht E, de Vos AM, Sprang SR. J Biol Chem 1992;267:2119–2122.
34. Weare JA, Reichert LE Jr. J Biol Chem 1979;254:6972–6979.

35. Keutmann HT, Ratanabanangkoon K, Pierce MW, Kitzmann K, Ryan RJ. J Biol Chem 1983;258: 14521–14526.
36. Santa Coloma TA, Reichert LE Jr. J Biol Chem 1990;265:5037–5042.
37. Strickland TW, Puett D. Endocrinology 1981;109:1933–1942.
38. Hojo H, Ryan, RJ. Endocrinology 1985;117:2428–2434.

New recombinant hCG analogs with potent FSH activity in vivo

Yanhong Wang[1], Yi Han[1], Rebecca V. Myers[1], Gordon J. Macdonald[2] and William R. Moyle[2]

[1]*Department of OBGYN;* [2]*Department of Neuroscience and Cell Biology, Robert Wood Johnson Medical School, Piscataway, NJ 08854, USA*

Human luteinizing hormone (LH), follicle-stimulating hormone (FSH) and chorionic gonadotropin (hCG) are gonadotropins essential for reproduction. In women, FSH and LH promote follicle development and ovulation. hCG signals that conception has occurred and, through its actions on the corpus luteum, maintains the initial stages of pregnancy. In men, LH is needed for androgen secretion by the testes. FSH is essential for the onset of spermatogenesis. All three hormones have been used to stimulate human fertility (reviewed in [1]).

The physiological actions of these hormones depend on their specific interactions with either LH or FSH receptors [2]. hLH and hCG interact with LH receptors; hFSH interacts with FSH receptors. The mechanism by which binding specificity is controlled will not be known until the structures of the hormones and the receptors are known in detail. However, portions of the hormones that modulate binding specificity have been identified beginning with studies reported in the late 1960s [3]. The gonadotropins are α,β heterodimers in which the smaller α subunit has the same amino acid sequence in hLH, hFSH and hCG. Each of the larger β subunits of these hormones has a different amino acid sequence and is responsible for the abilities of the hormones to bind specific receptors. The observation that both hCG and hLH bind to LH receptors is explained by the similarities in their β subunits. While the hLHβ subunit has 114 amino acids and the hCGβ subunit has 145 amino acids, only 17 amino acids of the first 114 in hCG differ from those of hLHβ subunit. Amino acids 115–145 of hCG appear to stabilize its biological half-life and have long been postulated to enhance its activity in vivo. They do not appear to have a role in hormone binding specificity or affinity of hCG for LH receptors. The β subunit of hFSH contains only 111 amino acids and differs considerably from that of hCG and hLH, particularly in the regions found between cysteines 5 and 6 and between cysteine 10 and the carboxyterminus. In spite of these differences, similarities in the relative locations of the 12 cysteine residues in hFSH, hLH and hCG suggest that the gonadotropin β subunits have the same overall folding pattern. This explains the abilities of the β subunits of LH, hCG and hFSH to combine with the α subunit.

Experiments to identify portions of the β subunits that participate in receptor binding specificity involved interchanging portions of the β subunits from hCG and hFSH to form analogs termed hCG/hFSH chimeras [4]. The observations that these chimeras fold similar to the β subunit and can combine with the α subunit to yield active hormone analogs support the notion that the β subunit folding patterns in hFSH and hCG are very similar. Surprisingly, only a few amino acids of the β subunit control the abilities of the gonadotropins to distinguish LH and FSH receptors [4]. Thus, an α,β heterodimer containing a chimeric 117 residue β subunit composed of hCGβ subunit residues 1—93 and hFSHβ subunit residues 88—111 had high affinity for FSH receptors and low affinity for LH receptors. In addition, this analog had nearly the same ability as hFSH to stimulate steroidogenesis in granulosa cells. This suggested that only about one-fifth of the hFSHβ subunit is needed for receptor binding specificity. Indeed, further studies revealed that substitution of even fewer hFSHβ subunit residues for their hCGβ subunit homologs was sufficient to permit binding to FSH receptors. Thus, substitution of only eight hFSH residues found between the eleventh and twelfth cysteines is sufficient to enable hCG to bind to FSH receptors [5]. Surprisingly, analogs containing hCGβ subunit residues between cysteines 10 and 11 and hFSHβ subunit residues between cysteines 11 and 12 bind to both LH and FSH receptors. Thus, receptor binding specificity appears to be controlled by very small portions of the β subunit.

The development of hCG analogs with FSH activity in vitro has potential implications for treatments that are designed to induce human fertility. Because hCG has a longer biological half-life than hFSH [6—8], analogs of hCG that had FSH activity might also have longer half-lives. Thus, they would be expected to be more potent than hFSH for ovulation induction or enhancement of spermatogenesis. In addition, since their structures differ substantially from that of hFSH, administration of these hormones to humans will not interfere with measurements of endogenous hFSH levels. This would permit the physiological assessment of the feedback relationships between FSH and gonadal function in persons (or animals) after stimulation of their gonads with a hormone that has FSH activity. Here, we describe the structures and activities in vivo of two hCG analogs that are highly effective in stimulating ovarian weight gain in rodents.

Materials and Methods

The structures of the analogs are illustrated in Fig. 1. Procedures used to prepare and characterize CF94—117 β subunit have been described [4]. CFC94—114 β subunit was prepared by polymerase chain reaction directed mutagenesis using the hCGβ subunit as a template and standard cloning methods. The sequence encoding CF94—117 β subunit was cloned into the XhoI site of pBMT2x [9] obtained from Dr George Pavlakis (NCI, Frederick Cancer Research Facility, MD) downstream of the mouse metalothioneine promoter to give pBMT2x-CF94—117 β. The sequence encoding CFC94—114 β subunit was cloned into pLEN obtained from Dr Peter Kushner (UCSF, San Francisco, CA) to give pLEN-CFC94—114β. The cDNA of the human α subunit [10], obtained from Dr John Fiddes (California Biotechnology, Inc., Mountain View, CA), was cloned into pBMT2x and pLEN to give pBMT2x-hCGα

Analog	β subunit amino acid sequence

```
              1              2  3           4    5                         6
hCG       skeplrprcrpinatlavekegcpvcitvntticagycptmtrvlqgvlpalpqvvcny
hfsh             nsceltnitiavekegcgfcitinttwcagycytrdlvykdparpkiqktctf
cf94-117  skeplrprcrpinatlavekegcpvcitvntticagycptmtrvlqgvlpalpqvvcny
cfc94-114 skeplrprcrpinatlavekegcpvcitvntticagycptmtrvlqgvlpalpqvvcny

                      7              8 9 10        11             12
hCG       rdvrfesirlpgcprgvnpvvsyavalscqcalcrrsttdcggpkdhpltcddprfqds
hFSH      kelvyetvrvpgcahhadslytypvatqchcgkcdsdstdctvrglgpsycsfgemke
CF94-117  rdvrfesirlpgcprgvnpvvsyavalscqcalcDSDSTDCTVRGLGPSYCSFGEMKE
CFC94-114 rdvrfesirlpgcprgvnpvvsyavalscqcalcDSDSTDCTVRGLGPSYCSFGEfqds

hCG       ssskapppslpspsrlpgpsdtpilpq
hFSH
CF94-117
CFC94-114 ssskapppslpspsrlpgpsdtpilpq
```

Fig. 1. Primary amino acid sequences of hCG, CF94–117, CFC94–114, and hFSHβ subunits. The amino acids are written in the single letter amino acid code which is: A, alanine; C, cysteine; D, aspartic acid; E, glutamic acid; F, phenylalanine; G, glycine; H, histidine; I, isoleucine; K, lysine; L, leucine; M, methionine; N, asparagine; P, proline; Q, glutamine; R, arginine; S, serine; T, threonine; V, valine; W, tryptophan; Y, tyrosine. For emphasis, all residues are illustrated in lower case except those derived from the hFSHβ subunit that are substituted for their hCGβ subunit homologs. The numbers refer to the conserved cysteine residues.

and pLEN-hCGα, respectively. The pBMT2x vectors were transfected into C127 cells and pLEN vectors were transfected into CHO cells to create tissue culture cell lines that stably secreted heterodimers composed of human-α plus CF94–117β and human-α plus CFC94–114β. Henceforth, these will be termed CF94–117 and CFC94–114, respectively.

The proteins secreted into the culture medium were concentrated and analyzed by sandwich immunoassays similar to those that have been published [11] except that antibody A113 was used as a capture agent and radiolabeled antibody B105 was used as a detection agent. These assays measure the materials in the medium by virtue of their hCG structures. Because we have not prepared purified CF94–117 and CFC94–114 for use as standards, we also characterized their activities in FSH radioligand receptor assays against a highly purified FSH standard. This was a gift of Dr Scott Chappel (Ares Advanced Technology, Randolph, MA). These assays were performed by monitoring the abilities of CF94–117 and CFC94–114 to prevent binding of radioiodinated hFSH to CHO cells that expressed the human FSH receptor.

The in vivo activities of CF94–117 and CFC94–114 were measured using a modified Steelman-Pohley assay [12]. This assay depends on the ability of hFSH to induce ovarian weight gain in sexually immature rats. To perform the assay, we mixed 0, 0.1, 0.3, 1, or 3 µg hFSH with 50 IU of hCG and injected one-sixth of this mixture subcutaneously into 21-day-old rats twice per day for 3 days. The rats were sacrificed on the 4th day and their ovaries were weighed. Similar concentrations of CF94–117 or CFC94–114 were substituted for those of hFSH.

Results and Discussion

C127 and CHO cells transfected with genes encoding the human α subunit and genes encoding CF94–117 or CFC94–114 β subunits secreted these proteins into the medium. The α,β heterodimers were readily detected using the A113–B105 sandwich assay indicating that the α and β subunits combined as had been expected based on previous observations for CF94–117 expressed in COS-7 cells [4]. Both analogs gave parallel dose response curves with hFSH in the FSH radioreceptor assays (Fig. 2) suggesting that they bound to human FSH receptors like hFSH. Administration of these analogs to immature rats led to an increase in the weights of the rat ovaries (Fig. 3). In these assays CFC94–114 appeared to be approximately 3–4 times more active than hFSH or CF94–117 based on its FSH activity in vitro. CF94–117 appeared to be equally as active as hFSH.

These observations suggest that analogs of hCG having hFSHβ subunit residues substituted for hCGβ subunit residues 94–114 or 94–117 bind to FSH receptors like FSH. The hormone analogs are potent inducers of FSH activity in vivo. Although we have not tested the activities of these analogs in women, the observations that they bind to human FSH receptors in vitro and that they are active in rodents suggests that they are likely to be active in people. Thus, we anticipate that they would be useful

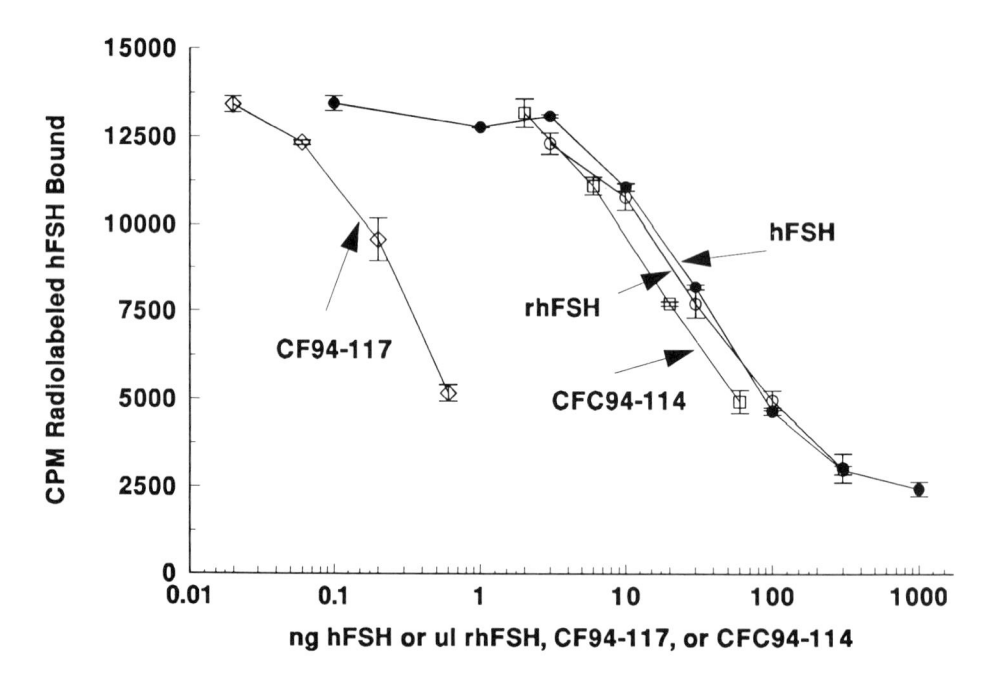

Fig. 2. Assay of the hFSH receptor binding potency of CF94–117 and CFC94–114. hFSH or medium containing CF94–117 or CFC94–114 were added to ^{125}I-hFSH prior to adding the mixture to CHO cells expressing human FSH receptors. After 1 h at 37°C, the cell suspensions were diluted with 2 ml of 0.9% NaCl solution containing 1 mg bovine serum albumin/ml. The mixtures were centrifuged at 2000 ×g, the supernatants aspirated, and the radioactivity in the pellet measured in a γ counter.

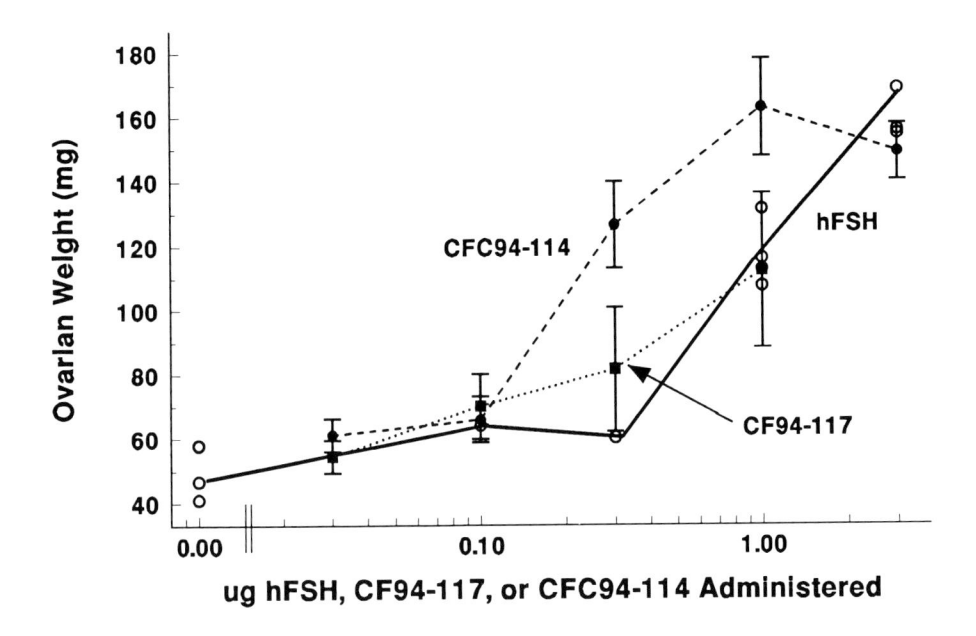

Fig. 3. Ovarian weight augmentation assay of CFC94−114 and CF94−117. Either hFSH, CFC94−114, or CF94−117 were mixed with hCG and administered to sexually immature rats as described in the text. Values illustrated represent four different dose response curves (hFSH) or the responses to CFC94−114 and CF94−117. Values extend to the limits of the SEM.

for inducing follicle development in women or for enhancing spermatogenesis in men.

The data of Figs. 2 and 3 suggest that CFC94−114 is more active than CF94−117. This is most likely explained by the presence of the additional residues of hCG found in CFC94−114. Addition of this region of the hCGβ subunit to the hFSHβ subunit has been shown to increase the biological activity of FSH [13].

Approximately 0.05 ng of either CF94−117 or CFC94−114 can readily be detected in the A113−B105 sandwich immunoassay. Since B105 does not bind to hFSH, hFSH does not interfere with measurements of either CF94−117 or CFC94−114 in this assay. Conversely, hFSH is readily detected in a sandwich immunoassay employing A113 and radioiodinated B602. Since B602 does not bind hCG, CF94−117 or CFC94−114, the presence of hFSH does not interfere with measurements of these compounds. Consequently, it should be feasible to measure plasma levels of hFSH and CF94−117 or CFC94−114 following stimulation of ovarian or testicular function with CF94−117 or CFC94− 114. This will permit monitoring of the feedback effects of ovarian and testicular secretions on hFSH secretion following stimulation of their FSH receptors.

We have monitored the immunological activities of CF94−117 and CF101−109 in mice. CF101−109 is an analog of hCG that contains only 114 amino acids and contains hFSHβ subunit residues 95−104 in place of hCGβ subunit residues 101−109

[5]. This analog binds to both LH and FSH receptors. As will be published in detail elsewhere, immunization of mice with either CF94–117 or CF101–109 in Freund's adjuvant led to the development of antibodies that would immunoprecipitate hCG and hFSH. This was expected since the structures of hCG and mouse LH are very different. Thus, these analogs would be foreign proteins to the mouse. To determine whether these antibodies recognized a conformation of the protein that was not found in hCG, we attempted to prevent the immunoprecipitation of radioiodinated hFSH with hCG or the human α subunit. In all but one animal, we observed that we were able to completely prevent the immunoprecipitation of hFSH using hCG or α subunit. This suggested that the regions of the molecules that are unique to FSH are not antigenic and that the antigenicity of the chimeras was due primarily to their content of hCG residues. Since hCG is not antigenic in humans, we anticipate that these analogs will not be antigenic in either men or women.

Acknowledgements

We thank Dr Robert Canfield (Columbia University, New York, NY) for the highly purified hCG and B105. We thank Drs Robert Wolfert and Glenn Armstrong (Hybritech Inc., San Diego, CA) for antibodies A113 and B602. We thank Dr George Pavlakis for the pBM2x vector used to express CF94–117. We thank Dr Peter Kushner, for pLEN used to express CFC94–114. We thank Dr Scott Chappel for the highly purified recombinant hFSH used as a standard in these studies. And we thank the NICHD for financial support. These studies were supported by NIH grants HD24650 and HD15454.

References

1. Moyle WR, Campbell RK. In: DeGroot LJ, Endocrinology, 3rd edn, Philadelphia: Saunders, 1994 (in press).
2. Moyle WR. 1980. In: Finn CA (ed) Oxford Reviews of Reproductive Biology, vol 2, New York: Oxford University Press, 1980;123–204.
3. Pierce JG, Parsons TF. Annu Rev Biochem 1981;50:465–495.
4. Campbell RK, Dean Emig DM, Moyle WR. Proc Natl Acad Sci USA 1991;88:760–764.
5. Moyle W R, Campbell RK, Myers RV, Bernard MP, Han Y, Wang X. Nature 1994 (in press).
6. Yen SSC, Llerena LA, Pearson OH, Littell AS. J Clin Endocrinol Metab 1970;30:325–329.
7. Urban RJ, Padmanabhan V, Beitins I, Veldhuis JD. J Clin Endocrinol Metab 1991;73:818–823.
8. Damewood MD, Shen W, Zacur HA, Schlaff WD, Rock JA, Wallach EE. Fertil Steril 1989;52:398–400.
9. Pavlakis GN, Felber BK, Wright CM, Papamatheakis J, Tse T. In: Miller JH, Calos MP (eds) Gene Transfer Vectors for Mammalian Cells. Cold Spring Harbor: Cold Spring Harbor Press, 1987;29–38.
10. Fiddes JC, Goodman HM. Nature 1979;281:351–356.
11. Moyle WR, Ehrlich PH, Canfield RE. Proc Natl Acad Sci USA 1982;79:2245–2249.
12. Steelman SL, Pohley FM. Endocrinology 1953;53:604–616.
13. Fares FA, Suganuma N, Nishimori K, LaPolt PS, Hsueh AJ, Boime I. Proc Natl Acad Sci USA 1992; 89:4304–4308.

Recombinant gonadotropins: clinical aspects

Pharmacokinetics of natural/recombinant FSH (follitropin) and some analogs

M.R. Sairam* and K. Sebok

Reproduction Research Laboratory, Clinical Research Institute of Montreal, Montreal, Québec, Canada

Abstract. Follicle-stimulating hormone (FSH), follitropin, is a critical factor in determining folliculogenesis and forms an important part of many treatments of infertility in women (and men). It is also important in many veterinary applications. Numerous studies have paved the way for commercial production of genetically engineered hormone and the era of recombinant FSH therapy has arrived. Recombinant FSH is free of luteinizing hormone (LH) contamination and any residual activity seen should be regarded as intrinsic to the molecule. The new preparations display pharmacokinetic properties closely resembling clinical grade urinary FSH. Limited phase 1 studies have shown the product to be safe, but potential long-term complications such as antibody formation, if any, remain to be evaluated. Thus, the future of gonadotropin therapy in assisted reproductive technology will likely be with the production of large and uniform batches of recombinant hFSH having high biochemical purity and biological activity.

Introduction

Pituitary follicle-stimulating hormone (FSH), follitropin, plays a critical role in male and female reproductive function by regulating the growth, differentiation, maturation and secretory activities of Sertoli cells in the testis and granulosa cells in the ovary. The hormone exerts its effects by first binding to specific receptors located on the cell membrane and subsequent activation of second messenger systems like cyclic AMP. In the male the hormones' action leads to a functional seminiferous epithelium and maintenance of spermatogenesis, whereas in the female it becomes responsible for follicular maturation and development of the ovum.

FSH belongs to the glycoprotein hormone family which consists of the two pituitary gonadotropins (FSH and luteinizing hormone, LH), the placental chorionic gonadotropins (CG) and pituitary thyroid-stimulating hormone (TSH, Thyrotropin). All these hormones are composed of two nonidentical subunits which are assembled by noncovalent forces into a unique three-dimensional structure, each capable of interacting with their own receptors in the target cells. Remarkably, the α subunits are identical with a unique β subunit, in each case contributing to the overall specificity required for selective interaction with a receptor and activation of the cell [1–3]. Oligosaccharides which are present in both subunits, or added co/post-

---

Address for correspondence: Dr. M.R. Sairam, Reproduction Research Laboratory, Clinical Research Institute of Montreal, 110 Pine Ave. W., Montreal, Québec, Canada H2W 1R7.

translationally, are required for full hormonal function [4,5]. Numerous studies have reported (see [5]) that the biological activity of gonadotropins may vary with the endocrine status of the individual and it is therefore important to understand the final form of the hormone that interacts with the gonadal cells.

Gonadotropins, being complex glycoprotein hormones with high carbohydrate content, remain in blood circulation longer than most simple peptide and protein hormones. As substantial amounts of these hormones are also excreted in the urine, this has been an important source for the preparation of clinically useful formulations.

The first pregnancy after treatment of an infertile patient with partially purified human pituitary FSH was reported in 1960. Since then, ovarian stimulation and testicular development in deficient patients has been achieved by the use of crude or partially purified menopausal urinary preparations. FSH extracted from the urine and hCG from pregnant women have become standard therapies in infertility clinics around the world. However, with the emergence of biotechnological methods of producing gonadotropins, the picture might change quite rapidly in the field of assisted reproductive technology. It thus becomes necessary to evaluate the pharmacokinetics of new recombinant FSH in particular and compare it with existing materials. In this article we review the structural basis of the metabolic behavior of natural FSH, and genetically engineered hormones that are expressed in mammalian cells and in recombinant analogs created in the laboratory, starting from natural hormones.

Methods and Results

Preparations

Human or animal pituitary FSH have been isolated to different degrees of purity by many investigators and some of their pharmacokinetic properties have been evaluated. There are no recent reports using pure human pituitary FSH preparations. Partially purified urinary FSH preparations (pergonal) or highly purified ones like Metrodin are made by suppliers such as Serono labs, USA. Recombinant human FSH has been prepared by two research laboratories [6,7] and two commercial suppliers. A product under the name Gonal F has been developed by Serono, and Organon, the Netherlands, labels its product Org32489. The purified FSH investigated in our laboratory is of ovine origin and two of its analogs consist of removal of terminal sialic acid by enzymatic treatment and a recombinant hormone in which the natural α subunit has been selectively depleted of sugars before reassociation with the natural β subunit [8]. This should not be confused with genetically engineered FSH. One group has engineered hFSH with an extended β subunit with the intention of prolonging the circulatory half-life of the hormone [9].

Evaluations

Ideally, for calculation of the pharmacokinetic parameters of the hormone, an intravenous application is desirable and this has been recently done with Metrodin HP in women [10]. In this approach following administration, the early phase, called the distribution phase, represents the distribution of the hormone to the well-perfused organs, including the liver and the kidney. This phase primarily determines the rapid decline in plasma concentrations of the hormone, reflecting movement of the hormone within rather than elimination from the body. With time, the distribution equilibrium is established with more tissues and the changes in plasma concentrations eventually reflect a proportional change in the amount of the hormone in the body. This proportionality phase is linear and reflects elimination of the hormone from the body.

In clinical practice, most administrations are done by the parenteral route and in such cases pharmacokinetics are influenced by considerations such as dose, site of administration, body weight, etc. Earlier pharmacokinetic studies where a single type of radioimmunoassay was feasible did not always reflect intact undissociated and biologically active hormone in circulation. However, more recent work, including those on rhFSH preparations, employ more refined, sensitive and carefully validated immunoradiometric assays (IRMAs) using two types of antibodies and an in vitro bioassay. For the latter, either the Sertoli cells or granulosa cells are utilised with estradiol production where the sample is an index of FSH activity [11]. The pharmacodynamic properties of the hormone reflect subsequent short/long-term actions such as increase in size and number of follicles, estradiol levels in serum or a rise in proteins such as inhibin.

Pharmacokinetic parameters are derived by analyzing serum hormone levels by software programs developed for microcomputers. Most such programs use least squares minimization parameters, assuming that serum hormone levels follow the sum of two or more exponentials.

Owing to differing degrees of N-glycosylation, all hFSH preparations including recombinant hormones are very heterogeneous. As many as 15—20 molecular species may be present in human pituitary [12,13] or purified Metrodin preparations [14] and several of these species differ greatly in biological activity [12], despite being highly purified. The proportion of the different components from the two sources as revealed by chromato-focussing is not identical and consequently the type of the hormone reaching the ovary during treatment will never be the same as in a normal cycle.

The pharmacokinetic parameters determined for pituitary FSH and urinary FSH are compared in Table 1 from a study performed in rats. The excreted FSH isoforms are more acidic than those released from the pituitary and survive the longest in circulation. It is pertinent to note in this context that the relative abundance of different FSH isoforms of circulating FSH changes according to the stage of the menstrual cycle, especially at midcycle during which isoforms around pI 4.8 increase [15]. The pituitary of elderly women contains and secretes more acidic isoforms in comparison to glands of fertile women [16,17] and consequently postmenopausal FSH tends to be more acidic in nature. Thus, although FSH preparations like Metrodin or recombinant FSH are bioactive, one cannot be certain that the stimulating signal that interacts with the ovary in the treatment cycle is the same as in the natural state.

Table 1. Apparent isoelectric points and pharmacokinetic parameters of h pituitary FSH and urinary FSH as determined in rats

pI range	PCR (ml/min)	MRT (min)	$t_{1/2}$ (min)
7.6–7.1 (P)	0.102	221.6	147.2
5.9–5.3 (P)	0.789	44.8	35.4
5.5–5.1 (U)	0.589	28.4	56.6
5.0–4.7 (P)	0.349	63.9	43.8
5.0–4.6 (U)	0.321	84.6	58.4
4.5–4.1 (P)	0.23	112.0	76.2
4.5–4.3 (U)	0.374	113.5	77.1
3.9–3.8 (P)	0.349	95.9	66.4
4.1 (U)	0.254	102.4	69.1
Salt peak (P)	0.104	150.9	101.2
Salt peak (U)	0.115	184.6	123.5

Data compiled from [13] and [14]. P = pituitary; U = urinary. Note that the pI segregation is not identical. PCR = plasma clearance rate; MRT = mean residence time; $t_{1/2}$ = half-life.

Pharmacokinetics of urinary FSH in women and men

The pharmacokinetics of Metrodin and Metrodin HP have been studied in healthy female and male volunteers without or with suppression of endogenous FSH by suitable drug treatment. In one study [10], female volunteers were administered FSH by the i.v. route and males were treated with a single i.m. or s.c. dose of the hormone. In women the pharmacokinetic parameters determined by immunoassays and in vitro bioassays appeared to be somewhat different. However, the authors caution about the higher variability of the bioassay (Table 2). In general, the true terminal half-life was about 1 day and approximately 25% of the administered hormone was excreted in the urine. Whether this was bioactive or not is not known. There is fairly good agreement between two independent studies [10,18] evaluating Metrodin in men (Table 3). The terminal half-life of the hormone was ~1.5 days, with one study [18] reporting higher C_{max} and AUC when 450 IU hormone was injected. There is a discrepancy, however, in the degree of testicular stimulation observed following the injection of the hormone. Le Cotonnec et al. [10] report a rise in plasma inhibin after 24 h, which apparently was sustained up to 72 h with both Metrodin and Metrodin HP (150 IU) in men. Another group has concluded that a slight increase seen 36 h postinjection was not statistically significant from baseline

Table 2. Kinetics parameters of urinary FSH (Metrodin HP) following i.v. administration in women

	AUC (IU/l/h)	C_{max} (IU/l/h)	MRT (h)	$t_{1/2}$ (h)
Immunoassay	316 ± 48	25 ± 6	22 ± 6	18 ± 6
Bioassay	2,100 ± 700	86 ± 17	43 ± 18	36 ± 15

Data from [10]. Women received a single dose of 150 IU FSH-HP with serum values determined by IRMA. Similar results have been reported with standard (Metrodin) FSH.

Table 3. Pharmacokinetic parameters of two clinically-used human urinary preparations in men

	AUC (IU/l/h)	C_{max} (IU/l/h)	T_{max} (h)	$t_{1/2}$ (h)
uFSH (i.m.)	339 ± 125	4.7 ± 1.8	10	36 ± 8
uFSH-HP (i.m.)[a]	245 ± 84	3.8 ± 1.7	13	39 ± 15
uFSH-HP (s.c.)[a]	283 ± 96	3.3 ± 1.7	18	45 ± 21
uFSH (i.m.) 150 IU[b]	162	3.8	9.7	24.6
uFSH (i.m.) 450 IU[b]	605	10.4	9.8	36.2

Adapted from [a][10](150 IU) and [b][18] (150 IU and 450 IU). AUC = Area under the curve; C_{max} = peak of FSH concentration; T_{max} = time of C_{max}; and $t_{1/2}$ = half-life.

values before treatment [18]. This would suggest that injections of 150 IU FSH, the dose currently employed for treatment in males for hypogonadotropic hypogonadism, may be inadequate as the serum FSH levels can be maintained in the normal range only for less than 13 h. These studies have important implications for the treatment of male infertility, because sustained availability of bioactive FSH may be critical for restoration of spermatogenesis.

Pharmacokinetics and pharmacodynamics of recombinant hFSH in men and women
The results of a multicenter study evaluating the safety and pharmacokinetic and pharmacodynamic properties of Organon's rhFSH have been published [19] (Table 4). The prospective study was done in 15 gonadotropin-deficient men and women who were given a single bolus therapeutic dose (300 IU) of rhFSH (Organon 32489) by i.m. injection. Blood samples were taken hourly for the first 12 h and thereafter regularly up to 11 days. Levels of serum FSH, LH, inhibin, estradiol (female) and testosterone (male) were measured.

This single injection was well-tolerated with no incidents of drug-related adverse effects. Comparison of pre- and posttreatment values of the blood chemistry revealed no changes of clinical relevance. Serum FSH levels rose 30 min after injection and returned to baseline values by about 264 h. Half-life of rhFSH was comparable with that seen for urinary FSH (Table 3). Elimination half-lives were also comparable, being 44 ± 14 h in men and 32 ± 12 h in women. Interestingly, peak FSH values were significantly lower in women than men (4.3 vs. 7.4 IU/l) and the time required to attain peak hormone concentration, C_{max}, was much longer in women (27 h vs. 14

Table 4. Mean pharmacokinetic parameters of Organon rhFSH in women and men

	AUC (IU/l/h)	C_{max} (IU/l/h)	T_{max} (h)	$t_{1/2}$ (h)
Women (n = 8)	339 ± 105	4.3 ± 1.7	27 ± 5[b]	44 ± 14
Men (n = 6)	452 ± 183	7.4 ± 28[a]	14 ± 8	32 ± 12

Adapted from [19]. Subjects received 300 IU rhFSH in a single i.m. injection in the gluteal area. Immunoassay of serum FSH was used to calculate parameters. AUC = area under the curve; C_{max} = peak FSH concentration; T_{max} = time at which it occurred; and $t_{1/2}$ = elimination half-time.
[a]Significantly higher in men; [b]significantly later in women.

h). In both sexes there appeared to be a negative correlation between body weight and hormone levels attained in serum. Serum inhibin levels rose in some men but not women, 3 days after hormone injection. It was concluded that rhFSH is a safe drug with pharmacokinetic properties comparable with those previously reported for natural urinary FSH. Larger and more detailed studies will further clarify the safety of rhFSH.

The same group of investigators has extended this study in two gonadotropin-deficient women and evaluated the induction of follicular growth [20]. In this phase in one multiple-increasing dose study, rhFSH was administered i.m. once per day for 3 weeks, at 75 IU/day in the first week, 150 IU/day in the 2nd week, followed by 225 IU/day during the final 3rd week. An i.m. injection resulted in dose-related increases in serum FSH. Both subjects showed follicular growth (17 mm diameter). Steady-state serum levels of FSH were reached in 3—5 days, and the pharmacokinetics were linear in the dose ranges tested. The FSH treatment induced normal follicular development without causing high elevation in estradiol levels. Hence complete steroidogenesis requires the synergistic action of the LH (CG as administered in the clinical setting).

In neither studies were anti-rhFSH antibodies detectable, suggesting that at least under these conditions the preparation was not immunogenic. However, further testing on a larger scale, especially in men who may require long-term treatment for induction of spermatogenesis, will be required before drawing final conclusions.

Successful in vitro fertilization and embryo transfer [21] including the first established pregnancy and birth of a baby girl [22] following treatment with rhFSH has been reported recently. Other positive cases have been noted but not yet published.

Plasma survival of recombinant FSH analogs
It has long been known that the total content as well as the nature of the carbohydrate residues on glycoproteins markedly affect their metabolic fate in circulation and consequently their biological activity. In this context we will consider two sets of studies involving preparation of FSH analogs with opposite effects on their pharmacokinetics.

In an experimental investigation we have compared the pharmacokinetics of the plasma disappearance of purified ovine FSH and three of its analogs [8]. Besides the natural hormone, oFSH, which is structurally and functionally similar to hFSH, we employed asial-oFSH, deglycosylated (DG-)oFSH, and DG-$\alpha+\beta$ recombinant hormones. These three analogs differ from oFSH in the following ways. In asial-oFSH terminal sialic acids have been removed; in DG-oFSH nearly 75% of the sugars have been depleted by selective chemical treatment; and in DG-$\alpha+\beta$ the recombinant sugars in the α subunit only are affected. A comparison of the time course of hormone disappearance following a single intracardiac bolus of 2.5 µg hormone or analog is shown in Fig. 1. In each sample there was a rapid initial decline phase followed by a slower linear terminal phase. This biexponential decline in plasma hormone levels is consistent with the pharmacokinetic two-compartment open model.

FSH DISAPPEARANCE

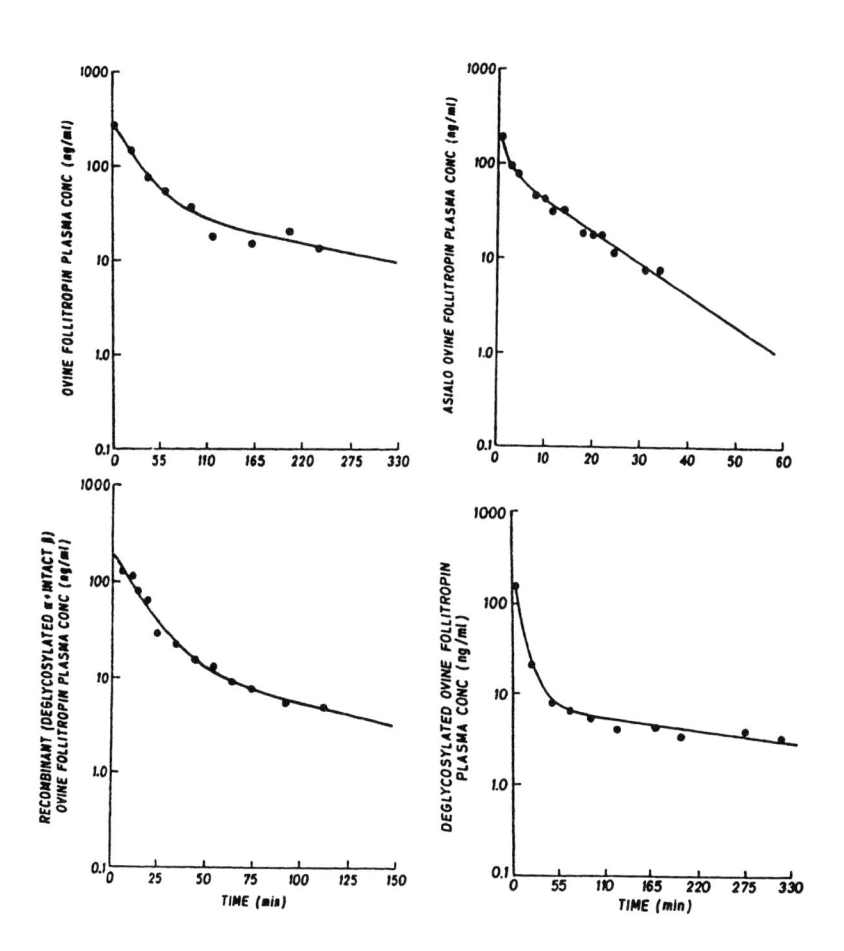

Fig. 1. Diminution in plasma concentrations (ng/ml) of oFSH and its analogs.

Table 5. Parameters of the two-component exponential plasma disappearance curves of oFSH and analogs after a single bolus injection

	$t_{1/2}$ (min)		MCR (ml/min/kg)	Volume of distribution[a] (ml/kg)
	Distribution	Elimination		
oFSH	23	565	0.56	31.1
asial-oFSH	3.4 ± 1.4[b]	32 ± 15[b]	8.1 ± 0.5	45.7
DG-α+β	7.7 ± 0.5[b]	67 ± 8[b]	2.4 ± 0.5	52.3
DG-oFSH	5.2[b]	251	4.0	36.9

[a] Calculated from the extrapolated "zero time" plasma concentrations.
[b] Denotes significant difference compared to oFSH control ($p < 0.05$).

The mean parameters are summarized in Table 5. Overall, the native hormone disappears the slowest from the blood as reflected by its $t_{1/2}$ for distribution and elimination as well as its MCR value. Asial-oFSH, DG-α+β and DG-oFSH exhibited shorter $t_{1/2}$ for distribution. The highest MCR value was observed for asial-oFSH, DG-oFSH, DG-α+β and finally, oFSH. The high clearance rate of asial-oFSH and DG-α+β is reflected in their rapid elimination phase. DG-oFSH on the contrary, like oFSH, has a much longer $t_{1/2}$ for elimination. Based on these data it is reasonable to argue that sialic acid residues are not the only sugars regulating clearance of FSH in vivo. Removal of a large part of oligosaccharides or sialic acid accelerates distribution of hormonal analogs and alters their metabolism and/or excretion.

An important issue that dictates the success of clinical application of rhFSH is the potential short half-life in vivo, even though it is about 1.5 days, requiring frequent administration as shown in examples of recent work [20,22]. In the hope that the availability of long-acting FSH agonists may help better clinical protocols and contribute to the increased efficiency of ART procedures, Fares et al. [9] have come up with clever designs by gene manipulation. In these studies the gene of the FSH β subunit was reconstructed to add at the c-terminal one or two copies of the carboxyterminal peptide of the placental hormonal hCG-β subunit. When such a modified FSH β gene is coexpressed with the α gene in CHO cells, a new analog of FSH containing one or two additional sequences at the c-terminal portions is created. This region, which undergoes extensive glycosylation in nature, has now been shown to contribute additional glycosylation (up to eight sites) and enhance survival in circulation. In animal studies the results have been very encouraging. Thus, an FSH analog bearing (CTP) 2 extensions in the β subunit had about 10-fold greater half-life in rats [9]. The ovulatory potential of these agonists in rats was also enhanced [23]. Furthermore, it has been indicated that prolonged action of these agonistic forms may not cause significant desensitization or impairment of ovarian responses. However, the finding that daily injections of FSH CTP1 agonist are more effective than a single large dose of the new hormone suggests a note of caution requiring further investigation. Studies in patients with these and other analogs will be forthcoming and these will be very useful in developing new therapeutic regimens. It must be noted that hCG which contains the extended carboxylterminus functions in a state where immune suppressive functions are operating. As these conditions are not likely to be encountered in treatment of infertile patients (especially men), careful immunological analysis following repeated injections of analogs such as (FSH)-CTP$_2$ become very important in establishing safety.

Conclusions and Comments

After more than a quarter century of the use of urinary FSH preparations in their various forms for clinical application, the era of recombinant genetically engineered hormones for treatment of infertility has finally arrived. It is gratifying to observe that the basic studies on hormone purification, structure, action and gene cloning have finally paved the way for production on a large scale. The product has been successfully used in volunteers and patients and the birth of a baby girl has been recorded in a recent publication. The pharmacokinetic parameters of the new preparations are similar to those currently on the market. However, glycoproteins produced in CHO cells are still heterogeneous and somewhat different in their periphery when compared to natural hormone. An area of particular concern is that there may be large batch-to-batch variations in production, as has been recently noted in the case of rhTSH [24]. Whether these differences, if found for FSH, present any long-term complications such as induction of resistance by formation of antibodies remains an open issue. However, long-term studies with recombinant erythropoietin in humans has not resulted in antibodies following chronic use over 18 months [25], and represent an encouraging sign. There will undoubtedly be a host of novel investigations, both basic and clinical, striving to produce new and more effective formulations. The pharmaceutical industry might be able to exploit differences in sugar composition to produce new analogs of value.

Acknowledgements

Our research has been supported by MRC of Canada. We thank Ashwin Sairam and Isabelle Blain for help in manuscript preparation.

References

1. Pierce JG, Parsons TF. Ann Rev Biochem 1981;50:465–495.
2. Sairam MR. In: Li CH (eds) Hormonal proteins and peptides, vol 11. New York: Academic Press, 1983;1–79.
3. Hartree AS, Renwick AGC. Biochem J 1992;287:664–679.
4. Sairam MR. FASEB J 1989;3:1915–1926.
5. Wilson CA, Leigh AJ, Chapman J. Endocrinology 1990;125:3–14.
6. Keene JF, Matzuk MM, Otani T, Fauser BCJM, Galway AB, Hsueh AJW, Boime I. J Biol Chem 1989;264:4769–4775.
7. Cerpa-Poljak A, Bishop LA, Hort YJ, Chin CKH, Dekroon R, Mahler SM, Smith GM, Stuart MC, Schofield PR. Endocrinology 1993;132:351–356.
8. Sebok K, Meloche S, Sairam MR. Life Sci 1990;46:927–934.
9. Fares FA, Suganuma N, Nishimori K, Lapolt PS, Hsueh AJW, Boime I. Proc Natl Acad Sci 1992;89:4304–4308.
10. le Cotonnec JY, Porchet HC, Beltrami V, Howles C. Hum Reprod 1993;8:1604–1611.
11. Wang C. Endocrine Rev 1988;9:374–377.
12. Stanton PG, Robertson DM, Burgon PG, Schmauk-White B, Hearn MTW. Endocrinology 1992;130:2820–2832.
13. Ulloa-Aguirre A, Cravioto A, Damain-Matsumura P, Jiménez M, Zambrano E, Diaz-Sánchez V. Hum Reprod 1992;7:23–30.
14. Ulloa-Aguirre A, Damian-Matsumura P, Jiménez M, Zambrano E, Diaz-Sánchez V. Hum Reprod 1992;7:1371–1378.
15. Padmanabhan V, Lang LL, Sonstein J, Kelch RP, Beitins IZ. J Clin Endocrinol 1988;61:465–473.
16. Wide L. J Clin Endocrinol Metab 1982;55:652–688.

17. Wide L. Acta Endocrinol 1989;123:519−529.
18. Jockenhövel F, Fingscheidt U, Khan SA, Behre HM, Nieschlag E. Clin Endocrinol 1990;33:573−584.
19. Mannaerts B, Shoham Z, Schoot D, Bouchard P, Harlin J, Fauser B, Jacobs H, Rombout F, Bennick HC. Fertil Steril 1993;59:108−114.
20. Shoham Z, Mannaerts B, Insler V, Bennink HC. Fertil Steril 1993;59:738−742.
21. Germond M, Dessole S, Senn A, Loumaye E, Howles C, Beltrami V. Lancet 1992;339:1170.
22. Devroey P, Mannaerts B, Smitz J, Bennink HC, Van Steirteghem A. Hum Reprod 1993;8:863−865.
23. Lapolt PS, Nishimori K, Fares FA, Perlas E, Boime I, Hsueh AJW. Endocrinology 1992;131:2514−2520.
24. Szkudlinski MW, Thotakura NR, Bucci I, Joshi LR, Tsai A, Palmer JE, Shidoach J, Weintraub BD. Endocrinology 1993;133:1490−1503.
25. Canaud B, Polito-Bouloux C, Garred LJ, Rivory JP, Donadieu P, Taib J, Florence P, Mion C. Am J Kidney Dis 1990;15:169−175.

Biological action of recombinant human FSH (Puregon®) during induction of multiple follicular growth

B. Mannaerts[1]*, R. de Leeuw[1] and P. Devroey[2]

[1]*Scientific Development Group, Organon International BV, Oss, The Netherlands;* and [2]*Centre for Reproductive Medicine, Dutch-speaking Brussels Free University, Brussels, Belgium*

Abstract. Recombinant human FSH (recFSH, Puregon®) was applied for the induction of multiple follicular growth in preclinical and clinical experimental models in which endogenous FSH and LH were absent, relatively low, or relatively high. In hypophysectomised rats recFSH induced follicular growth up to preovulatory sizes and prevented small antral follicles from atresia. Supplementation with small amounts of hCG only increased the percentage of healthy follicles. Patients treated with buserelin in a short protocol required less recFSH for superovulation than patients treated with triptorelin in a long protocol. Accordingly, in the latter group rises of oestradiol and inhibin were noted at least 4 treatment-days later. No clear correlation between endogenous LH levels and the number of ampoules required was evident and the initial gonadotrophin flare-up in the short protocol is thought to contribute mostly to the favourable outcome of this regimen.

Introduction

The biological action of FSH is determined by its structure and is influenced by other endocrine factors (Fig. 1). Three main properties that are determined by hormone molecule structure are receptor affinity, intrinsic bioactivity and bioavailability. For therapeutic preparations the latter depends on absorption and excretion processes, which are responsible for the amount and duration that FSH remains available to the target organ. After interaction with the target cell receptor, other endocrine and paracrine factors are known to modulate FSH-induced responses. Such factors, acting directly or indirectly, include LH, GnRH, insulin, GH, IGFs, inhibin and activin [1–4].

So far, the biological activity of FSH has been studied in animals and man by means of natural FSH preparations of urinary or pituitary origin. Possible contamination of these preparations with other hormones like LH complicates the interpretation of these experiments and is probably the cause of contradictory study results. In contrast, recombinant human FSH (Puregon®, Org 32489, Organon International) is guaranteed free from intrinsic LH activity [5] and is therefore an excellent research tool that enables one to distinguish the effects of FSH and LH on the ovary.

Address for correspondence: Bernadette Mannaerts, Medical R&D Unit, Organon International BV, PO Box 20, 5340 BH Oss, The Netherlands. Tel.: +31-4120-61828. Fax: +31-4120-62617/62555.

```
        ┌─────────────────────┐
        │  biological action  │
        └─────────────────────┘
                 ↑      ┌──────────────┐
                 │ ←─── │  endocrine   │
                 │ +/-  │  environment │
                 │      └──────────────┘
        ┌─────────────────────┐
        │  receptor affinity  │
        │  signal transduction│
        │  bioavailability    │
        └─────────────────────┘
                 ↑
                 │
        ┌─────────────────────┐
        │      structure      │
        └─────────────────────┘
```

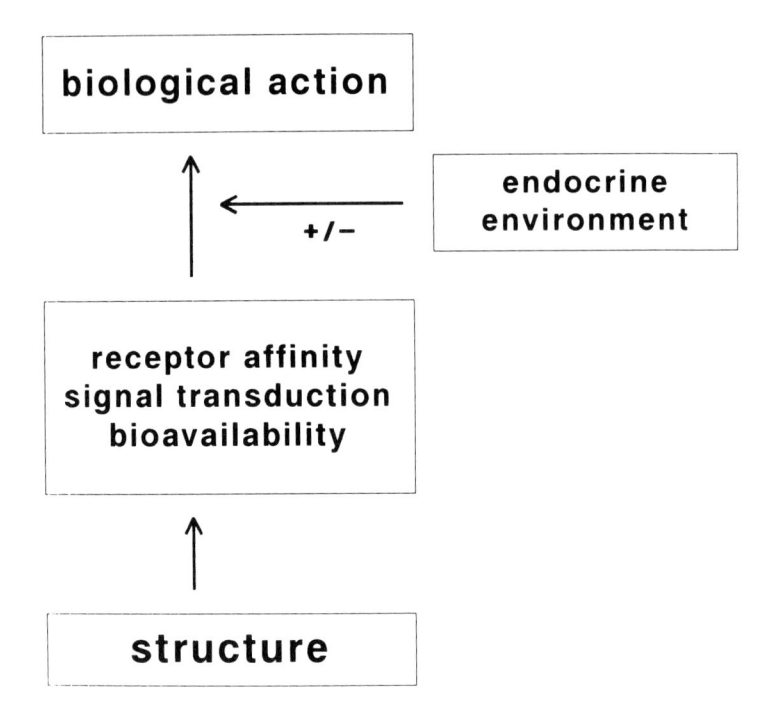

Fig. 1. Schematic presentation of factors determining biological FSH action.

Previous comparative studies have focussed on the biological profiling of Puregon®, and include its chromatofocussing profile, receptor affinity, intrinsic bioactivity and pharmacokinetic properties [5–10]. The current proceedings summarise some main findings using Puregon® as a research tool in experimental models in which endogenous FSH and LH is i) absent, ii) relatively low, or iii) relatively high. The data were obtained by using Puregon® for induction of multiple follicular growth in immature hypophysectomised (hypox) rats, in patients concomitantly treated with triptorelin (depot) in a long protocol, and in patients treated with buserelin in a short protocol, respectively.

Multiple follicular growth in hypox rats

Previous comparative experiments in hypox rats were designed to re-examine the two-cell two-gonadotrophin theory [5]. These studies showed that recFSH is able to induce follicular growth up to the preovulatory stage without increasing plasma oestradiol levels. Supplementation of recFSH with small amounts of hCG augmented ovarian weight responses, ovarian aromatase and largely increased circulating oestradiol.

In subsequent experiments [11], the role of FSH and LH in follicular growth and atresia and simultaneous uterine development was investigated by treating immature hypox rats with either increasing doses of 0 to 40 IU recFSH or with one submaximal dose of 8 IU recFSH supplemented with increasing doses of 0 to 5 IU hCG. Animals were treated for 4 days by twice daily s.c. injections. The total number of antral follicles (diameter >275 μm) and the incidence of atresia in these follicles were evaluated as described by Meijs-Roelofs and colleagues [12] and Osman [13].

In the complete absence of LH activity, recFSH caused dose-dependent increases of ovarian weight and uterine weight, whereas serum oestradiol remained unchanged at the baseline (see Fig. 2). Minimal doses of recFSH required to cause a significant increase ($p < 0.05$) of ovarian and uterine weight were 2.5 and 10 IU, respectively. So far, reports on uterine weight after recFSH treatment are contradictory. After 2 days of recFSH treatment (total dose 72 IU/hypox rat), Whitelaw and co-workers [14] found that uterine weights were not different from controls. However, in our study

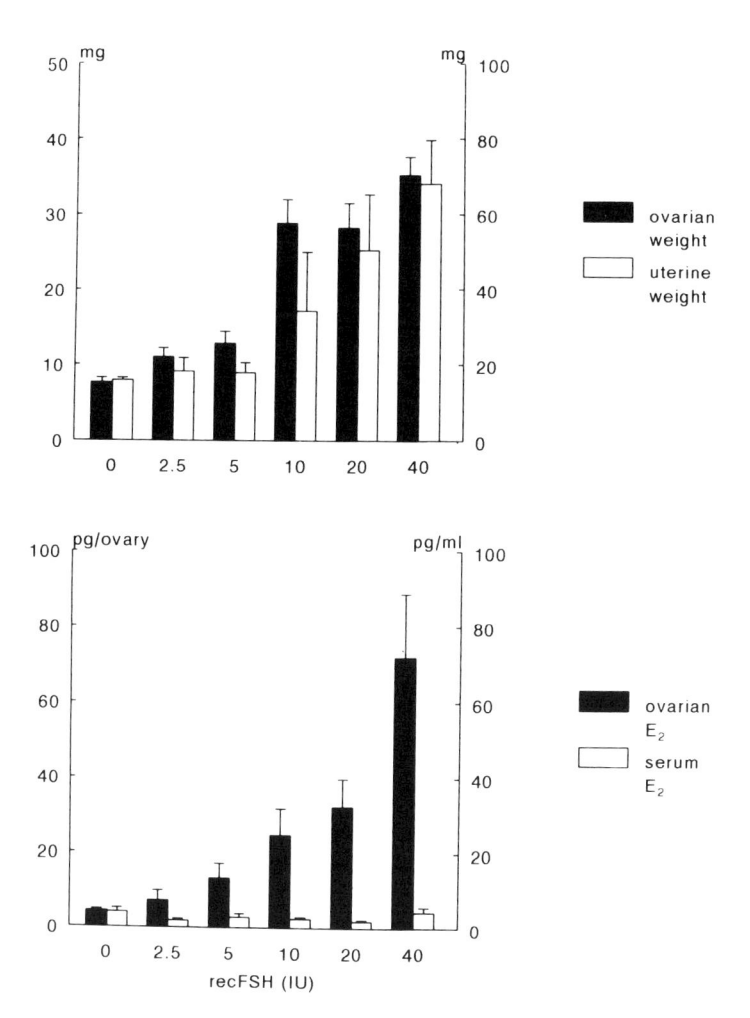

Fig. 2. Ovarian and uterine weight (A) and intraovarian and serum oestradiol concentrations (B) of immature hypox rats after treatment for 4 days with increasing doses of recFSH (Puregon®).

treatment for 4 days with at least 10 IU recFSH per animal significantly increased uterine weight and caused endometrial proliferative growth. Increases of uterine weight were also reported in adult hypox mice following recFSH treatment [15]. Retrospective measurements of intraovarian and intrauterine oestradiol revealed in both organs small, recFSH dose-related increases [16]. The ovarian oestradiol levels are included in Fig. 2B. Together, these data indicate that the rat uterus is highly sensitive to oestrogens which might bypass the central circulation and/or bind to a uterine protein. Like ovarian weight responses, the number of antral follicles increased in a recFSH dose-dependent manner (Table 1). A gradual shift of small antral follicles to large preovulatory follicles was noted. The latter ovulated after a single bolus injection of 10 IU hCG. In comparison to hypox vehicle-treated animals, the incidence of atresia diminished, especially in the smallest size class of antral follicles. However, after treatment with 40 IU recFSH, 26% of all antral follicles exhibited loosely arranged granulosa cells around the oocyte and antral layer, a phenomenon that could be interpreted as an early phase of atresia [17].

When a submaximal dose of 8 IU recFSH was supplemented with hCG, ovarian weight was augmented in a hCG dose-dependent fashion, but no further increases of total number of antral follicles were noted, with the exception of the highest hCG dose (5 IU) given (Table 1). However, addition of relatively low doses of hCG caused considerable shifts of small follicles to large, preovulatory follicles. Furthermore, supplementation with hCG reduced the incidence of atresia in antral follicles of all size classes, especially after administration of low dosages hCG (0.2 and 0.5 IU). Higher doses of hCG (2 and 5 IU) caused granulosa cell dispersion in a comparable amount and fashion as treatment with 40 IU recFSH only. To conclude, these data suggest that small amounts of LH activity support the growth of small antral follicles to healthy preovulatory follicles, but that too high doses of LH (or FSH) activity are detrimental for normal follicular development.

Table 1. Total number and quality of antral follicles ($\varnothing$ > 275 µm) per ovary of immature, hypox rats treated twice daily for 4 days

RecFSH (IU)	hCG (IU)	N	Antral follicles	Atresia (%)	Dispersion (%)
0	–	6	11 ± 4	69 ± 15	–
2.5	–	5	36 ± 4	45 ± 8	–
5	–	4	52 ± 12	44 ± 9	–
10	–	5	99 ± 6	44 ± 3	–
20	–	4	85 ± 14	31 ± 9	–
40	–	6	80 ± 7	6 ± 3	26 ± 3
8	0	4	65 ± 8	58 ± 2	–
8	0.2	3	89 ± 15	20 ± 8	–
8	0.5	3	54 ± 14	2 ± 1	–
8	2	3	67 ± 12	6 ± 3	25 ± 11
8	5	5	105 ± 11	6 ± 2	29 ± 8
0	5	3	–	–	–

Controlled superovulation in pituitary-suppressed patients

Hormonal profiles in relation to clinical outcome were studied in patients undergoing IVF/ET and participating in a pilot efficacy study on recFSH combined with various GnRH agonist regimens [18]. With respect to the amount of endogenous LH, large differences were noted between patients (n = 9) treated with recFSH in conjunction with buserelin intranasal spray (4 × 150 µg/day, Suprecur®, Hoechst) and those (n = 11) treated with recFSH in conjunction with i.m. administered triptorelin (3.75 mg, Decapeptyl® CR, Ferring). Therefore, these two groups were evaluated in further detail. All patients started GnRH agonist treatment on the first day of the menstrual cycle. Patients treated with buserelin in a short protocol started recFSH treatment 2 days later, whereas those treated with triptorelin started after approximately 2 weeks after pituitary desensitization was established. The daily dose of recFSH was started with one ampoule (75 IU) for those treated with buserelin in a short protocol, and with two ampoules for those treated with triptorelin in a long protocol. After 3 days of treatment the doses were adjusted per patient. hCG (10,000 IU) was administered when at least three follicles ≥17 mm were detectable. The two groups of patients had normal ovulatory cycles and their age ranged between 23 and 38 years. Causes of infertility were tubal (n = 6), andrological (n = 6), unexplained (n = 6) or endometriotic (n = 2).

In patients treated with buserelin in a short protocol, the initial flare-up of endogenous LH caused relatively high serum LH levels during recFSH treatment (Fig. 3). Individual LH levels largely varied between subjects and median (range) levels were 8 (2.6–24) IU/l after 4 days of recFSH treatment, and 2.3 (<0.5–12.0) IU/l on the day of hCG administration. In comparison, serum LH levels during recFSH treatment of patients in whom pituitary suppression was accomplished by triptorelin in a long protocol were very low (2.8 (2.3–4.9) IU/l) at the start of recFSH treatment, and even lower (1.2 (0.8–3.5) IU/l) on the day of hCG administration.

In each treatment group ovarian response as reflected by levels of serum oestradiol largely varied between patients (Fig. 4). However, patients with significant rises of serum oestradiol were first noted after 4 days of recFSH treatment in association with buserelin in a short protocol, whereas such increases required at least 4 additional treatment days with recFSH in patients pituitary-suppressed by triptorelin.

In response to ovarian stimulation by recFSH, serum immunoactive inhibin (LH-independent) rose in parallel and at the same time as serum oestradiol (LH-dependent) regardless of GnRH agonist treatment. Intraindividual comparison of serum oestradiol and inhibin revealed a positive, linear relationship between these response parameters (Fig. 5). The curve-fit coefficients (r) were 0.8 and 0.9 in the groups treated with buserelin and triptorelin, respectively. Since previous studies have indicated that inhibin is an equally good [19] or even better marker [20] of granulosa cell maturity, these data indicate that recFSH induces normal follicular maturation and that oestrogen biosynthesis is not impaired, not even after severe suppression by triptorelin.

On the day of hCG administration, follicular growth and serum oestradiol levels

Table 2. Main clinical findings in IVF patients treated with two different GnRH agonist/recFSH regimens

	Buserelin short (n = 9)	Triptorelin long (n = 11)
Ampoules	22 (7–50)	35 (24–81)
Treatment days	12 (7–17)	14 (12–18)
FSH[a] (IU/l)	13 (4–17)	17 (9–27)
Oestradiol[a] (pg/ml)	1899 (948–2640)	1768 (781–2952)
Oocytes/retrieval	9 (6–13)	10 (4–20)
Ongoing pregnancies	3/7	2/8

[a]On the day of hCG administration.

were comparable in the two treatment groups (Table 2). However, to accomplish this degree of ovarian stimulation, a total of (median) 35 ampoules of recFSH were required in patients treated with triptorelin (Decapeptyl® CR) whereas only 22 ampoules were sufficient in patients treated with buserelin in a short protocol. In

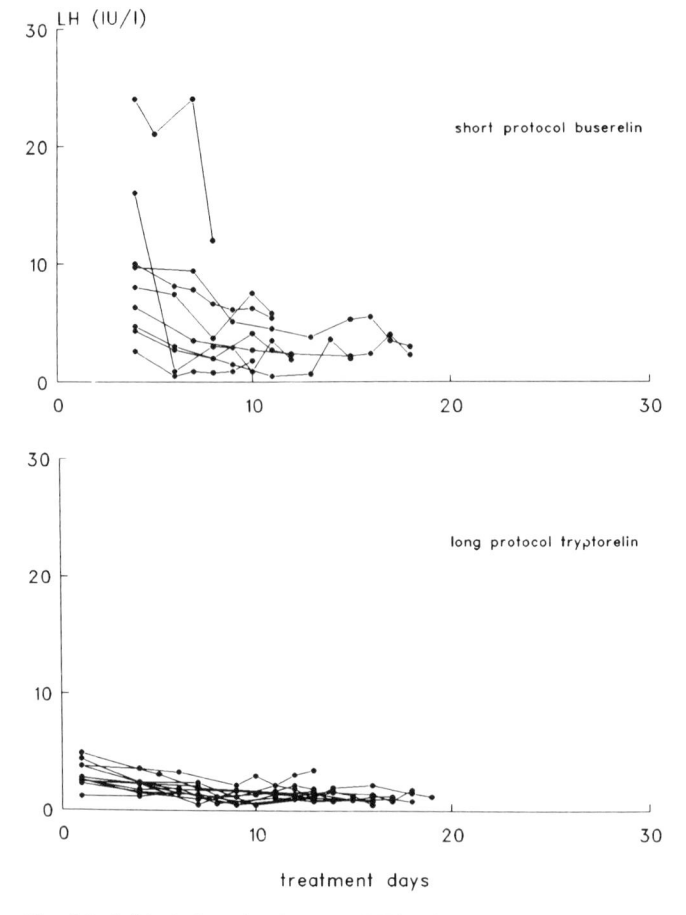

Fig. 3. Individual plots of endogenous LH levels measured in IVF patients during ovarian stimulation with recFSH in combination with buserelin in a short protocol (A) or with triptorelin in a long protocol (B).

accordance with the higher daily dosages administered, serum FSH levels were higher in those treated with triptorelin (see also Table 2). However, no clear correlation was evident between the amount of endogenous LH and the number of recFSH ampoules required. Therefore, the observed difference might be explained by the fact that in the short protocol, follicles were recruited and prevented from atresia by the initial FSH flare-up, whereas endogenous LH facilitated FSH action. In contrast, during pretreatment with triptorelin, antral follicles became atretic and recFSH had to initiate follicle recruitment from the early antral stage.

In both treatment groups comparable number of oocytes were retrieved indicating equal efficacy of both regimens. Ongoing pregnancies [21–22] were established in both groups i.e., 3 out of 7 transfers and 2 out of 8 transfers in those treated with recFSH in association with buserelin and triptorelin, respectively.

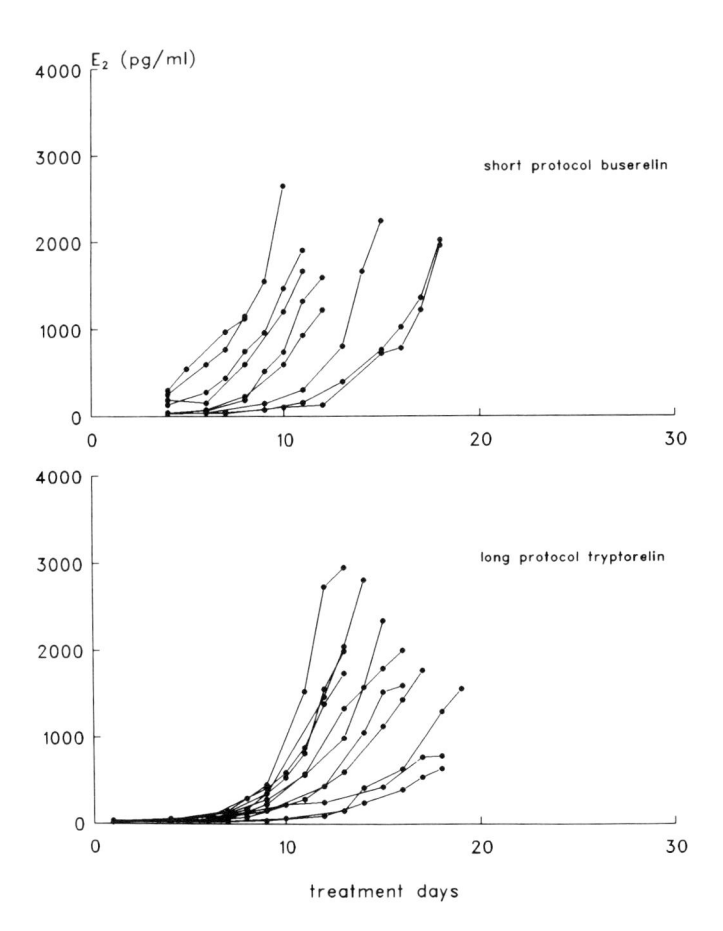

Fig. 4. Individual plots of serum oestradiol measured in IVF patients during ovarian stimulation with recFSH in combination with buserelin in a short protocol (A) or with triptorelin in a long protocol (B).

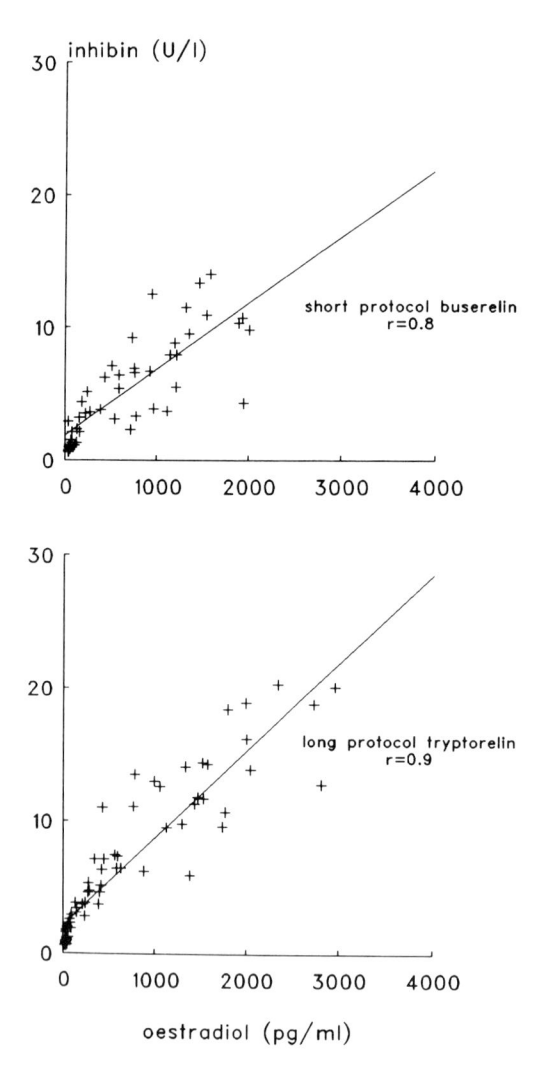

Fig. 5. Correlation of serum inhibin with serum oestradiol levels induced by recFSH treatment in combination with buserelin in a short protocol (A) or with triptorelin in a long protocol (B).

Acknowledgements

Histological evaluation of rat ovaries was performed by Dr J. Uilenbroek and colleagues from the Department of Endocrinology and Reproduction, Rotterdam, The Netherlands. The clinical study on Puregon® was under the responsibility of Prof Devroey, Prof van Steirteghem and Dr Smitz from Free University of Brussels, Brussels, Belgium.

References

1. Hsueh AJW, Adashi EY, Jones PBC, Welsh TH. Endocrine Rev 1984;5:76—127.
2. Hsueh AJW, Dahl KD, Vaughan J, Tucker E, Rivier J, Bardin CW, Vale W. Proc Natl Acad Sci USA 1987;84:5082—5086.
3. Adashi EY, Resnick CE, Hurwitz A, Ricciarellie E, Hernandez ER, Roberts CT, Leroith D, Rosenfeld R. Growth Reg 1992;2:10—15.
4. Chappel SC, Howles C. Hum Reprod 1991;6:1206—1212.
5. Mannaerts B, De Leeuw R, Geelen J, Van Ravenstein A, Van Wezenbeek P, Schuurs A, Kloosterboer L. Endocrinology 1992;129:2623—2630.
6. De Boer W, Mannaerts B. In: Crommelin DJA, Schellekens H (eds) From Clone to Clinic, Developments in Biotherapy. Kluwer Academic Publishers, 1990;1:253—259.
7. Mannaerts B, De Leeuw R. Proceedings of the Fourth Symposium on Reproductive Endocrine Disorders — Control and Stimulation of Follicular Growth, 29—30th September, 1992, Bristol, UK. In: Advances in Reproductive Endocrinology, 1993;1—11.
8. Mason HD, Mannaerts B, De Leeuw R, Willis SD, Franks S. Hum Reprod 1993;8:1823—1827.
9. Mannaerts B, Shoham Z, Schoot D, Bouchard P, Harlin J, Fauser B, Jacobs H, Rombout F, Coelingh Bennink H. Fertil Steril 1993;59:108—114.
10. Matikainen T, De Leeuw R, Mannaerts B, Huhtaniemi I. Circulating bioactive and immunoreactive recombinant human follicle stimulating hormone (Org 32489) after administration to gonadotropin-deficient subjects. Fertil Steril 1993; (accepted).
11. Mannaerts B, Uilenbroek J, Schot P, De Leeuw R. Folliculogenesis in hypophysectomized rats after treatment with recombinant human FSH. Biol Reprod 1994 (in press).
12. Meijs-Roelofs HMA, Osman P, Kramer P. J Endocrinol 1982;92:341—349.
13. Osman P. J Reprod Fert 1985;73:261—270.
14. Whitelaw PF, Smyth CD, Howles CM, Hillier SG. J Mol Endocrinol 1993;9:309—312.
15. Wang X, Greenwald GS. Endocrinology 1993;132:2009—2016.
16. De Leeuw R, Van Ravestein A, Geelen J, Mannaerts B, Kloosterboer H. Pharmacodynamics of recombinant FSH in immature, hypophysectomized female rats. Abstract 107 of the 8th Annual Meeting of the ESHRE, The Hague, 1992.
17. Bogovich K. Biol Reprod 1992;47:149—161.
18. Devroey P, Mannaerts B, Smitz J, Coelingh Bennink H, Van Steirteghem A. Clinical outcome of a pilot efficacy study on recombinant human FSH (Org 32489) combined with various GnRH agonist regimens. Hum Reprod 1994 (in press).
19. Matson PL, Morris ID, Sun JG, Ibrahim ZHZ, Lieberman BA. Horm Res 1991;35:173—177.
20. Buckler HM, Robertson WR, Sun JG, Morris ID. Clin Endocrinol 1992;37:552—557.
21. Devroey P, Van Steirteghem A, Mannaerts B, Coelingh Bennink H. Lancet 1992;339:1170—1171.
22. Devroey P, Van Steirteghem A, Mannaerts B, Coelingh Bennink H. Lancet 1992;340:1108.

Potential clinical applications of recombinant FSH

Herjan J.T. Coelingh Bennink[1]*, Philippe Bouchard[2], Paul Devroey[3], Bart C.J.M. Fauser[4], Jonas Harlin[5] and Zeev Shoham[6]

[1]*Scientific Development Group, NV Organon, Oss, the Netherlands;* [2]*Service d'Endocrinologie, Hôpital Saint-Antoine, Paris, France;* [3]*Centre for Reproductive Medicine, Free University Brussels, Belgium;* [4]*Department of Obstetrics and Gynaecology, Dijkzigt University Hospital, Rotterdam, the Netherlands;* [5]*Department of Obstetrics and Gynaecology, Karolinska Hospital, Stockholm, Sweden;* [6]*Department of Obstetrics and Gynaecology, Kaplan Hospital, Rehovot, Israel*

Abstract. The availability of recFSH has allowed us to study the ovarian response during FSH treatment in conditions characterized by low LH levels. Based on such studies it appears that the lower LH threshold for normal steroidogenesis may be in the range of 0.5—0.8 IU/l. Below this LH level steroidogenesis is compromised. Ovarian inhibin synthesis and follicle growth seem to be normal under such low LH level conditions. The clinical implications of these studies are that recFSH will be able to replace urinary FSH containing gonadotropin preparations without problems, except in women with profound hypogonadotropic hypogonadism, who may require additional LH treatment.

Introduction

Potential clinical applications of recombinant human FSH (recFSH) are the same as those of urinary FSH preparations such as human menopausal gonadotropin (hMG) or urinary FSH (uFSH). These are indicated for the induction of ovulation in hypo- or normogonadotropic women, controlled ovarian hyperstimulation (COH) for assisted reproduction techniques (ART), and induction of spermatogenesis in hypogonadotropic men.

Safety and efficacy of recFSH and natural FSH are not expected to differ, because the polypeptide backbone of the molecules is identical and the carbohydrate side chains are very similar. The major safety concern related to the clinical use of recFSH would be that the minor differences of these side chains may theoretically give rise to antibody formation. However, no anti-recFSH antibodies have been found in more than 700 women treated with Org 32489 (recFSH) because of infertility by induction of ovulation or COH for ART.

A major difference between recombinant and urinary FSH preparations, that might have implications for efficacy, is the lack of LH-activity of recFSH. In this paper two

---

Address for correspondence: Herjan J.T. Coelingh Bennink, Scientific Development Group, Medical Research & Development Unit, NV Organon, P.O. Box 20, 5340 BH Oss, The Netherlands. Tel. +31-4120-62635. Fax +31-4120-62555.

studies are summarized and compared, addressing the role of LH during treatment with recFSH (Org 32489). Both studies have been accepted for publication [1,2]. The first study by Schoot et al. [1] shows the ovarian response during recFSH treatment in extreme gonadotropin-deficient women, lacking LH almost completely. The second study by Devroey et al. [2] shows the efficacy of recFSH in women treated by in vitro fertilization and embryo transfer (IVF-ET) after pituitary desensitization with a gonadotropin-releasing hormone agonist (GnRH-a) according to a long protocol, resulting in suppressed LH levels.

Study I: recFSH in gonadotropin-deficient women

Seven females suffering from hypogonadism due to previous hypophysectomy, isolated gonadotropin deficiency, or Kallmann syndrome (mean age 39, range 24—45 yrs), volunteered to participate in a study to assess ovarian response following multiple dose administration of recFSH (Org 32489). Baseline serum FSH and LH levels were 0.25 (<0.05—1.15) IU/l and 0.06 (<0.05—0.37) IU/l, respectively. Subjects received daily i.m. injections of recFSH for 3 weeks (week 1: 75 IU/d; week 2: 150 IU/d; week 3: 225 IU/d). Blood sampling and sonographic investigations were performed on alternate days. Steady-state FSH concentrations were reached approximately 3 to 5 days after alterations of the doses administered. Maximum FSH levels were between 7.1 and 11.8 IU/l, whereas serum LH concentrations remained low and unchanged (Table 1) due to absent follicle development and lack of a rise in immunoreactive inhibin (INH) (response failure possibly due to early ovarian failure or resistant ovary syndrome) in two subjects; analysis of ovarian response was restricted to five volunteers. Serum androstenedione (AD) and testosterone (T) levels showed no significant changes during recFSH administration (Table 1). Although serum immunoreactive INH concentrations reached normal late follicular phase levels (659 U/l, range 388—993), serum estradiol (E_2) revealed only a minor increase (77

Table 1. Effect of recFSH on androgen synthesis. Pretreatment and maximal A, T and LH levels during recFSH treatment

	Androstenedione (nmol/l)		Testosterone (nmol/l)		LH (IU/l)	
	Pretreatment	Maximum	Pretreatment	Maximum	Pretreatment	Maximum
Hypophysectomy						
1	0.08	0.27	<0.38	<0.38	0.09	0.13
2	0.20	0.15	<0.38	<0.38	0.06	0.08
3	1.16	1.95	<0.38	0.52	<0.05	0.13
Idiopathic						
1	2.05	1.92	0.57	0.50	0.37	0.38
2	3.31	3.26	0.55	0.64	0.06	0.08
3	4.23	4.14	0.36	0.43	0.23	0.47
4	7.76	4.73	0.69	0.50	<0.05	0.05

Table 2. Effect of recFSH on estradiol, inhibin and follicle growth. Maximal FSH, estradiol and inhibin levels and maximum mean follicular diameter and age during recFSH treatment

	FSH (IU/l)	Estradiol (pmol/l)	Inhibin (IU/l)	Follicular diameter (mm)	Age (yrs)
Hypophysectomy					
1	9.9	49	143	no follicles	36
2	8.8	18	69	<8	45
3	8.3	112	993	12	42
Idiopathic					
1	10.1	140	659	>16	38
2	11.8	77	581	>16	39
3	8.5	210	659	>16	39
4	7.1	43	388	15	24

pmol/l, range 18–210), whereas growth of (multiple) ovarian follicles was observed up to preovulatory sizes (>15 mm) in these patients (Table 2). From this study it was concluded, that:

1. recFSH exhibits no intrinsic LH activity;
2. recFSH stimulation in hypogonadotropic women results in an immunoreactive INH rise which is similar as compared to normal, whereas in contrast only a minor increase in E_2 concentrations is observed, suggesting normal granulosa cell function and low availability of androgens as a substrate for aromatization, and
3. despite the minimal E_2 increase, ovarian follicles developed normally to a preovulatory size.

Study II: recFSH after GnRH-a downregulation in IVF

In total, 50 couples participated in a study evaluating the efficacy of various regimens of a GnRH-a in association with recFSH in women undergoing IVF-ET. The patients were treated with recFSH alone (group I), or with recFSH in conjunction with pituitary desensitization using a buserelin intranasal spray, 4 × 150 µg/day in a short protocol (group II) or in a long protocol (group III), or using tryptorelin in a long protocol, giving a single dose of 3.75 mg intramuscularly (group IV) or daily subcutaneous injections of 200 µg (group V).

Table 3. Endocrine results IVF-GnRH-a study. Median values at the day of hCG administration

	Treatment group				
	I	II	III	IV	V
FSH (IU/l)	21	13	15	17	17
LH (IU/l)	5.1	2.3	1.3	1.2	1.6
E_2 (pg/ml)	1101	1899	1773	1768	1531
Inhibin (IU/l)	9.7	10.3	9.0	13.5	18.5

Table 4. Clinical results IVF-GnRH-a study

	Treatment group				
	I	II	III	IV	V
Follicles punctured (median)	14	11	11	14	12
Oocytes recovered (median)	7	9	11	10	11
Transfers	7	7	11	8	10
Embryos/transfer (mean)	2.3	2.8	2.7	2.6	2.5
Clinical pregnancies	0	3	2	4	1
Ongoing pregnancies	0	3	2	2	1
Ampoules (median)	21	22	36	35	32
Treatment days (median)	7	12	14	14	13
Ampoules/day (mean)	3	1.8	2.6	2.5	2.5

Treatment with recFSH resulted in all women in multiple follicular growth and "normal" rises of serum INH and E_2 (Table 3). On the day of hCG administration, endogenous LH was most profoundly suppressed in subjects treated with tryptorelin (Table 3). The median number of ampoules and treatment days required in the various treatment groups varied from 21 to 36 ampoules and from 7 to 14 days, respectively (Table 4). The median number of oocytes per group ranged from 7 to 11; and all cumulus-corona-oocyte complexes, with the exception of two, were classified as mature. The median fertilization and cleavage rates ranged between the treatment groups from 40 to 73% and from 73 to 100%, respectively (Table 4). Fertilization failure of retrieved oocytes occurred in six couples with andrological or unexplained infertility. One patient had no transfer because of insufficient embryo quality. Finally, 43 couples had an embryo transfer (maximally 3 per transfer). Clinical pregnancies were established in 10 women, of whom two had a miscarriage resulting in eight ongoing pregnancies (18.6% per transfer) and the birth of 9 healthy children (Table 4).

From this study it was concluded that recFSH treatment is effective in women undergoing IVF-ET after pituitary desensitization by receptor downregulation with a GnRH-a according to a long protocol with concomitantly low LH levels.

LH levels and ovarian response

Comparing the ovarian responses in study I and study II with special emphasis on the low LH levels it could be concluded that follicle growth as well as inhibin secretion induced by recFSH were normal in hypogonadotropic as well as in downregulated women.

In Fig. 1 the E_2 and LH levels are compared before and after recFSH treatment in the seven hypogonadotropic women from study I and the 30 long protocol GnRH-a downregulated women from study II (groups III, IV and V). Whereas the E_2 levels showed only a minor rise in hypogonadotropic women, a normal rise was observed in downregulated women. However, although in both groups the LH levels were low, the LH levels in the hypogonadotropic women were much lower (<0.05–0.47 IU/l) compared to the LH levels in the downregulated women (2.3–4.9 IU/l at the start of recFSH decreasing to 0.8–3.5 IU/l after completion of COH). It may be concluded that the lower LH threshold for normal E_2 biosynthesis is not surpassed by GnRH-a downregulation for a period of up to 6 weeks, whereas in extreme hypogonadotropic women LH levels are indeed below this LH threshold.

Discussion

According to the two-cell two-gonadotropin concept the normal physiology of the ovary requires LH to stimulate the synthesis of androgens, especially A by theca cells. Aromatization of these androgens is then induced by FSH resulting in biosynthesis of estrogens, especially E_2. The availability of recFSH has enabled the confirmation of this concept in in vitro experiments with rat granulosa cells by Mannaerts et al. [3]. Evidence to support this concept in the human came from studies by Couzinet et al. [4] and Shoham et al. [5]. Both studies in rather extreme hypogonadotropic women demonstrated that treatment with uFSH induced normal follicle growth with suboptimal E_2. It was speculated that the suboptimal E_2 levels were due to the low endogenous LH levels, whereas hardly any exogenous LH had been administered, because uFSH contains less than 1 IU LH per 75 IU FSH. This observation was confirmed in the human for recFSH in a case report published by Schoot et al. [6] who also showed that follicle growth does not require high intrafollicular E_2 concentrations. This case is one of the seven hypogonadotropic women presented in this paper in study I. This study demonstrated that recFSH is devoid of any LH activity, as shown by the absence of any change in the levels of A, T and LH during recFSH treatment. Interestingly, recFSH induced normal follicle growth up to preovulatory size follicles, whereas due to the lack of androgen substrate, E_2 levels hardly showed any rise. Apparently the LH levels in these individuals are below the lower threshold for LH to induce androgen synthesis by theca cells. It seems that follicular steroidogenesis and mitogenesis are differentially regulated with steroidogenesis requiring FSH and LH, whereas follicle growth seems to require FSH only. This has also been demonstrated by a case report by Rabinovici et al. [7], dealing with a patient with 17-α-hydroxylase deficiency and therefore incapable of producing estrogens. Exogenous gonadotropins were able to induce growth of follicles up to preovulatory size in this patient and oocytes could be fertilized in vitro. The conclusion that the too-low LH levels are responsible for the compromised steroidogenesis in hypogonadotropic women is supported by the normal inhibin levels found in these women, demonstrating normal granulosa cell function

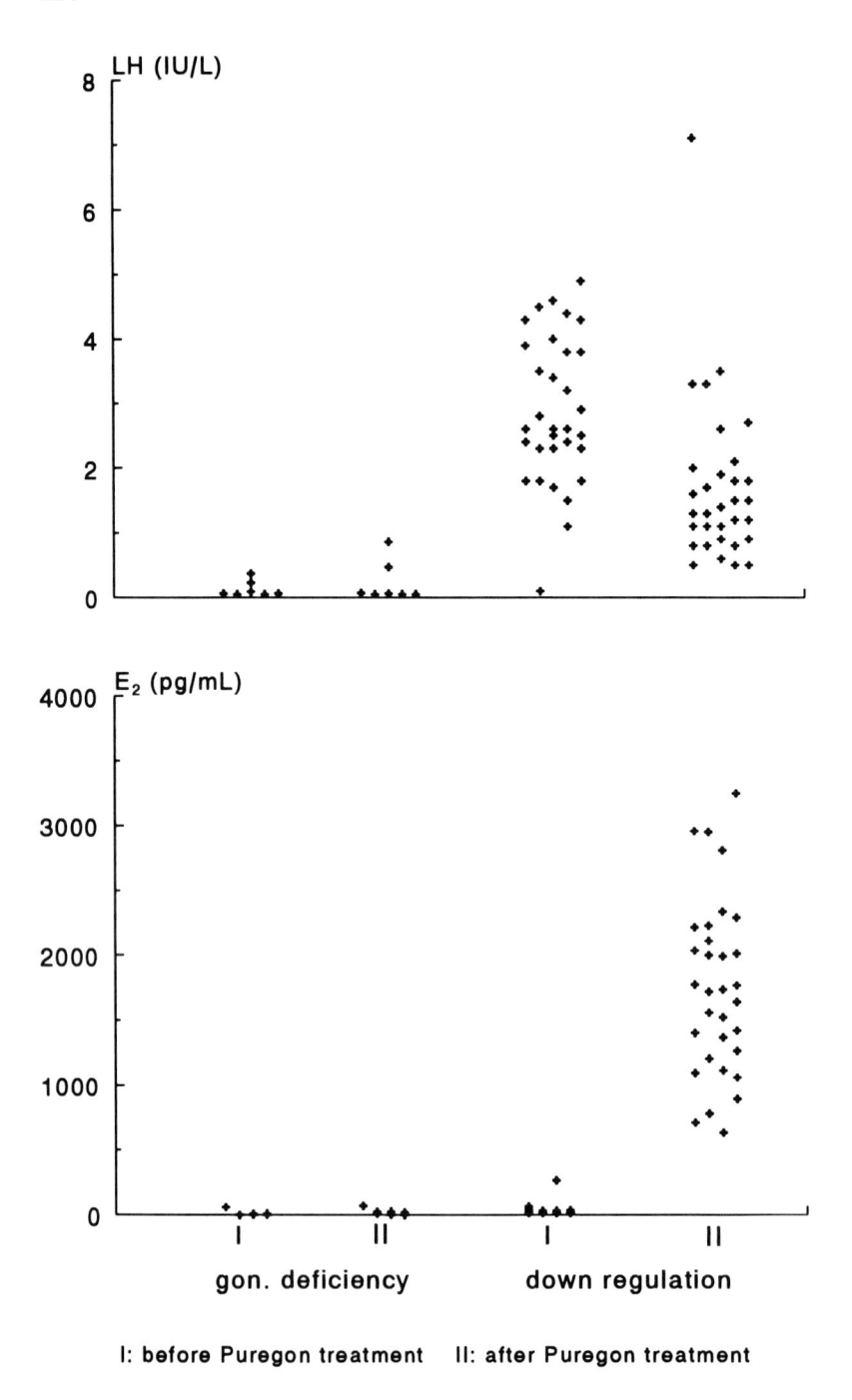

Fig. 1. Serum LH and E$_2$ in gonadotropin-deficient women and in women with suppressed gonadotropins after downregulation with GnRH-a.

in terms of FSH-induced inhibin synthesis. Furthermore, four out of five women showing follicular growth had experienced effective induction of ovulation with urinary gonadotropins, resulting in three women having been pregnant. Contrary to the results in study I, estradiol biosynthesis in study II reflecting granulosa cell function stimulated by recFSH during downregulation with a GnRH-a, appeared to be normal. As shown by the LH levels in these women in Fig. 1, apparently downregulation of LH is incomplete and enough LH is left to induce effective synthesis of androgen precursors. Comparison of the results of the two studies presented suggests that the lower LH threshold for normal E_2 biosynthesis is in the range of 0.5—0.8 IU/l.

The results presented in this paper may have implications for the clinical application of recFSH. First of all it can be concluded that recFSH is effective in COH, even in combination with GnRH-a downregulation. Administration of additional LH activity is not necessary in this situation. Also, in induction of ovulation in chronic anovulation (polycystic ovarian syndrome, PCOS) it is highly unlikely that the efficacy of recFSH will differ from uFSH because PCOS is characterized by either normal or increased LH levels. Those LH levels are certainly higher than those observed in the downregulated women in study II. However, in extreme hypogonadotropic women requiring induction of ovulation for infertility treatment, the addition of some LH activity during recFSH treatment may be necessary to achieve adequate E_2 biosynthesis, although this may not be required for normal follicle growth. Further clinical studies may demonstrate whether an LH level of around 0.5—0.8 IU/l can be used as a lower LH threshold level to decide upon the need for additional treatment with a compound delivering LH activity. Male infertility caused by hypogonadotropic hypogonadism is routinely treated with a combination of FSH and hCG and therefore recFSH is expected to be able to replace uFSH without any problems in this condition.

References

1. Schoot DC, Harlin J, Shoham Z, Mannaerts BMJL, Lahlou N, Bouchard P, Coelingh Bennink HJT, Fauser BCJM. Human recombinant follicle stimulating hormone and ovarian response in gonadotropin deficient women. Hum Reprod (in press).
2. Devroey P, Mannaerts BMJL, Smitz J, Coelingh Bennink HJT, Van Steirteghem A. Clinical outcome of a pilot efficacy study on recombinant human FSH (Org 32489) combined with various GnRH agonist regimens. Hum Reprod (in press).
3. Mannaerts BMJL, De Leeuw R, Geelen J, Van Ravenstein A, Van Wezenbeek P, Schuurs A and Kloosterboer H. Endocrinology 1991;129:2623—2630.
4. Couzinet B, Lestrat N, Brailly S, Forest M, Schaison G. J Clin Endocrinol Metab 1988;66:552—556.
5. Shoham Z, Balen A, Patel A, Jacobs HS. Fertil Steril 1991;56:1048—1053.
6. Schoot DC, Coelingh Bennink HJT, Mannaerts BMJL, Lamberts SWJ, Bouchard P, Fauser BCJM. J Clin Endocrinol Metab 1992;74:1471—1473.
7. Rabinovici J, Blankstein J, Goldman B, Rudak E, Dor Y, Pariente C, Geier A, Lunenfeld B, Mashiach S. J Clin Endocrinol Metab 1991;68:693—697.

Ovulation induction with recombinant human follicle-stimulating hormone and luteinizing hormone

Ernest Loumaye[1]*, Hervé C. Porchet[1], Vanya Beltrami[1], Danièle Giroud[1], Jean-Yves Le Cotonnec[1], Louis O'Dea[2], Angela Piazzi[1], Colin M. Howles[1] and Andrew Galazka[1]

[1]*Ares Serono R&D, CH 1211 Geneva, Switzerland; and* [2]*Serono Inc, Norwell, MA 02061, USA*

Abstract. Pharmaceutical preparations of recombinant FSH and LH produced in vitro by genetically engineered CHO cells are currently available for clinical assessment. Both recombinant gonadotropins have been shown to have pharmacokinetic characteristics very similar to their urinary equivalent. r-hFSH alone is effective and safe for stimulating multiple follicular development in ovulatory patients undergoing assisted reproductive technology treatment, even when endogenous LH secretion is suppressed by administration of a GnRH agonist. r-hFSH alone is effective and safe for stimulating follicular development in WHO group II anovulatory patients (PCOD). In hypogonadotropic hypogonadic females, r-hFSH is not sufficient for achieving successful follicular development. Preliminary data suggest that r-hLH would be an ideal adjunctive therapy to r-hFSH in this indication.

Introduction

Menotropin (hMG) was developed more than 30 years ago and urofollitropin (Metrodin®) was introduced in clinics 10 years ago.

In 1984, Chappel et al. at Integrated Genetics, successfully cloned and expressed human CG, FSH and LH [1]. Since then, several other groups have also expressed hFSH [2,3]. In 1991, a pharmaceutical preparation of recombinant human FSH (r-hFSH) produced in vitro by genetically engineered Chinese hamster ovary cells (CHO cells) became available for clinical assessment (Gonal-F™, Serono, Aubonne, Switzerland). More recently, a pharmaceutical preparation of recombinant human LH (r-hLH) also produced in vitro by genetically engineered CHO cells has entered a stage of clinical assessment (LHadi™, Serono, Aubonne, Switzerland).

The aim of this paper is to highlight salient differences between currently used hMG/FSH preparations and r-hFSH, review the clinical indications for r-hFSH in female patients and summarize some aspects of the clinical experience gained with r-hFSH in these indications. In addition, the characteristics of r-hLH will briefly be presented and the anticipated main clinical indications for r-hLH will be discussed.

Address for correspondence: E. Loumaye, Ares Serono R&D, 15bis Chemin des Mines, CH 1211 Geneva, Switzerland.

FSH production by recombinant DNA technology

The differences between r-hFSH preparations and u-hFSH preparations (including HMG) are presented in Table 1. These differences can be summarized as follows:

1. Source of bulk materials: In contrast with u-FSH, the production of r-hFSH is no longer dependent on urine collection and extraction. Currently, yearly collection of urine for worldwide gonadotropin supply represents tens of millions of liters, and hundreds of thousands donors are participating in these programs. Being independent of this source minimizes the risk of shortage of FSH for clinical use due to lack of raw materials. Further, it removes concerns about infectious agents, drugs or drug metabolites derived from the human-recovered raw materials. Finally, since cells derived from a single transfected cell will be used to supply FSH for decades, recombinant technology should offer a long-term consistency in product characteristics.
2. Purity and specific activity: Since the production of r-hFSH has been coupled with an effective purification process, the r-hFSH preparation has a high specific activity (~10,000 IU FSH/mg of protein). Practically, this means that a 75 IU ampoule of r-hFSH contains around 10 µg of FSH which accounts for >99% of the preparation's protein content. This contrasts with current hMG and u-hFSH preparation-specific activities which are around 75–150 IU FSH/mg of protein. This means that an average hMG ampoule contains about 500 µg of nonspecific copurified urinary proteins and around 10 µg of bioactive FSH. The high purity of u-hFSH favours good local tolerance to injections and low immunogenicity when administered subcutaneously (s.c.). It also means that physicochemical characterization of the product can be used for quality control and product specification purpose.
3. LH activity: In contrast to u-hFSH and hMG, the r-hFSH preparation is free of LH activity providing a monotherapeutic agent for clinical use.

Table 1. Preparations of human FSH

Preparation	Commercial name	Source of FSH	FSH activity (IU)	LH activity (IU)	FSH-specific activity (FSH IU/mg protein)	Copurified nonFSH human proteins
hMG	Pergonal®	Urine	75	75	75–150	>95%
u-hFSH	Metrodin®	Urine	75	<0.7	100–150	>95%
u-hFSH HP[a]	Metrodin HP®	Urine	75–150	<0.001	~10,000	<1%
r-hFSH	Gonal-F®	CHO cells	75–150	none	~10,000	none

[a]Highly purified u-hFSH

Clinical pharmacology assessment of r-hFSH

Several studies have been conducted in nonhuman primates and human volunteers to determine r-hFSH pharmacokinetic characteristics. Despite their limitations, FSH immunoassays have been used as the primary tool for characterizing hFSH pharmacokinetics. In some studies, however, an in vitro FSH bioassay has also been used (rat granulosa cell bioassay, GAB) and results compared with the immunoassay data [4].

In nonhumans primates, r-hFSH pharmacokinetic characteristics have been shown to be similar to u-hFSH characteristics [5].

In human female volunteers, pretreated with a GnRH agonist (Goserelin, Zoladex® depot, Zeneca, UK) for suppressing endogenous secretion of gonadotropins, the total clearance of the r-hFSH and u-hFSH preparations were found to be comparable. The volumes of distribution at steady state (11 l) were similar and represent the extracellular body water. Further, the distribution half-life was close to 2 h and the terminal half-life was nearly 1 day when estimated by modeling the intravenous (i.v.) data [4]. After a single i.m. and s.c. injection, the absolute bioavailability of Gonal-F® following intramuscular (i.m.) and s.c. administration was about 70%. After repeated s.c. administration of 150 IU r-hFSH for 7 days, the accumulation factor for repeated s.c. administration was around 3 when steady-state was reached [4]. The measure of serum FSH levels with the in vitro bioassay (GAB assay) essentially confirm the similarity of r-hFSH and u-hFSH pharmacokinetic characteristics.

During repeated administration (7 days) of a fixed daily dose of Gonal-F® (150 IU s.c./day), a majority of volunteers developed significant follicular growth, inhibin and E_2 secretion. The first pharmacodynamic marker of the ovarian response to FSH was serum-immunoreactive inhibin, followed by plasma E_2 and then follicular growth (in this case measured by total volume of follicles >10 mm diameter). No correlation was found between maximal serum FSH concentrations during Gonal-F® administration and the maximal E_2 responses, inhibin responses and follicular growth responses [6].

Apparent terminal half-life after s.c. and i.m. administration of r-hFSH and of several u-hFSH preparations are summarized in Table 2.

Together, these data indicate that the pharmacokinetic characteristics of currently tested r-hFSH preparations are essentially similar to those of u-hFSH preparations. For clinicians, this means that r-hFSH can be used with the current regimes and doses applied to u-hFSH.

Clinical assessment of r-hFSH

r-hFSH assessment in patients undergoing superovulation for ART

The benefit of stimulating multiple follicular development in ovulatory patients undergoing ART is well established [7]. hMG has been used as the primary pharmacological agent to achieve this objective [8]. Subsequently, treatment with u-hFSH preparations devoid of significant LH activity has been demonstrated [9–17] to be as

Table 2. Estimated apparent terminal half-lives for r-hFSH and different u-hFSH preparations administered i.m. or s.c.

References	No. of subjects (sex)	FSH preparation (IU)[a]	Estimated terminal half-life (h)
[18]	3 (female)	hMG (600)[a] (i.m.)	35
[19]	5 (female)	hMG (150)[b] (i.m.)	48
[20]	7 (male)	u-hFSH (150)[a] (i.m.)	25
	5 (male)	u-hFSH (450)[a] (i.m.)	36
[21]	16 (male)	u-hFSH (150)[a] (i.m.)	36 ± 16^c
[22]	12 (male)	u-hFSH (150)[a] (i.m.)	36 ± 8^c
		u-hFSH HP (150)[a] (i.m.)	39 ± 15^c
		u-hFSH HP (150)[a] (s.c.)	45 ± 21^c
[4(I)]	12 (female)[d]	r-hFSH[f] (150)[a] (i.m.)	37 ± 25^c
		r-hFSH[f] (150)[a,b] (s.c.)	37 ± 28^c
[23]	8 (female)[e]	r-hFSH[g] (300)[a] (i.m.)	44 ± 14^c
	7 (male)[e]	r-hFSH[g] (300)[a] (i.m.)	32 ± 12^c

[a]Single administration; [b]repeated administration (150 IU/day for 7 days); [c]±SD; [d]volunteers were pretreated with a GnRH agonist (Zoladex Depot); [e]hypogonadotropic hypogonadal patients; [f]Gonal-F® — Serono, Aubonne, Switzerland; [g]Org32489 — Organon, Oss, the Netherlands.

effective as hMG therapy for stimulating multiple follicular development for assisted reproductive technologies (ART) (Table 3). This indicates that the active LH component of hMG is unnecessary in this indication, even when endogenous LH

Table 3. Overall results from clinical studies comparing u-hFSH with hMG to stimulate multiple follicular development for ART

Cycle pretreatment	Studies reviewed	Treatment	Patients treated	Pregnancy	Pregnancy/ cycle (%)	Pregnancy/ OPU (%)	Pregnancy/ ET (%)
None	Four	hMG	117	11	9.4	12.3	16.3[a]
		u-hFSH	107	14	13.0	14.7	15.6
GnRH-A Flare-up	Two	hMG	65	15	23.0	23.8	26.3
		u-hFSH	77	11	14.3	15.7	17.8
GnRH-A Desensitization	Four	hMG	133	35	26.3	26.7	29.0
		u-hFSH	144	40	27.8	28.4	31.5
Overall	Ten	hMG	315	61	19.4	21.5	25.6[b]
		u-hFSH	328	65	19.9	21.2	24.5

[a]Data only available for two studies; [b]data only available for eight studies.

secretion is suppressed by administration of a GnRH agonist.

r-hFSH has been evaluated in ART. Preliminary reports have indicated that r-hFSH can successfully stimulate multiple ovarian follicular growth and estradiol secretion in patients undergoing IVF-ET who were pretreated with a GnRH agonist [24–27]. Further, a comparative, nonrandomized pilot study assessing the role of GnRH agonist pretreatment on the endocrine response and IVF outcome of r-hFSH-induced superovulation (Org 32489) has been reported [28]. One group of patients were not treated with an agonist, and four groups were treated with different agonist regimens, namely 1) a flare-up protocol; 2) a pituitary desensitization protocol using nasally administered buserelin; 3) a desensitization protocol using s.c. administration of triptorelin; and 4) a desensitization protocol using a depot preparation of triptorelin. Different degrees of LH suppression were achieved, but this did not appear to significantly influence r-hFSH-induced follicular development.

A prospective, randomized, parallel group open study has been completed in accordance with EEC GCP guidelines for comparing r-hFSH (Gonal-F®) administered s.c. with u-hFSH (Metrodin®) administered i.m. in women undergoing IVF-ET. In this study all patients were pretreated with buserelin (200 µg/s.c./day) for inducing pituitary desensitization prior to stimulation with FSH. Sixty patients were treated with r-hFSH and 63 with u-hFSH. No significant difference was observed in the mean number of growing follicles, retrieved oocytes and cleaved embryos (Table 4). The duration of FSH treatment to achieve full follicular development was 9.9 ± 2.3 and 9.4 ± 1.8 days, for r-hFSH and u-hFSH, respectively ($p = 0.21$) and the average dose of FSH to reach this stage was $2,270 \pm 714$ and $2,095 \pm 591$ IU of FSH, for r-hFSH and u-hFSH, respectively ($p = 0.16$). Eighty-three and 82% of the patients achieved embryo transfer in the r-hFSH and u-hFSH group, respectively. The achieved pregnancy rates are described in Table 5. In terms of safety, no difference was

Table 4. Follicular development, OPU and IVF results

Variables	r-hFSH		u-hFSH		Tests and p values
	n	mean ± SD	n	mean ± SD	
No. of follicles >10 mm on the day of hCG	60	10.3 ± 4.9	63	11.2 ± 5.2	ANOVA[a]: 0.177
No. of follicles ≥14 mm on the day of hCG	60	7.8 ± 3.6	63	9.2 ± 4.5	ANOVA[a]: 0.037
No. of oocytes recovered	55	9.3 ± 5.0	59	10.7 ± 5.3	ANOVA[a]: 0.35
No. of cleaved embryos	53	5.0 ± 3.0	52	6.1 ± 3.4	ANOVA[a]: 0.12
No. of patients for each no. of transferred embryos	r-hFSH		u-hFSH		Tests and p values
1	0		4 (8%)		CMH[b]: 0.77
2	12 (24%)		6 (11.5%)		
3	34 (68%)		35 (67%)		
4	4 (8%)		6 (11.5%)		
5	0		1 (2%)		

[a]ANOVA: analysis of variance; [b]CMH: Cochran-Mantel-Haenszel test.

Table 5. Number of pregnancies, deliveries, and pregnancy rates[a]

Variables	Number (n)		Pregnancy/cycle (%)		Pregnancy/OPU (%)		Pregnancy/ET (%)	
	r-hFSH	u-hFSH	r-hFSH	u-hFSH	r-hFSH	u-hFSH	r-hFSH	u-hFSH
All pregnancies	13	11	22	17	24	19	26	21
Clinical pregnancies	13	10	20	16	22	17	24	19
Delivery of ≥ one live baby	9	8	15	13	16	14	18	15

[a]fresh embryo transfer only

recorded between the groups. Gonal-F® was not found to be immunogenic. Local tolerance to s.c. injection for Gonal-F® was good and did not differ significantly from local tolerance to i.m. injection of Metrodin®.

r-hFSH assessment in WHO group II anovulation

The most frequent type of anovulation is characterized by asynchronous gonadotropin and estrogen production and normal levels of prolactin (PRL). These patients present with a variety of menstrual disorders, ranging from regular but anovulatory cycles to oligomenorrhea and amenorrhea. The persistence of estrogen production is demonstrated by the presence of spontaneous bleeding or progesterone-induced withdrawal bleeding. This corresponds to the group II in the WHO classification of anovulation [29]. These anovulations are often (>90%), but not always, associated with features of the polycystic ovarian disease (PCOD) when morphology of the ovary is assessed by ultrasound [30,31].

In this indication, treatment with u-hFSH preparations devoid of significant LH activity (Metrodin®) has been demonstrated to be as effective as hMG therapy for stimulating (single) follicular development and achieving ovulation and pregnancy after hCG administration [32–39] (Table 6). Recently, it has also been shown that the FSH threshold concentration to initiate follicular growth with u-hFSH is not influenced by coadministration of LH [40]. Finally, in a multicenter randomized, parallel group clinical trial comparing u-hFSH (Metrodin®) with highly purified u-hFSH (Metrodin HP®), in WHO group II anovulation, it has been shown that u-hFSH achieves similar levels of efficacy and safety whether associated with high or low

Table 6. Overall results from eight clinical studies comparing u-hFSH with hMG for stimulation of follicular development in WHO group II anovulatory women

Treatment	Patients treated	Treatment cycles	Ovulatory cycles	Pregnancy/ cycle	Pregnancy/ ovulation	Miscarriage rate
hMG	109	325	241/325 (74%)	36/325 (11%)	36/241 (15%)	13/30 (43%)
u-hFSH	136	309	214/309 (69%)	33/309 (11%)	33/214 (15%)	10/29 (34%)

serum levels of LH on baseline evaluation (O'Dea, personal communication). Together, these data confirm that addition of LH to FSH is unnecessary in this indication.

r-hFSH has been evaluated in this indication. The earliest results to be published indicate that r-hFSH alone is effective in stimulating follicular development and when hCG is administered ovulation is achieved and pregnancy obtained [41,42]. Further, it shows that in this population r-hFSH-induced follicular growth is characterized by a clear-cut increase in serum estradiol and inhibin levels [42].

More recently, a partial analysis of a multinational, prospective, open, randomized, parallel group study comparing the efficacy of r-hFSH (Gonal-F®) with u-hFSH (Metrodin®) for inducing ovulation in WHO group II anovulatory patients has been presented [43]. Using a chronic low dose protocol, the ovulation rate per initiated cycle was 58% and 64%; the pregnancy rate per ovulatory cycle was 18% and 21%; and per initiated cycle 11% and 12% for Gonal-F® and Metrodin®, respectively.

These preliminary results need further confirmation by analyzing final study data to provide an appropriate power to detect putative differences. However, so far r-hFSH appears to be at least as effective as u-hFSH for restoring fertility in this population.

r-hFSH assessment in WHO group I anovulation

A much less frequently encountered anovulation is WHO group I anovulation [29]. It is also named central failure or hypogonadotropic hypogonadism and is characterised by reduced hypothalamic or pituitary activity. As a consequence, serum gonadotropins are abnormally low and estrogen activity is negligible.

In some WHO group I anovulatory patients, coadministration of LH appears to be required during FSH therapy to obtain optimal follicular development. This is supported by the following clinical evidence:
1. Couzinet et al. compared, in a crossover design, u-hFSH with hMG in 10 hypogonadotropic hypogonadal patients. Ovulation was assessed by luteal phase progesterone (P_4) levels and ultrasonography. During the hMG treatment, two cycles were cancelled because of risk of ovarian hyperstimulation syndrome (OHSS), and ovulation occurred in the eight other cycles. During FSH treatment, one cycle was cancelled for risk of OHSS, and ovulation occurred in six out of the nine remaining cycles. Preovulatory E_2 levels were, on average, 3 times lower with FSH than with hMG [44].
2. Shoham et al. reported a similar crossover study comparing FSH to hMG in nine hypogonadotropic hypogonadal patients. Ovulation was assessed by measuring luteal phase P_4 and ultrasonographic appearance of the corpus luteum (CL). All hMG-treated cycles led to ovulation and only three out of nine FSH-treated cycles led to ovulation. Moreover, in FSH-treated cycles mean preovulator/y E_2 levels were 3 times lower and endometrial thickness was significantly reduced by almost 30% when compared with hMG-treated cycles [45].

These observations indicated that in the hypogonadotropic hypogonadal female population, a significant proportion of patients do not have the threshold level of endogenous LH required to achieve optimal follicular development and steroidogenesis during therapy with pure FSH.

The availability of r-hFSH definitively devoid of any residual LH activity has prompted a reappraisal of this question. The first case of hypogonadotropic hypogonadism treated with r-hFSH (Org 32489) is described below. Multiple follicular development (defined as fluid cavities in the ovaries, visualized with ultrasound) was achieved while the E_2 level remained very low (about 4 times lower than the expected average value). Follicular fluid E_2 concentrations were 1,500 times lower than expected. Serum P_4 showed no elevation following hCG administration [46]. This first observation has been recently confirmed in 12 patients. Some follicular development was recorded in all patients, E_2 secretion was consistently low, and immunoreactive inhibin secretion did not appear to be impaired (Bouchard et al., personal communication).

These data suggest that in this population, r-hFSH is not sufficient for achieving successful follicular development and that exogenous administration of LH will be required in at least some patients. r-hLH will be an ideal adjunctive therapy to r-hFSH in this indication.

LH production by recombinant DNA technology

Recombinant human LH is produced by CHO cells in which DNAs encoding the α and β LH subunits have been introduced. The r-hLH secreted in vitro is purified and formulated to yield a pharmaceutical preparation with high specific activity (LHadi™, Serono, Aubonne, Switzerland). This new source of materials, independent of urine collection and extraction, will provide unlimited materials for clinical use.

Clinical pharmacological assessment of r-hLH

A crossover pharmacokinetic study in nonhuman primates performed to assess and compare pituitary, urinary and recombinant human LH has been reported by Le Cotonnec and Porchet [47]. After i.v. administration of p-hLH, u-hLH and r-hLH, the mean concentration time curves were parallel. After normalization by the immunological dose the mean $AUC_{0-\infty}$ were not different. The mean clearance estimates (around 0.05 l/h/kg), and the volume of distribution at steady-state (around 0.14 l/kg, which coincides to the extracellular fluid volume) were similar for the three LHs. Similarly, the distribution half-lives were about 0.7 h and the terminal half-lives were around 10 h.

Clinical assessment of r-hLH

r-hLH's efficacy and safety is currently being evaluated as support of r-hFSH-induced follicular development in LH and FSH deficient anovulatory women (WHO group I). Preliminary data indicate that s.c. administration of LHadi™ leads to a significant increase in serum LH levels and promotes estradiol secretion.

Conclusions

Human FSH produced by recombinant DNA technology is different from urinary-derived FSH in terms of source of bulk materials. Moreover, the production has been coupled with an effective purification process leading to a level of purity about 60 times higher than standard hMG/FSH preparations. The product characteristics speak in favor of a safer and more consistent preparation. In clinics, r-hFSH has been found to be at least as effective and safe as currently available u-hFSH. The s.c. route of administration is effective and well-tolerated, allowing convenient self-administration by the patient. At this stage of assessment of the r-hFSH preparation, it is already quite apparent that r-hFSH will replace urinary-derived FSH preparations.

A pharmaceutical preparation of r-hLH is currently under clinical investigation. It is anticipated that the main indication for r-LH will be the coadministration of r-hLH during r-hFSH treatment in patients with profound LH deficiency.

References

1. Chappel S, Kelton C, Nugent N. In: Genazzi AR, Petraglia F (eds) Proceedings of the 3rd Congress on Gynecological Endocrinology. Cranforth, UK: The Parthenon Publishing Group, 1992;179–184.
2. Keene JL, Matzuk MM, Otani T, Fauser BCJM, Galway AB, Hsueh AJW, Boime I. J Biol Chem 1989;264:4769–4775.
3. Mannaerts B, De Leeuw R, Geelen J, Van Raicustein A, Van Wezenbeek P, Schruurs A, Kloosterboer H. Endocrinology 1991;129:2623–2630.
4. Le Cotonnec J-Y, Porchet HC, Beltrami V, Khan A, Toon S, Rowland M. Clinical pharmacology of recombinant human follicle stimulating hormone: I. Single doses and steady state pharmacokinetics. Fertil Steril 1994 (in press). II. Comparative pharmacokinetics with urinary hFSH. Fertil Steril 1994 (in press).
5. Porchet HC, Le Cotonnec J-Y, Canali S, Zanolo G, Drug Metab Dispos 1993;21144–21150.
6. Porchet HC, Loumaye E, Le Cotonnec J-Y. Clinical pharmacology studies of recombinant human follicle stimulating hormone: pharmacokinetic-pharmacodynamic modeling after repeated subcutaneous administration. Fertil Steril 1994 (in press).
7. Wood C, McMaster R, Rennie G, Trounson A, Leeton J. Fertil Steril 1985;43:245.
8. Jones HW Jr, Jones SG, Andrews MC et al. Fertil Steril 1982;38:14.
9. Russell J, Polan M, Decherney A. Fertil Steril 1986;45:829.
10. Scoccia B, Blumenthal P, Wagner C, Prins G, Scommegna A, Marut E. Fertil Steril 1987;46:446–449.
11. Frydman R, Forman R, Belaisch-Allart J, Hazout A, Parneik I, Testart J. Fertil Steril 1988;50:471–475.
12. Quigley M, Collins RM, Blankstein J. Fertil Steril 1988;50:562.

13. Lavy G, Pellicer A, Diamond M, Decherney A. Fertil Steril 1988;50:74.
14. Edelstein M, Brzyski R, Jones G, Simonetti S, Muasher S. Fertil Steril 1990;53:103.
15. Fries N, Hedon B, Audibert E et al. Randomized study of pure FSH versus hMG in ovarian agonist stimulation (long Protocol). (Abstract no. 7—8) Contraception-fertilité-sexualité 1990;18:670 (with English translation).
16. Tanbo T, Dale P, Haug E, Abyholm T, Kjekshus E. Fertil Steril 1990;53:798.
17. Török A, Hamori M, Tinneberg HR, Cledon P, Gagsteiger F, Hanf V. Hum Reprod 1991;6:922.
18. Flamigni C, Venturoli S, Paradisi R. Contracept Fertil Sexual 1985;13:1097.
19. Diczfalusy E. and Harlin J. Hum Reprod 1988;3:21—27.
20. Jockenhövel F, Fingscheidt U, Khan SA, Behre HM, Nieschlag E. Clin Endocrinol 1990;33:573—584.
21. Mizunuma H, Takagi T, Honjyo S, Ibuki Y, Igarashi M. Fertil Steril 1990;53:440—445.
22. Le Cotonnec J-Y, Porchet H.C, Beltrami V, Howles CM. Hum Reprod 1993;8:1604—1611.
23. Mannaerts B, Shoham Z, Schoot D, Bouchard P, Harlin J, Fauser B, Jacobs H, Rombout F, Coelingh Bennink H. Fertil Steril 1993;59:108—114.
24. Germond M, Dessole S, Senn A, Loumaye E, Howles C, Beltrami V. Lancet 1992;338:1170.
25. Devroey P, Van Steirteghem A, Mannaerts B, Coelingh Bennink H. Lancet 1992;339:1170—1171.
26. Loumaye E, Alvarez S, Barlow D, Barri P.N, Beltrami V, Bergh T, Demoulin A, Dessole V, Egan D, Fanchin R, Frydman R, Germond M, Gudmundsson J, Hazout A, Howles CM, Hull M, Salat-Baroux J. In: Jacobs HS (ed) The new frontier in ovulation induction. Cranforth, UK: The Parthenon Publishing Group, 1993;27—38.
27. O'Dea L, Loumaye E, Liu H. Fertil Steril 1993(suppl);0—106,950.
28. Devroey P, Mannaerts B, Smitz J, Coelingh Bennink H, Van Steirteghem A. Hum Reprod 1993;8(suppl. 1):A34.
29. WHO. Wld Hlth Org Techn Rep Ser 1973;514.
30. Franks S. Clin Endocrinol 1989;31:87.
31. Fox R, Corrigan E, Thomas P, Hull M. Clin Endocrinol 1991;34:127—131.
32. Seibel MM, McArdle C, Smith D, Taymor ML, Fertil Steril 1985;43:703.
33. Venturoli S, Paradisi R, Fabbri R, Porcu E, Orsini LF, Flamigni C. Int J Fertil 1987;32:66.
34. Butt W.R. Acta Endocrinol 1988;288:51.
35. Homburg R, Eshel A, Kilborn J, Adams J, Jacobs HS. Human Reprod 1990;5:32.
36. Fulghesu AM, Guida C, Nicoletti CL et al. In: Adashi E.Y. and Mancuso S (eds) Serono Symposia vol. 73: Major Advances in Human Female Reproduction. New York: Raven Press, 1990;389.
37. Gadir AA, Mowafi RS, Alnaser HMI et al. Clin Endocrinol 1990;33:585.
38. Larsen T, Larsen JF, Schioler V, Bostofte E, Felding C. Fertil Steril 1990;53:426.
39. Sagle MA, Hamilton-Fairley D, Kiddy D, Franks S. Fertil Steril 1991;55:56.
40. van Weissenbruch MM, Schoemaker HC, Drexhage HA, Schoemaker J. Hum Reprod 1993;8:813—818.
41. Donderwinkel PFJ, Schoot DC, Coelingh Bennink HJT, Fauser BCJM. Lancet 1992;340:983.
42. Hornnes P, Giroud D, Howles C, Loumaye E. Fertil Steril 1993;60:724—726.
43. Jacobs H, Birkhauser M, Cittadini E, Crosignani G, Flamigni C, Hornnes P, Templeton A, Balasch J, Braendle W, Buvat J, De Cecco L, Demoulin A, Dellenbach P, Emperaire J, Homburg R, Jansson P, Kahn J, Koninckx P, Lehmann F, Pellicer A, Rabinovici J, Romeu A, Ron El R, Salat-Baroux J, Yates R, Zorn J, Giroud D, Howles C, Loumaye E. Hum Reprod 1993;8(suppl. 1):A241.
44. Couzinet B, Lestrat N, Brailly S, Forest M, Schaison G. J Clin Endocrinol Metab 1988;66:552.
45. Shoham Z, Balen A, Patel A, Jacobs H. Fertil Steril 1991;56:1048.
46. Schoot DC, Coeling Bennink HTJ, Mannaerts BMJL, Lamberts SWJ, Bouchard P, Fauser BCJM. J Clin Endocrinol Metab 1992;74:1471—1473.
47. Le Cotonnec J-Y, Porchet HC. In: Emperaire JC (ed) The triggering of ovulation in stimualted cycles: hCG or LH. Cranforth, UK: The Parthenon Publishing Group, 1994.

Ovulation induction with pulsatile GnRH

Use of GnRH and its analogs in the treatment of ovulatory disorders: an overview

Marco Filicori*

Reproductive Endocrinology Center, University of Bologna, Bologna, Italy

Abstract. In this overview we report clinical results obtained in more than 1,000 treatment cycles conducted in different centers. Ovulatory and pregnancy rates obtained with pulsatile GnRH in different reproductive disorders vary between 70–93% and 18–29%, respectively. Spontaneous abortion occurs in 10–29% of pregnancies, while the incidence of multiple pregnancy is below 14% and can be further reduced to 8% or less by the use of low-dose pulsatile GnRH; moreover, multiple pregnancy can be virtually eliminated by GnRH agonist pretreatment of selected patients. Ovarian hyperstimulation is not a complication of pulsatile GnRH. Thus, pulsatile GnRH can be effectively and safely applied to anovulatory patients.

Introduction

Pulsatile gonadotropin-releasing hormone (GnRH) has been used for over a decade for effective and safe ovulation induction in anovulatory women and to achieve normal testicular function in hypogonadotropic males [1]. This chapter will review the most relevant aspects of this form of treatment in women.

Basic characteristics

When administered to hypogonadotropic women with intact pituitary and gonadal function (i.e., patients with a selective deficit of endogenous GnRH secretion) pulsatile GnRH is capable of fully restoring the normal pattern of gonadotropin and gonadal steroid secretion of the spontaneous menstrual cycle [1,2]. If a low GnRH dose (2.5–5.0 µg/bolus) is employed the development of a single dominant follicle is usually observed ultrasonographically. The risk of ovarian hyperstimulation is virtually nonexistent with pulsatile GnRH, and the incidence of multiple pregnancy is markedly reduced when compared to gonadotropin administration [3,4]. Therefore, endocrine monitoring with daily estrogens is not required with pulsatile GnRH, and pelvic ultrasound is needed mostly for the identification of the preovulatory period

---

Requests for reprints: Dr Marco Filicori, Clinica Ostetrica e Ginecologica, via Massarenti 13, 40138 Bologna, Italy. Fax: +39-51-222101.

and to target intercourse or artificial insemination. Basal body temperature (BBT) measurements nicely overlap with endogenous progesterone secretion after ovulation is induced with pulsatile GnRH and can be effectively used to monitor efficacy of this form of treatment. Pulsatile GnRH administration can be continued with the same regimen throughout the luteal phase; if menses do not occur within 2 weeks after the presumed ovulation and the BBT remains elevated βhCG determinations are warranted to diagnose pregnancy. Alternatively, exogenous hCG administration (1—2,000 units every 3 days, thrice daily) can be employed for corpus luteum support, but in this case serum βhCG determinations as a pregnancy test must be delayed until exogenous hCG has been cleared (at least 1—2 weeks).

Regimens of GnRH administration

In general, pulsatile GnRH is administered at a dose per bolus of between 2.5—20.0 µg given at 60—90-min intervals [3]. We recently showed [5] that a low GnRH dose of 2.5—5.0 µg given at 60 min intervals is associated with a remarkably low incidence of multiple pregnancy and should thus be preferred, particularly as a first course of treatment. An automatic pump is required for pulsatile GnRH administration. Although several manufacturers produce infusion devices that can be adapted, the Ferring Zyklomat pump appears to be optimal for this form of treatment. Older Zyklomat models were fitted with soft plastic reservoirs containing the GnRH solution (about 10 ml); occasional reservoir leaking could damage the electric and mechanical components of the pump. Furthermore, administration regimens were limited both in terms of bolus volume (50 µl) and frequency of administration (90- or 120-min intervals); GnRH bolus dose could only be changed by varying GnRH concentration in the infusion fluid, while GnRH pulse frequency could not be modified beyond the two preset values. These frequency limitations were particularly severe in the treatment of anovulatory women as the physiologic circhoral frequency of spontaneous follicular phase LH peaks [6] could not be exactly reproduced. Although increasing the GnRH dose is capable of limiting the negative impact of a suboptimal GnRH frequency [7], excessive GnRH dosages should be avoided as they are associated with a greater risk of multiple conception [8]. The new Zyklomat pump that was recently made available in Europe is manufactured by Disetronic Medical Systems, weighs only 90 g and has dimensions of 84 × 54 × 19 mm. The GnRH solution is contained in a rigid vial hermetically separated from the electronic and mechanical apparatus. GnRH dose and frequency of administration can respectively vary between 1—50 µg (at 1 µg steps) and between 5—240 min (at 5 min steps), thus allowing an extremely flexible range of regimens.

Prognostic factors

Although the majority of anovulatory women without ovarian failure will eventually ovulate, certain endocrine and clinical features may predispose patients to better or worse response to pulsatile GnRH. As shown by us and other groups [2,5,9] the better candidates for pulsatile GnRH are represented by hypogonadotropic women of normal or low weight. In most of these subjects reduced pituitary and gonadal function is related to inadequate endogenous GnRH secretion; thus, that pulsatile GnRH will correct their fundamental endocrine disturbance and ovulatory rates of 85% per cycle or more can be expected. Paradoxically, optimal restoration of menstrual cycle endocrine dynamics can be achieved in those hypogonadotropic patients with the most severe reductions in endogenous GnRH secretion (women with primary hypogonadotropic amenorrhea) [2]. Other patients with less severe hypogonadotropic disorders (secondary amenorrhea or oligomenorrhea) respond equally well in terms of ovulatory rates but may be exposed to a greater risk of multiple conception [5], probably in relation to maintained or enhanced pituitary gonadotropin reserve [2].

Conversely, hyperandrogenic women are less responsive to pulsatile GnRH and ovulation may be achieved in 60% or less of cycles [5,9]. Other negative prognostic parameters include elevated LH and insulin as well as excessive weight [5]. Reduced response in hyperandrogenic subjects may be related to high intraovarian androgen levels, a condition associated with increased follicular atresia and dysfunctional follicular development [10]. Obesity compounds problems in hyperandrogenism and it is not uncommon that less than 40% of cycles in these patients result in ovulation. GnRH agonist pretreatment improves response in hyperandrogenic patients with polycystic ovaries (PCO) as will be discussed later in this chapter but obesity negatively affects treatment even after this combined regimen [11].

Women with multifollicular ovaries (MFO) are often mistaken for PCO patients although MFO subjects are not hyperandrogenic. Pulsatile GnRH is an excellent treatment option for MFO patients, and ovulatory and pregnancy rates comparable to the ones of hypogonadotropic subjects can be expected [5,12].

Clinical results and complications

We recently completed the evaluation of 600 consecutive pulsatile GnRH treatment cycles in 292 patients [5] which represents the largest series so far reported by a single group. This and other recent large studies [4,8,9] provide a consistent picture of the clinical results that can be achieved with this form of treatment (Table 1).

In the general patient population, the mean ovulatory rates obtainable with pulsatile GnRH are in the range of 70–75% [5,9]. Better results (80–95% ovulatory rates) can be achieved when treating hypogonadotropic patients [4,5,9] while PCO subjects do not appear to respond in more than 40–50% of cycles [5,9]. General pregnancy rates per treatment cycle range between 18–23% [5,9]; higher and lower pregnancy rates per cycle can be expected in hypogonadotropic and PCO patients, respectively [4,5,9]. However, we showed [5] that once ovulation is achieved, no significant difference in the pregnancy rate existed among the different disorder

Table 1. Clinical results obtained with pulsatile GnRH ovulation induction in four recent large studies

	Homburg et al. [9]	Braat et al. [8]	Martin et al. [4]	Filicori et al. [5]
Patients	118	NR	41	292
Cycles	434	NR	118	600
Pregnancies	100	223	NR	105
Ovulatory rates (%)	70	NR	93	75
Pregnancy rates per treatment cycle (%)	23	NR	29	18
Multiple pregnancy rates (%)	7.0	13.5	8.3	3.8
Abortion rates (%)	28.0	10.3	23.8	29.5

NR: not reported.

groups. In the same study we also demonstrated that ovulatory rates were improved in the hyperandrogenic patients by pretreatment with a GnRH agonist (Buserelin, 300 µg, s.c. twice a day for 4–8 weeks). We hypothesize that such regimen reduces not only serum [11,13] but also intraovarian androgen levels, thus creating an ovarian environment more conducive to normal folliculogenesis [10]; once ovulation is achieved, however, conception is not affected by this regimen.

A wide range of multiple pregnancy rates (3.8 to 13.5%) has been reported (Table 1); several factors may affect the occurrence of this complication. Patients with less severe forms of hypogonadotropic hypogonadism (not primary amenorrhea) run the greater risk of multiple conception (about 8%) [4,5,8,9]. The incidence of multiple pregnancy (Table 1) is also influenced by GnRH dose, as indicated in the multicenter study of Braat et al. [8]; when a low GnRH dose (5 µg/bolus or less) is applied the risk of multiple pregnancy is 8.3% or less. Other factors can be relevant as showed in our recent study [5]: only a total of one multiple pregnancy occurred in our primary hypogonadotropic amenorrhea group (31 pregnancies in 161 cycles), and in pulsatile GnRH cycles performed in various disorders after GnRH agonist suppression (38 pregnancies in 228 cycles). Thus, our data suggest that in patients with spontaneous (primary amenorrhea) or induced (with GnRH agonist) profound hypogonadotropic hypogonadism, the risk of pulsatile GnRH-induced multiple pregnancy (one out of 69) is comparable to that of spontaneous unstimulated cycles [14].

Pulsatile GnRH is associated with a risk of spontaneous abortion of around 20–30% per pregnancy (Table 1). Braat et al. [8] reported a lower (10.3%) rate but in their study miscarriages occurring before the 4th week from ovulation were not counted. Particularly in PCO patients this complication appears to be common (40–45%) and to occur very early in pregnancy [3,9]. The pathogenesis of spontaneous abortion is not clear although it was suggested that high follicular phase LH levels may be detrimental [15]. Nevertheless, we were not able to find a relationship between high LH and spontaneous abortion [5,11].

Conclusions

The extensive experience accrued in these years permits to conclude that pulsatile GnRH is effective and safe for the treatment of anovulation in infertile women. The absence of ovarian hyperstimulation and the low incidence of multiple pregnancy permits one to limit monitoring of pulsatile GnRH to ovarian ultrasound while avoiding daily estrogen determinations. Thus, pulsatile GnRH should be considered the first treatment option after clomiphene in the management of ovulatory disorders.

Acknowledgements

I wish to thank Mrs. Silvia Arsento for outstanding secretarial assistance.

References

1. Crowley WF Jr, Filicori M, Spratt DI, Santoro NF. Rec Prog Horm Res 1985;41:473–531.
2. Filicori M, Flamigni C, Meriggiola MC, Ferrari P, Michelacci L, Campaniello E, Valdiserri A, Cognigni G. J Clin Endocrinol Metab 1991;72:965–972.
3. Filicori M, Flamigni C, Meriggiola MC, Cognigni G, Valdiserri A, Ferrari P, Campaniello E. Fertil Steril 1991;56:1–13.
4. Martin KA, Hall JE, Adams JM, Crowley WF Jr. J Clin Endocrinol Metab 1993;77:125–129.
5. Filicori M, Flamigni C, Dellai P, Cognigni G, Michelacci L, Arnone R, Sambataro M, Falbo A. Treatment of anovulation with pulsatile GnRH: prognostic factors and clinical results in 600 cycles. J Clin Endocrinol Metab 1994 (in press).
6. Filicori M, Santoro NF, Merriam GR, Crowley WF Jr. J Clin Endocrinol Metab 1986;62:1136–1144.
7. Filicori M, Flamigni C, Campaniello E, Ferrari P, Meriggiola MC, Michelacci L, Pareschi A, Valdiserri A. Am J Physiol 1989;257:E930–E936.
8. Braat DDM, Ayalon D, Blunt SM Bogchelmant D, Coelingh Bennink HJT, Handelsman DJ, Heineman MJ, Lappöhn RE, Lorijn RHW, Rolland R, Willemsen WMP, Schoemaker J. Gynecol Endocrinol 1989;3:35–44.
9. Homburg R, Eshel A, Armar NA, Tucker M, Mason PW, Adams J, Kilborn J, Sutherland IA. Br Med J 1989;298:809–812.
10. Louvet JP, Harman SM, Schreiber JR, Ross GT. Endocrinology 1975;97:366–72.
11. Filicori M, Flamigni C, Campaniello E, Valdiserri A, Ferrari P, Meriggiola MC, Michelacci L, Pareschi A. J Clin Endocrinol Metab 1989;69:825–831.
12. Adams J, Franks S, Polson DW, Mason HD, Abdulwahid N, Tucker M. Lancet 1985;2:1375–1379.
13. Filicori M, Campaniello E, Michelacci L, Pareschi A, Ferrari P, Bolelli GF, Flamigni C. J Clin Endocrinol Metab 1988;66:327–333.
14. Benirschke K, Kim CK. N Engl J Med 1973;288:1276–1284.
15. Shoham Z, Jacobs HS, Insler V. Fertil Steril 1993;59:1153–1161.

Appropriate regimens of pulsatile gonadotropin-releasing hormone (GnRH) administration

Gilbert B. Wilshire and Nanette Santoro*

Department of Obstetrics and Gynecology, UMDNJ — New Jersey Medical School, 185 South Orange Avenue, Newark, NJ 07103-2714, USA

Abstract. Various indications and methodologies for the pulsatile administration of GnRH are reviewed. Normal hypothalamic-pituitary physiology is explained and the relevant pharmacology of GnRH therapies are discussed. Ovulation induction requires closely reproducing the normal GnRH pulsatility seen in menstruating women. Intravenous administration of GnRH with a portable pump appears to be the most effective method of inducing ovulation in a large number of scenarios. Proper patient selection may also maximize successes with the subcutaneous injection route as well. Current treatment systems are very safe, effective and have a high level of patient acceptance.

Introduction

The pulsatile administration of GnRH for the correction of hypogonadotropic hypogonadism is a therapy which developed rapidly from studies of primate physiology. After the pioneering work of Ernst Knobil and co-workers in the 1970s, human pregnancies were soon reported by Leyendecker and colleagues by mimicking the innate pulsatility of hypothalamic GnRH with an automated intravenous pump [1–4]. Soon thereafter a number of groups around the world were reporting successful ovulation induction and pregnancies in women with hypothalamic amenorrhea (HA) [5–7]. Therapeutic pulsatile GnRH administration is now a proven therapy for HA. Most groups induce ovulation in well over 90% of attempted cycles [5,8,9]. Other indications for this therapy now include ovulation induction for women with hyperprolactinemia, oligo-ovulation (polycystic ovarian syndrome — PCOS), and both sexes for delayed puberty or Kallmann syndrome [10–14].

Physiology of GnRH administration

Because it is not practical to measure GnRH directly from the hypophyseal portal system of humans, investigators have relied upon the measurement of peripheral LH as a surrogate marker of central GnRH activity. Luteinizing hormone's accessibility

---

Address for reprints: Nanette Santoro, Department of Obstetrics and Gynecology, UMDNJ — New Jersey Medical School, 185 South Orange Avenue, Newark, NJ 07103-2714, USA.

from the peripheral circulation and its short half-life make its measurement practical and accurate. The frequency of LH pulsations gives us precise information regarding the frequency of hypothalamic electrical activity but reveals little information regarding the quantity of portal GnRH secreted per pulse [15]. It is important to keep this distinction in mind when evaluating the following physiological data and treatment modalities.

In the early follicular phase of the human menstrual cycle, LH pulsations are observed at roughly 90-min intervals. They then increase in frequency to approximately every 60–70 min in the late follicular phase. After ovulation, LH pulsations decrease to a frequency of every 100 min and then further decrease to a frequency of roughly every 200 min by the late luteal phase [16]. Treatment regimens which have imitated this physiologic pulse frequency have met with excellent success; however, other regimens which have used different fixed dosing schedules (e.g., pulses every 60, 90, 120 min or even twice a day) have also fostered pregnancies [17–20]. A minimum frequency of 2 h appears to be required for women with complete absence of endogenous gonadotropin-releasing hormone secretion [18]. Nonetheless, the hypothalamic-pituitary axis does not require strict adherence to a specific pulse frequency pattern to perform. Evidence indicates that pulse shape and hormone concentration play a large role in determining pituitary response [21–23]. Pulses which display a waveform with a steep, brief rise in hormone concentration are the most effective in producing pulsatile LH secretion [24]. Continuous GnRH infusion or pulse frequencies faster than every 30 min uniformly decrease pituitary gonadotropin secretion [1,14]. Higher doses result in a preferential increase in LH secretion and less frequent pulses can result in preferred secretion of FSH [14,15]. Pulsatile GnRH most efficiently causes gonadotropin release when it is given at frequent, hourly intervals. Less frequent administration schedules can also be effective, however, if pulse doses are increased disproportionately [18,20].

Body composition has a significant impact on GnRH distribution volume and half-life, therefore, therapeutic effectiveness. Women of normal body weight demonstrate a half-life for exogenously administered GnRH of 5.6 min with an apparent volume of distribution of 12 l. Obese women (>50% overweight) demonstrate an approximate doubling of their GnRH distribution volumes to 20.6 l with no significant changes in hormonal half-life. Anorexic women (approximately 60% normal body weight) display a halving of the distribution volume to 6.5 liters and a significant increase in half-life to 7.3 min [25]. These findings indicate that obese women require higher doses whereas slender women require lower doses of hormone to produce equivalent serum gonadotropin concentrations.

Routes of GnRH administration

Synthetic GnRH has been administered via the intravenous (IV), subcutaneous (SC), intranasal (IN) and the transdermal (TD) routes [9,26–28]. Presently, only the IV and SC routes have successful track records and both are viable treatment options in selected patients.

Peripheral IV administration of pulsatile GnRH results in pituitary portal vein hormone concentrations which are similar to those which result from endogenous hypothalamic secretion. This pulsatile therapy can produce menstrual cycles which are indistinguishable from normal, spontaneous menstrual cycles [29,30]. IV administration of any medication, however, is dependent on ease of venous access, the ability to maintain the line, and the presence of any contraindications to indwelling IV catheters. Studies which employed the use of peripheral IV catheters demonstrated the safety of these devices. One study (which used fastidious care of IV sites and a closed infusion system) reported the results from 1958 catheter-days. Catheter-tip and blood cultures were taken after the discontinuation of every line. There were no episodes of fever, only three catheters were removed because of signs of local inflammation, and 11% of the catheter tips grew bacteria in culture. An important finding was that the chance of infection at the IV site actually decreased with insertion times greater than 7 days. Two patients with positive blood cultures for *S. epidermidis* also had positive catheter-tip cultures for this organism. These authors concluded that long-term IV GnRH administration is safe in the vast majority of individuals but those patients with cardiac lesions who are susceptible to endocardial infection should either employ very short-term (i.e., 48 h) IV catheterization with frequent changing of sites or consider another route of administration [31]. Another study observed no case of regional cellulitis out of 63 consecutive cycles although 24% of the catheters were changed for reasons of local inflammation or pain [19].

In general, it is our experience that women tolerate IV GnRH therapy very well and its use is simpler than it originally appears. The portable GnRH pump (Lutrepulse; Ferring Laboratories, Suffern, NY) is easily concealed under most clothing, and daily activities are not curtailed. Activities such as showering can be performed after wrapping the IV site with plastic wrap and placing the pump just outside the shower stall. Virtually any outdoor activity can be performed as long as the pump is well supported (usually around the waist with an elastic belt). Occasionally an Orthodox Jewish patient is not permitted to maintain an IV line during the Mikvah ritual but if the line can be restarted within several hours this has not affected the success of the treatment.

An alternative to IV GnRH administration is the SC route. Because the drug must pass through interstitial and capillary tissues the mechanisms of SC absorption should be contemplated before deciding to use this route of administration. Medications which are injected into the SC space undergo a two-step process of absorption. First, the medication solution must be injected at a pressure sufficient to break open the subdermal connective tissue (usually 30–40 mm water) and infiltrate the area as a functional depot injection. The efficiency of this step can be decreased if significant degradation of the compound occurs within the tissue. The second step requires the transcapillary absorption of the material into the blood. This step is directly proportional to the amount of vascular membrane within the tissue and is highly variable from person to person and between anatomical areas. Some clinical evidence indicates that SC injection in the upper arm at the base of the deltoid muscle is absorbed most effectively [32]. Histamines which increase outward vascular permeability clearly decrease rates of absorption. Lymphatic absorption appears to be negligible [33].

Clinical observations after SC GnRH administration are consistent with the mechanisms of SC absorption discussed above. Protease activity consumes approximately one third of the peptide before capillary uptake can occur and GnRH pulse profiles exhibit a sinusoidal rather than a sharp pulse wave form. Studies in humans show that rapid bolus infusions of GnRH are the most effective way to achieve pulsatile gonadotropin secretion [21]. Therefore SC GnRH administration would appear to be less effective than the IV route for pituitary stimulation.

SC administration of GnRH, although relatively inefficient, has some advantages over the IV route and may be preferable in certain situations. The injection site (usually a butterfly-type needle placed near the umbilicus) can be changed by the patient or any properly instructed individual at home because the technique is so simple. This may allow women to have greater flexibility regarding physical activities since the pump can easily be disconnected during swimming, for example, and restarted with little or no interruption in drug administration. Patients with valvular heart lesions can also use the pump with safety because the capillary bed acts as a filter to bacterial contamination. This method is still a very effective treatment for the induction of puberty and the maintenance of spermatogenesis in men with Kallmann syndrome or idiopathic hypogonadotropic hypogonadism [12]. Studies involving treatment of anovulatory women with hypothalamic amenorrhea have reported ovulation success rates between 65 and 100% per cycle [6,7,34]. Some compensation for the SC route in the form of increased dosing appears to be necessary. Although these rates are overall lower than those reported from IV treatment, they are still successful in a majority of individuals. Theoretically, slender patients (because of their decreased volume of distribution and probable faster rate of SC absorption) should experience sharper GnRH concentration peaks and better gonadotropin responses than overweight patients. Clinically, these considerations would appear to be borne out.

Alternate modes of GnRH administration include the IN and TD routes. Both IN and TD routes can be expected to avoid any first-pass effects of liver metabolism. Although the IN route is appealing because of its nonreliance upon needles, in the only reported clinical use of the technique, inconsistent absorption and an obvious inability to use the medication during sleep was evident [27]. Although the continuous TD administration of steroids and anticholinergic medications is now common in medical practice, a method for the pulsatile TD administration of small charged peptides is still being developed. The stratum corneum of the dermis is 15–20 cells thick and is relatively impermeable to most compounds. The tissue is composed largely of lipids. The layer can be made semipermeable to charged molecules, however, with the application of low amperage, direct electrical current (iontophoresis). The administration of the peptide via this route can theoretically be precisely controlled by the timing and amount of current applied to skin patches. Early work with TD iontophoresis of the GnRH agonist leuprolide in human volunteers has met with success in acutely elevating serum LH levels. Patches were generally well tolerated and LH responses were seen as early as 60 min after current was applied. The effect of pulsatile current application was not reported [28]. Recent in vitro work with GnRH and its analogues in a mouse skin model confirms that native GnRH undergoes significant intradermal degradation. Pulsatile iontophoresis was successful with a protease-resistant superagonist, however, and clinical applications are awaited in the near future [35].

GnRH pulse frequencies and doses

The hypothalamic-pituitary-gonadal axis responds to a wide spectrum of exogenously administered GnRH pulse frequencies. The sexually immature male patient (due to idiopathic hypogonadotropic hypogonadism or Kallmann syndrome) responds successfully to hourly SC administration even when given only at night [36]. Pulses given every 2 h also appear effective in these individuals [12,37].

The process of ovulation in women appears to be more exacting in its requirements of GnRH pulsatility than does spermatogenesis and sexual maturation in men. As noted previously, women in the follicular phase demonstrate a GnRH pulse frequency between 60 to 90 min [15]. For this reason most studies have used pulse frequencies between 60 and 90 min with equivalent clinical results [5,19,29]. When a pulse frequency of 120 min was directly compared to a once-hourly pulse regimen, the faster physiological rate produced a significantly higher rate of ovulation (94% vs. 79%) and higher midcycle LH surges and luteal phase progesterone levels [18]. It was also noted that higher GnRH doses at slower rates of delivery could reduce the observed differences.

GnRH pulse frequency decreases significantly in the luteal phase but the hypothalamic-pituitary-ovarian axis appears capable of tolerating a wide range of pulse frequencies at this time. GnRH pumps are frequently left in place throughout the luteal phase with no adjustment of the 90-min pulse frequency. In clinical use, slowing the pulse frequency to once every 4 h provides equivalent luteal support and provides the potential for less drug use and cost savings [17,29,38]. GnRH pulse doses are frequently computed on a ng/kg or a total mass per bolus basis. Most IV GnRH treatment regimens use GnRH at a dose between 25 and 400 ng/kg or approximately 1 to 20 µg per bolus [11,29]. The large majority of normal weight women with pure HA respond well to doses of 5 µg per bolus or less; we routinely start most of our patients on this dose [18,29]. Growth of a single dominant follicle should be expected. Multiple gestations increase in frequency when the dose per bolus is increased to over 10 µg [9,39]. Oligo-ovulation associated with PCOD is also known to respond to pulsatile GnRH but it has a lower success rate per cycle and may require higher doses to be effective [12,40]. These findings are understandable from a physiological point of view because the defect in these women is not due to hypofunction of the hypothalamus but an increased or abnormal pulse frequency [41,42]. There is evidence that pituitary downregulation with long-term GnRH agonist suppression before pulsatile GnRH therapy is helpful in these patients [12]. Recent data indicates that pulsatile GnRH therapy, when given continually for 2 months, results in improved responses in the second cycle [43]. It is hypothesized that the inducement of ovarian progesterone secretion may slow hypothalamic activity and render the next cycle more conducive to ovulation. Both of the above modifications for women with PCOS may enable lower doses of medication to be effective.

Patient selection

The decision to employ gonadotropins (hMG) or pulsatile GnRH for ovulation induction should be made by the patient-physician team after considering the pros and cons of the two therapies. Pumps must be worn 24 h a day while hMG is usually given once a day. Neither regimen avoids injections but the pump can frequently be started and maintained with just one needle stick. Patients usually tolerate the pump quite well and make the proper adjustments in their activities easily. Because ovulation induction with the pump is associated with a normal rate of follicular growth and a trivial rate of hyperstimulation (when used alone), cycle monitoring with ultrasound scans and blood steroid levels can be minimized [38]. This can be an attractive option for busy patients who must frequently make short-notice changes in their schedules. In the absence of a significant infertility problem in the male partner, the couple can rely on timed intercourse to achieve pregnancy. This may further add to the flexibility of this treatment regimen. Patients must also be counselled as to the success rates which are typically seen with their particular diagnosis. Women with isolated HA as a cause of their infertility can expect a normal monthly fecundity rate (22%) with a >90% chance of pregnancy after 1 year [9]. Results in women with PCOS are significantly less successful (50—75% ovulation rate, 30—40% eventual pregnancy rate) although recent modifications in GnRH treatment may improve these odds [40].

The cost-effectiveness of hMG vs. pulsatile GnRH administration may also be an important consideration when choosing a particular treatment modality. Women with HA can expect to use low doses of GnRH and will usually be pregnant within 3 to 6 months. Pulsatile GnRH is the most economical treatment option for these women [29]. The cost to benefit ratio for couples with additional infertility factors is much less clear.

Clinical monitoring

Women undergoing their first cycle of pulsatile GnRH therapy may exhibit an accelerated ovarian response due to the additive effects of administered hormone to that from endogenous hypothalamic activity. Couples should be advised to have regular intercourse during these cycles because the follicular phase may be shortened and ovulation may occur earlier than expected. If subsequent cycles are attempted in a consecutive fashion they usually follow a more predictable pattern. Follicular monitoring can therefore be relaxed. We have monitored women with hypothalamic amenorrhea and even PCOS simply with home urine monitoring for the LH surge alone. When clinical data are confusing, serial sonographic and steroid level evaluations define the progress of the cycle in question.

Patients can also be instructed to inspect and care for the IV insertion site. Although the safety of long-term, closed-system IV catheters is well established, patients should be instructed to take their temperatures daily and call their doctors if the injection site appears at all suspicious for phlebitis. If a patient appears ill without an obvious alternative explanation, the physician should have a low threshold for removing the line and obtaining blood cultures.

On a practical note, patients using the Lutrepulse pump may sometimes experience a progressive back up of blood into their IV tubing. The cause for this may not be clear. The screen may stay lit even though the peristaltic pump is not working and a break in the system has been ruled out by inspection. This complication is usually due to an undetected exhaustion of the lithium battery, a separate battery from the 9 volt cell which directly powers the pumping mechanism. The patient changes the 9 volt cell every 1 to 2 weeks. Replacement of the lithium battery, which is located under the drug reservoir, is required every 2 years.

Alternate methodologies

Pulsatile GnRH therapy may be continued indefinitely until pregnancy is established. This type of treatment regimen mimics the physiological events which occur in a normal cycling woman. Unfortunately, it also requires that the patient wear the pump without a rest. An alternative to continuing the infusion throughout the luteal phase is the substitution of exogenous hCG for this purpose. The pump can be removed as soon as this hormone is provided. Luteal support with 500 to 1,500 IU of hCG given intramuscularly every 2 to 3 days appears to be adequate in maintaining the function of the corpus luteum [38,44]. This treatment option, although equally efficacious as pulsatile GnRH therapy, invalidates early pregnancy testing and requires reinsertion of the IV should the cycle not be successful in producing a pregnancy.

Some studies have been performed with pumps other than the Pulsamat, Zyklomat or Lutrepulse devices. If pulse-dose volumes are reasonably accurate and are similar to those tested in the original pumps (25–50 µl) then clinical results should be equivalent. Some home-care nursing agencies encourage the use of percutaneous intracardiac catheters (PICC lines) or other central lines in their patients who use long-term IV therapies. We do not use these types of delivery systems because of the unknown effect of dead space within the tubing. We are also hesitant to add additional hardware to a system that is elegant in its simplicity and already very safe in its present design.

References

1. Belchetz PE, Plant TM, Nakai Y, Keogh EJ, Knobil E. Science 1978;202:631–633.
2. Knobil E, Plant TM, Wildt L, Belchetz PE, Marshall G. Science 1980;207:1371–1373.
3. Knobil E. Biol Reprod 1981;24:44–49.
4. Leyendecker G, Wildt L, Hansmann M. J Clin Endocrinol Metab 1980;51:1214–1216.
5. Santoro N, Wierman ME, Filicori M et al. J Clin Endocrinol Metab 1986;62:109–116.
6. Reid RL, Leopold GR, Yen SSC. Fertil Steril 1981;36:553–559.
7. Hurley DM, Brian R, Outch K, Stockdale J, Fry A, Hackman C, Clarke I, Burger HG. N Engl J Med 1984;310:1069–1074.
8. Jansen RPS, Handelsman DJ, Boylan LM, Conway A, Shearman RP, Fraser IS. Fertil Steril 1987;48:33–38.
9. Braat DDM, Schoemaker R, Schoemaker J. Fertil Steril 1991;55:266–270.
10. Leyendecker G, Struve T, Plotz EJ. Arch Gynecol 1980;229:177–190.
11. Hurwitz A, Rosenn B, Palti Z, Ebstein B, Har-Nir R, Ron M. Fertil Steril 1986;46:378–384.
12. Filicori M, Campanillo E, Michelacci L, Pareschi A, Ferrari P, Bolelli G, Flamigni C. J Clin Endocrinol Metab 1988;66: 327–333.
13. Hoffman AR, Crowley WF. N Eng J Med 1982;307:1237–1241.
14. Delemarre-van de Waal HA, Schoemaker J. Acta Endocrinol (Kbh) 1983;102:603–609.
15. Wildt L, Hausler A, Marshall G, Hutchison JS, Plant TM, Belchetz PE, Knobil E. Endocrinology 1981;109:376–385.
16. Filicori M, Santoro N, Merriam G, Crowley WF. J Clin Endocrinol Metab 1986;62:1136–1144.
17. Braat DDM, Schoemaker J. Fertil Steril 1991;56:1054–1059.
18. Filicori M, Flamigni C, Campaniello E, Ferrari P, Meriggiola MC, Michelacci L, Pareschi A, Valdiserri A. Am J Physiol 1989;257:E930–E936.
19. Bringer J, Hedon B, Jaffiol C, Nicolau S, Gilbert F, Cristol P, Orsetti A, Viala J-L, Mirouze J. Fertil Steril 1985;44:42–48.
20. Hammond CB, Wiebe RH, Haney AF, Yancy SG. Am J Obstet Gynecol 1979;135:924–939.
21. Handelsman DJ, Boylan LM. J Clin Endocrinol Metab 1988;67:175–179.
22. Handelsman DJ, Jansen RPS, Boylan LM, Spaliviero JA, Turtle JR. J Clin Endocrinol Metab 1984;59:739–746.
23. Filicori M. Fertil Steril 1992;58:643.
24. McIntosh RP, McIntosh JEA. J Endocrinol 1983;98:411–421.
25. Chikamori K, Suehiro F, Ogawa T, Sato K, Mori H, Oshima I, Saito S. Acta Endocrinol (Kbh) 1981;96:1–6.
26. Seibel MM, Kamrava M, McArdle C, Taymor ML. Obstet Gynecol 1983;61:292–297.
27. Hanker JP, Bohnet HG, Schneider HPL. Neuroendocrinol Lett 1980;2:269.
28. Meyer BR, Kreis W, Eschbach J, O'Hara V, Rosen S, Sibalis D. Clin Pharmacol Ther 1988;44:607–612.
29. Martin K, Santoro N, Hall J, Filicori M, Wierman M, Crowley WF. J Clin Endocrinol Metab 1990;71:1081A–1081G.
30. Schriock ED, Jaffe RB. Obstet Gynecol Surv 1986;41:414–423.
31. Hopkins CC, Hall JE, Santoro NF, Martin KA, Filicori M, Crowley WF. Obstet Gynecol 1989;74:267–270.
32. Blunt SM, Menon BRK, Butt WR. In: Bloom SR, Jacobs HS (eds) Therapeutic applications of LHRH. London, Royal Society of Medicine Services, 1986:89–98.
33. Schou J. Pharmacol Rev 1961;13:441–464.
34. Mason P, Adams J, Morris DV, Tucker M, Price J, Voulgaris Z, Van Der Spuy ZM, Sutherland I, Chambers GR, White S, Wheeler MJ, Jacobs HS. Br Med J 1984;288:181–185.
35. Miller L, Kolaskie CJ, Smith GA, Rivier J. J Pharm Sci 1990;79:490–493.
36. Jacobson RI, Seyler LE, Tamborlane WV, Gertner JM, Genel M. J Clin Endocrinol Metab 1979;49:652–654.

37. Spratt DI, Crowley WF, Butler JP, Hoffman AR, Conn PM, Badger TM. J Clin Endocrinol Metab 1985;61:890–895.
38. Santoro N. Am J Obstet Gynecol 1990;163:1759–1764.
39. Braat DDM, Ayalon D, Blunt SM, Bogchelman D, Coelingh-Bennink HJT, Handelsman DJ, Heineman MJ, Lappohn RE, Lorijn RHW, Rolland R, Willemsen WMP, Schoemaker J. Gynecol Endocrinol 1989;3:35–44.
40. Filicori M, Flamigni C, Meriggiola MC, Cognigni G, Valdiserri A, Ferrari P, Campaniello E. Fertil Steril 1991;56:1–13.
41. Kazer RR, Kessel B, Yen SSC. J Clin Endocrinol Metab 1987;65:233.
42. Waldstreicher J, Santoro N, Hall JE, Filicori M, Crowley WF Jr. J Clin Endocrinol Metab 1988;66:165–172.
43. Corenthal L, Von Hagen S, Larkins D, Ibrahim J, Santoro N. Benefits of continuous physiologic pulsatile gonadotropin-releasing hormone therapy in women with polycystic ovarian syndrome. Fertil Steril 1994 (in press).
44. Santoro N, Elzahr D. Clin Obstet Gynecol 1993;36:727–736.

Pulsatile GnRH in hypogonadotropic hypogonadism

Kathryn A. Martin*, Janet Hall, Judith Adams and William F. Crowley Jr*

Reproductive Endocrine Unit, Department of Medicine, Massachusetts General Hospital, Boston, Massachusetts, USA

Introduction

Hypothalamic or hypogonadotropic amenorrhea is a disorder of ovulation, characterized by a spectrum of abnormal patterns of endogenous hypothalamic GnRH secretion, all of which are insufficient to sustain normal folliculogenesis and subsequent ovulation [1–3]. Therefore, these GnRH-deficient patients represent ideal candidates for exogenous GnRH replacement. However, until recently, only two agents were available for ovulation induction in these hypogonadotropic patients. Clomiphene citrate, whose mechanism of action is to increase FSH through blockade of estrogen negative feedback, is often ineffective in this hypoestrogenic group. Exogenous gonadotropins act directly on the ovary to stimulate folliculogenesis, resulting in high rates of ovulation and conception. However, gonadotropin therapy is associated with a significant risk of complications including multiple gestation, which is estimated to be as high as 24–50% for hypogonadotropic patients [4–6] and ovarian hyperstimulation syndrome, a potentially life-threatening complication [7].

The most recently available form of therapy for ovulation induction, intravenous pulsatile gonadotropin-releasing hormone (GnRH), was approved by the FDA in 1989 for use in women with primary amenorrhea. There are several theoretical advantages to pulsatile GnRH when compared to exogenous gonadotropin therapy. Exogenous pulsatile GnRH maintains normal pituitary-ovarian feedback mechanisms, employing rising levels of estradiol to restrain endogenous FSH secretion, resulting in the development of a single follicle [8]. With the potential decreased risk of multiple folliculogenesis, multiple gestation and ovarian hyperstimulation, a decreased need for intensive monitoring and possibly a decrease in cost would be anticipated.

Until recently, there had been no direct comparisons of these two forms of therapy using uniform diagnostic criteria and monitoring tools, and identified outcome measures to compare results. To explore issues of efficacy and safety with exogenous gonadotropins and pulsatile GnRH, we recently completed a retrospective analysis of patients with hypogonadotropic amenorrhea undergoing ovulation induction with a standard regimen of exogenous gonadotropins or pulsatile GnRH [9]. Outlined below

---

Request for reprint contact phone number: K.A. Martin MD and Crowley WF Jr. +31-617-726-8433.

is a review of 1) the clinical management of hypogonadotropic hypogonadal patients with pulsatile GnRH, including results of our dose experiments; and 2) a comparison of clinical results of pulsatile GnRH vs. exogenous gonadotropin therapy.

Pulsatile GnRH: protocol for administration

Route: i.v. vs. s.c.

We routinely use the intravenous route of administration, as more physiologic LH profiles when GnRH is administered intravenously when compared to the subcutaneous route [10]. In addition, ovulatory rates are significantly higher with i.v. GnRH. To date, over 300 cycles of subcutaneous pulsatile GnRH have been reported in patients with hypothalamic amenorrhea or idiopathic hypogonadotropic hypogonadism, with approximately 75% of cycles resulting in ovulation, and a 30% conception rate per ovulatory cycle [11]. In contrast, over 550 cycles of intravenous GnRH have been reported, with a considerably higher (90%) rate of ovulation, but a similar rate (27.6%) of conception per ovulatory cycle [11–14]. Although initial rates of ovulation are lower with the subcutaneous route, some investigators stress the convenience of this route as well as its relatively high rates of success, reserving intravenous GnRH only for those subjects who do not respond favorably. For clinical use, the FDA has thus far approved pulsatile GnRH only for the intravenous route because of the higher ovulatory rates.

When using the intravenous route, we use a 20 gauge 1¼ inch catheter inserted into a forearm vein using sterile technique. The catheter is then attached to a reservoir (Pulsamate™, Ferring Labs) filled with GnRH solution using a 60-inch microvolume extension set (Autosyringe Inc.). The catheter entry site is secured with a sterile transparent dressing (Tegaderm, 3M), and the GnRH solution is delivered using a portable peristaltic pump (Zyklomat™, Ferring). In our experience, patient's acceptance of the intravenous route has been excellent. When sterile technique is used, the line can be left in place for prolonged periods (up to 60 days) with a low risk of infection [15].

Frequency

The earliest reports using pulsatile administration of GnRH to induce ovulation were from women with hypothalamic amenorrhea and Kallmann syndrome [16,17]. In these instances, a fixed frequency of 90 and 120 min, respectively, proved successful in inducing ovulation. Since that time, numerous reports have been published utilizing a fixed frequency of 60 or 90 min with reasonable rates of success.

The frequencies of GnRH secretion that we have employed were derived from studies of normal women during 62 ovulatory cycles [18], and were tested prospectively as a regimen of pulsatile GnRH. A 90-min interval, reflective of the frequency of GnRH secretion of normal women in the early follicular phase, is used for the first week of folliculogenesis. This frequency is then increased to 60 min in the midfollicular phase of the induced cycle until there is clinical and/or ultrasonographic evidence of ovulation (i.e., disappearance of a dominant follicle by ultrasound, an LH surge by urinary monitoring, and/or a clear basal body temperature shift). The frequency of GnRH administration is then slowed to 90 min for one week after ovulation similar to normal women during the early luteal phase [18], and then to 4 h for the remainder of the luteal phase until menses or a positive pregnancy test intervenes.

To date, follicular phase frequencies of either 60 or 90 min in the early follicular phase have not resulted in any significant differences in sex steroid dynamics, ovulation, or pregnancy rates [13].

However, abnormalities have been described when a 60 min frequency is slowed to a 90 min frequency during the follicular phase [12]. This finding may not be surprising since the normal follicular phase is characterized by a speeding, not a slowing, of the hypothalamic secretion as follicular ripening develops. It has also been recently demonstrated that a 60-min frequency throughout the follicular phase is more effective than a 120-min frequency in inducing ovulation and a physiologic LH surge [19]. Taken together, these data suggest that the ovary is capable of tolerating a moderate range of GnRH-induced gonadotropin pulse frequencies for adequate follicular development and corpus luteum function, but that follicular phase frequencies slower than 90 min result in anovulation and abnormalities of the midcycle gonadotropin surge. Further testing will be needed to determine whether such close adherence to physiologic frequencies of GnRH is required for the highest rates of ovulation and/or pregnancy, or whether a fixed frequency of GnRH administration can suffice.

Ovulatory stimulus and luteal phase support

In most large series of GnRH administration, GnRH has been the sole ovulatory stimulus, i.e., human chorionic gonadotropin (hCG) is not required to rupture the ripened follicle since an endogenous LH surge can be induced. This feature of GnRH induction of ovulation is particularly attractive since it appears that large doses of hCG at midcycle appear to be essential to the subsequent development of the ovarian hyperstimulation syndrome occurring with gonadotropin therapy.

Two techniques have been described for supporting the corpus luteum in GnRH-treated women: continuation of pulsatile GnRH or the use of hCG. It has been suggested that there are no differences in pregnancy rates between GnRH or hCG as agents for support of the corpus luteum in an induced ovulatory cycle; however, this assertion has not yet been tested in a prospective fashion. Based upon our experience with continued GnRH administration in the luteal phase, there is no shortening of the luteal phase when GnRH pulse frequency is slowed to every 4 h, the average mid-to-late luteal phase pulse frequency documented in normal women. However, the ultimate selection of an approach to corpus luteum support may depend upon the practicalities of the clinical situation and available resources.

Dosage of pulsatile GnRH

Many studies using pulsatile GnRH have employed large doses. These regimens, involving the use of 10 to 20 µg of GnRH per bolus, yield satisfactory ovulatory rates overall. However, it must be recalled that these results are often obscured by the compounding variable of the subcutaneous route of administration, which generally requires larger doses of GnRH to attain the GnRH pharmacokinetics needed to achieve adequate folliculogenesis. Since subcutaneous GnRH results in distinctly unphysiologic GnRH and gonadotropin levels, the subsequent failure of ovulation may reflect the choice of the subcutaneous route and not merely the dosage employed. When the intravenous route is employed, considerably lower dosages of GnRH can be employed with no sacrifice in efficacy.

We have previously reported results from three doses of GnRH administered intravenously to GnRH-deficient women: 25 ng/kg (approximately 1 µg bolus), 75 ng/kg (3–4 µg) and 100 ng/kg (5 µg) [8,13]. Biochemical results are summarized in Fig. 1.

Results of 10 cycles using 25 ng/kg in seven patients demonstrated that only eight resulted in ovulation, with a single dominant follicle seen by ultrasound in each ovulatory cycle. While the pattern of daily estradiol and progesterone levels was similar to that seen in our normal women, the mean peak E2 level in the 25 ng/kg cycles was significantly lower than that of normal cycles, and integrated progesterone values (as an index of corpus luteum adequacy) were also significantly lower than in normal women. Therefore, 25 ng/kg appears to represent a threshold dose, resulting in an unacceptably low rate of ovulation (80%), and apparent luteal phase deficiency.

Using 75 ng/kg (31 cycles) resulted in midcycle estradiol levels and integrated

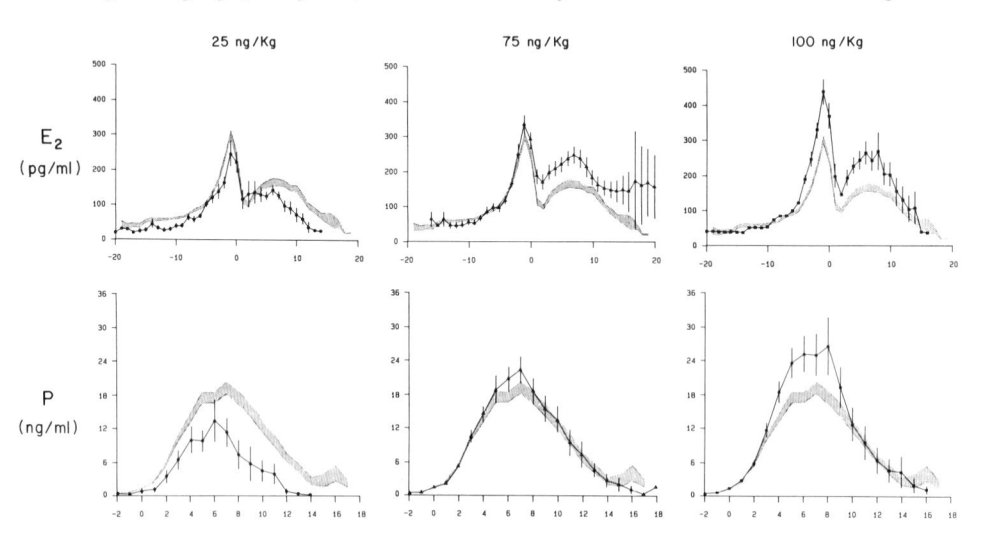

Fig. 1. Serum levels of E2 and progesterone (P) (mean ± SEM) during administration of varying doses of GnRH: 25 ng/kg (n = 10 cycles, 75 ng/kg (n = 31), and 100 ng/kg (n = 25) to women with disordered endogenous GnRH secretion. Mean ± SEM values in 62 normal ovulatory cycles are represented by the shaded areas with day 0 representing the day of the midcycle surge.

luteal phase progesterone levels which were indistinguishable from our normal population (Fig. 1). A single dominant follicle was seen by ultrasound in all ovulatory cycles, except one in which there was a double ovulation. The overall rate of ovulation in the 75 ng/kg group was 95%, which was higher than that seen in the 25 ng/kg group (80%), and similar to that seen in the 100 ng/kg group (93%).

Using 100 ng/kg (approximately 5 µg/bolus), resulted in a 93% ovulatory rate per cycle (14 women in 27 cycles). However, peak estradiol levels were significantly higher than those in either normal cycles or women receiving 25 ng/kg, and the integrated luteal phase progesterone values were significantly higher than those in the 25 ng/kg group.

In this dose study, only two patients failed to ovulate at doses of 75–100 ng/kg, both with complete GnRH deficiency. One who was not interested in fertility chose not to repeat the study at a higher dose, while the second patient subsequently ovulated when the dose was further increased to 100–250 ng/kg (Fig. 2). On 75 ng/kg, this patient appeared to initiate normal folliculogenesis as seen on serial ultrasound examinations, but failed to mount an adequate LH surge. What appeared clinically to be a dominant follicle regressed. When the GnRH dose was increased to 100 ng/kg, an LH surge and ovulation subsequently occurred. However, there was a shortened luteal phase suggestive of an inadequate luteal phase on this dose. In a subsequent 250 ng/kg cycle, the patient had normal folliculogenesis, ovulation and eventually conceived on this dose. Thus, while 75 ng/kg would appear to be the most physiologic dose of GnRH on average as evidenced by the mean gonadotropin and sex steroid levels, there may well be considerable individual variability in dose requirements.

Consequently, initiating therapy with 75 ng/kg of GnRH intravenously appears to mimic the hormonal dynamics of the normal menstrual cycle most closely, and has little risk of hyperstimulation or multiple gestation. Dosages can then be increased in those who fail to respond. In addition, considerable individual differences can also exist in requirements for GnRH. In obese women, for example, GnRH appears to be cleared from serum more rapidly than in their thin counterparts; therefore, larger GnRH doses may be required in obese subjects.

Pulsatile GnRH vs. exogenous gonadotropins

Subjects

Women with hypogonadotropic amenorrhea were defined by the absence of menses for at least 6 months, with low to normal gonadotropins compared to our normal population (n = 87). All patients were of normal body weight (between 10th and 90th percentile of height for weight by the Sargent scale), had no history of excessive exercise, and no evidence of androgen excess (no hirsutism or acne; and normal serum androgen levels when available). In addition, patients had normal TSH and PRL levels.

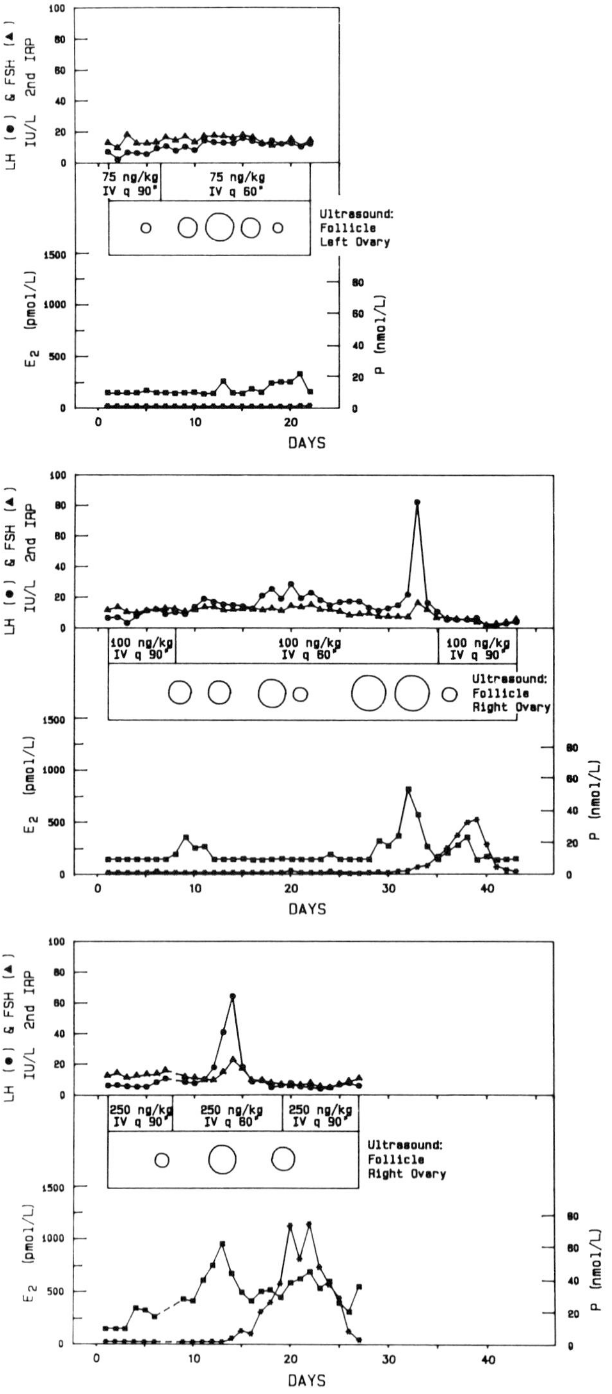

Fig. 2. Serum levels of LH (●–●), FSH (▲–▲), E2 (■–■), and progesterone P (✻–✻) in a patient with Kallmann's syndrome during serial increments of GnRH dosage: 75, 100 and 250 ng/kg (see text for details). Ultrasound data are depicted schematically for each dose.

We have now studied a total of 43 patients in 121 cycles of pulsatile GnRH, and 30 patients receiving exogenous gonadotropins for 111 cycles. Baseline clinical and biochemical characteristics were not different between the pulsatile GnRH and gonadotropin patients in terms of age, body mass index (BMI), LH, FSH, and E2. Hysterosalpingograms were obtained before treatment in both groups to verify tubal patency. Postcoital tests and/or semen analyses were performed routinely with normal parameters considered to be a sperm concentration >20 million/ml, with >50% motility. Patients considered to have male factor infertility were not included in this study with the exception of one couple in the exogenous gonadotropin group undergoing artificial insemination with donor sperm.

Protocol

Pulsatile GnRH was administered as outlined above. Only doses of 75–250 ng/kg were included in this analysis, as 25 ng/kg represents a subphysiologic dose. Exogenous gonadotropins were administered IM daily according to the protocol of Brown et al. [20], using a starting dose of 150 IU. If there was evidence of follicular development by plasma estradiol and ultrasound on day 5 of treatment, the same dose was continued until follicular diameter was greater than or equal to 1.8 cm, with a corresponding estradiol of approximately 734 pmol/l/follicle. If there was no evidence of follicular development, the dose was increased by approximately 30%. An ovulatory dose of hCG (3,000–5,000 units IM) was given at the time of follicular maturation, but was withheld (cycle cancelled), if E2 was >4405 pmol/l, or if there were more than three dominant follicles by ultrasound. Luteal phase ultrasound was performed 7 days after the ovulatory dose of hCG to determine if hyperstimulation was present, and small supplemental doses of IM hCG (500, 1,500, 500 units) were given for luteal phase support 7, 10, and 13 days, respectively, after ovulatory hCG. However, if midluteal ovarian diameter was greater than 6–7 cm, vaginal progesterone suppository supplements (25 mg b.i.d.) were administered instead of hCG.

Subjects in this study were monitored with serial pelvic ultrasounds (including one luteal phase ultrasound), performed using a 5 MHz transvaginal convex array probe or a 3.5–5 MHz transabdominal probe. Serum estradiol levels were monitored daily until ovulation in the gonadotropin group, and serum progesterone levels were drawn 7, 10 and 13 days after the ovulatory dose of hCG. Progesterone levels on day 7 were drawn prior to administration of hCG or progesterone supplements. In the pulsatile GnRH group, midcycle urinary LH monitoring was performed, and daily blood samples for estradiol (E2) and P were assayed at the completion of each treatment cycle.

Clinical results

Ovulatory rates (% of cycles resulting in ovulation) and conception rates (% conceptions per treatment cycle) are shown in Table 1. The overall ovulatory rate in the exogenous gonadotropin group was 97% compared to 93% in the pulsatile GnRH group (NS). Pulsatile GnRH conception rates per treatment cycle (31%) or per patient

Table 1. Clinical outcomes of pulsatile GnRH vs. exogenous gonadotropins in HA

	Pulsatile GnRH (75–250 ng/kg)	hMG
Ovulatory rate	93%	97%
Conception rate		
% cycles	31%	25%
% patients	76%	60%
Spontaneous abortion rate	25%	16.6%

(76%) were not significantly different from those seen with exogenous gonadotropins (25 and 60% respectively). Although the rate of spontaneous abortion appears to be higher in the pulsatile GnRH group (25 vs. 16.6%), this was not significantly different. The percentage of viable term pregnancies with exogenous gonadotropins was 21%, similar to the 23% seen with pulsatile GnRH (NS). Life table analysis of conceptions corrects for patients who conceive or discontinue therapy (Fig. 3). This analysis demonstrates that the cumulative chance of conceiving after 6 treatment cycles of pulsatile GnRH (96%) appears to be higher than that seen with exogenous gonadotropins (72%). The cumulative chance of conceiving appears to plateau after the fourth cycle of gonadotropin therapy, while that for pulsatile GnRH continues to increase through the sixth cycle.

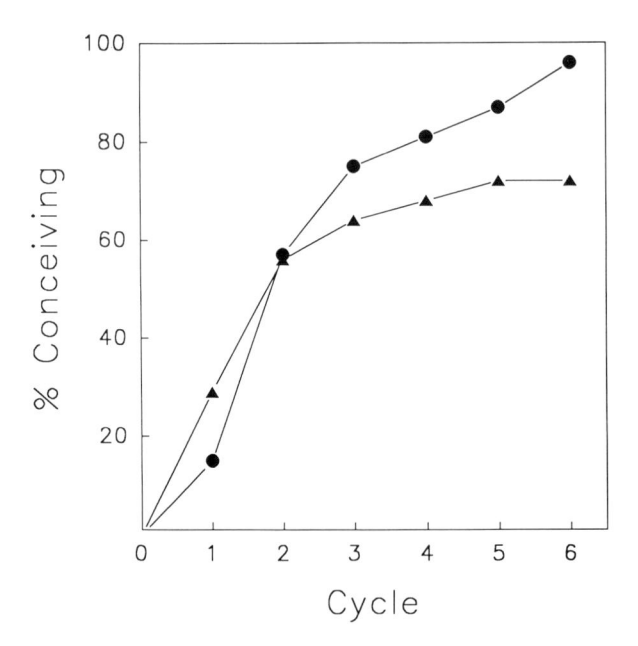

Fig. 3. Life-table analysis correcting for patients who conceive or discontinue therapy. The cumulative chance of conceiving after six treatment cycles of pulsatile GnRH (●—●) is 96% vs. 72% for exogenous gonadotropins (▲—▲).

Table 2. Multiple gestations with pulsatile GnRH vs. exogenous gonadotropins in HA

	Pulsatile GnRH (75–250 ng/kg)	hMG
Multiple gestations	10.7%	14.8%
Follicle number		
% > 2 folls	20.8%	47.6%[a]
% > 3 folls	5.2%	16.6%[a]

[a]$p < 0.05$.

Multiple gestations

The risk of multiple gestation, while higher in the gonadotropin group (14.8%) than with pulsatile GnRH (10.7%) was not significantly different (Table 2). All multiple gestations with pulsatile GnRH were twin pregnancies with no higher order multiples. In contrast, 75% of multiple gestations in the exogenous gonadotropin group were higher order pregnancies (triplets or more). Of note is that the incidence reported here for exogenous gonadotropins is lower than that previously noted for hypogonadotropic patients (24–50%) [4–6], possibly due to a conservative approach to gonadotropin dosing. It is possible that if a more aggressive gonadotropin regimen had been used or if a greater number of patients had been studied, a significant difference in multiple gestation risk from pulsatile GnRH would have been more evident.

More than two dominant follicles were seen on ultrasound in 47.6% of exogenous gonadotropin cycles, significantly higher than the 20.8% seen with pulsatile GnRH ($p < 0.01$). In addition, 16.6% of exogenous gonadotropin cycles resulted in more than three dominant follicles, significantly higher than the 5.2% seen with pulsatile GnRH ($p < 0.05$). It is striking that even with a conservative approach to ovulation induction with exogenous gonadotropins, multiple folliculogenesis is a frequent event. In contrast, when appropriate doses of GnRH are chosen (75–100 ng/kg), multiple folliculogenesis with pulsatile GnRH is far less common.

Midluteal ovarian size

There were no cases of severe ovarian hyperstimulation syndrome in either group using the criteria of Rabau [21]. However, mean maximum ovarian diameter on luteal phase ultrasound 7 days after the ovulatory dose of hCG (gonadotropin group) or LH surge (GnRH group) was significantly greater in the gonadotropin group when compared to the pulsatile GnRH group (6.2 x 5.5 cm vs. 3.3 x 2.8 cm; $p < 0.05$). presumably a reflection of the increased follicular number and therefore increased corpora lutea number with exogenous gonadotropins. Cycle cancellation rate for the exogenous gonadotropin group due to multiple follicular development and/or high serum estradiol levels was 4.5%, while no pulsatile GnRH cycles required cancellation ($p < 0.05$).

Biochemical evidence of hyperstimulation

Preovulatory serum estradiol levels, which have been shown to correlate with hyperstimulation risk [22], were supraphysiologic in the exogenous gonadotropin group when compared to our normal population, and were significantly higher than all GnRH treatment groups. Mean peak preovulatory E2 level (Fig. 4) for the exogenous gonadotropin group was 1684.5 ± 124.4 pmol/l, significantly higher than in normal women (1086.6 ± 38.5 pmol/l, $p < 0.01$), all doses of GnRH (1327.8 ± 74.2 pmol/l, $p < 0.05$), and GnRH 75 ng/kg (1230.8 ± 98.0 pmol/l, $p < 0.05$). Mean progesterone level 7 days after ovulatory hCG in the exogenous gonadotropin group was 84.9 ± 10.8 nmol/l, significantly higher than that seen in the normal women (61.1 ± 3.2 nmol/l, $p < 0.05$). Mean progesterone levels for all GnRH doses 70.6 ± 5.6 nmol/l), and GnRH 75 ng/kg (70.9 ± 6.9 nmol/l) appeared to be lower than in the gonadotropin group, although this did not reach statistical significance.

Economic implications

When comparing pulsatile GnRH to exogenous gonadotropin therapy, the issue of cost is frequently raised. Because of the apparent improved safety profile of pulsatile GnRH, ovulation induction does not require the intensity of monitoring that is key to the safe administration of exogenous gonadotropins. Therefore, in a therapeutic setting, we have previously estimated that the cost of ovulation induction could be considerably reduced with pulsatile GnRH in comparison with exogenous gonadotropins [8].

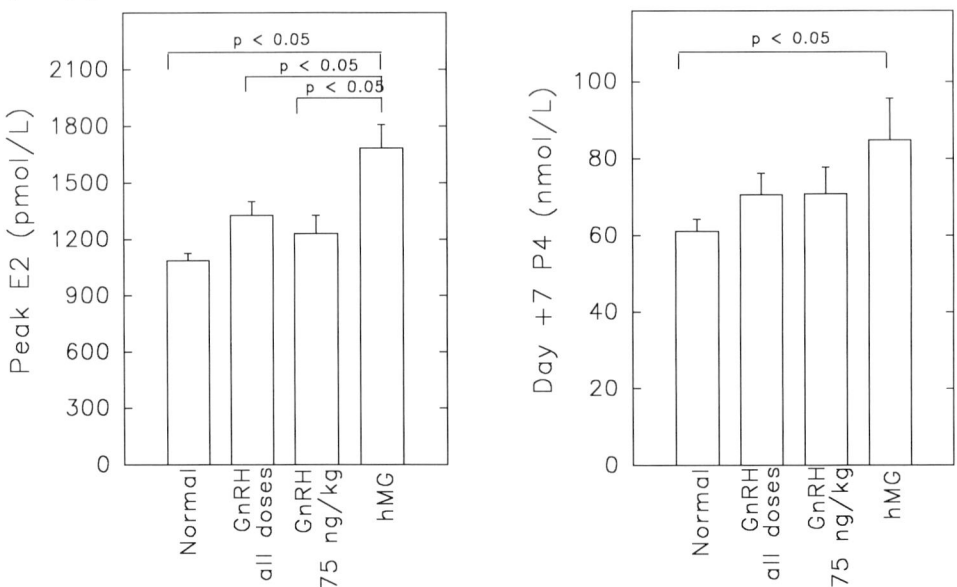

Fig. 4. Mean preovulatory serum estradiol (E2) (pmol/l) (left panel) and mean progesterone (P) levels (nmol/l) 1 week after ovulation or ovulatory hCG (right panel) for exogenous gonadotropins (hMG) vs. pulsatile GnRH and normals (n = 87).

Far more important is the potential economic impact of multiple gestations. We have recently reported that ovulation induction with exogenous gonadotropins either alone or in the setting of assisted reproductive technologies, has contributed significantly to the rising rate of multiple gestations [23]. In addition, Callahan has demonstrated that twin and triplet pregnancies result in a dramatic and disproportionate increase in hospital costs when compared to singleton pregnancies [23]. If pulsatile GnRH, on the other hand, is truly associated with a lowered risk of multiple gestation, as it appears to be, one would anticipate a substantial reduction in cost.

Conclusion

Pulsatile GnRH, when compared to exogenous gonadotropins, results in high rates of ovulation and conception, and a decreased risk of multiple folliculogenesis, higher order multiple gestations, ovarian enlargement, and cycle cancellation. In addition, pulsatile GnRH results in more physiologic preovulatory estradiol levels and luteal phase progesterone levels when compared to exogenous gonadotropins. Because of the improved safety profile, one would also anticipate a reduction in costs because of a decreased need for intensive monitoring. In addition, the apparent lowered risk of multiple gestations, particularly higher order multiples, would be anticipated to result in significant savings. A prospective, randomized trial with a carefully matched population is currently underway to further clarify these important issues.

Acknowledgements

Supported by grants HD 15080, HD-29164, FDU-00477 and RR 1066 from the National Institutes of Health.

This manuscript is largely based on previous work published previously by our group: 1) Martin KA, Hall JE, Adams JM, Crowley WF Jr. Comparison of exogenous gonadotropins and pulsatile gonadotropin-releasing hormone for induction of ovulation in hypogonadotropic amenorrhea. J Clin Endocrinol Metab 1993;77:125—129, and 2) Martin K, Santoro N, Hall J, Filicori M, Wierman M, Crowley WF Jr. Management of ovulatory disorders with pulsatile gonadotropin-releasing hormone. J Clin Endocrinol Metab 1990;71:1081A—1081G.

The authors wish to thank Helen Whitney, Janet Waldman and Veena Sharma for their meticulous care of the patients involved in these protocols.

References

1. Santoro N, Filicori M, Crowley WF Jr. Endocrine Rev 1986;7:11—23.
2. Reame NE, Sauder ED, Case GD, Kelch RP, Marshall JC. J Clin Endocrinol Metab 1985;61:851—858.
3. Martin KA, Hall JE, Santoro NF, Crowley WF Jr. Clin Res 1990;38:342A.

4. Caspi E, Ronen J, Schreyer P, Goldberg MD. Br J Obstet Gynaecol 1987;83:967—973.
5. Oelsner G, Serr DM, Mashiach S, Blankstein J, Snyder M, Lunenfeld B. Fertil Steril 1978;30:538—544.
6. Thompson CR, Hansen LM. Fertil Steril 1970;21:844—853.
7. Schenker JG, Weinstein D. Fertil Steril 1978;30:255—268.
8. Martin K, Santoro N, Hall J, Filicori M, Wierman M, Crowley WF Jr. J Clin Endocrinol Metab. 1990;71:1081A—1081G.
9. Martin KA, Hall JE, Adams JM, Crowley WF Jr. J Clin Endocrinol Metab 1993;77:125—129.
10. Spratt DI, Crowley WF Jr, Butler JP, Hoffman AR, Conn PM, Badger TM. J Clin Endocrinol Metab 1985;61:890—895.
11. Schriock ED, Jaffe RB. Obs Gyn Survey 1986;41:414—423.
12. Jansen RPS, Handelsman DJ, Boylan LM, Conway A, Shearman RP, Fraser IS. Fertil Steril 1987; 48:33—38.
13. Santoro N, Wierman ME, Filicori M, Waldstreicher J, Crowley WF Jr. Intravenous Administration of Pulsatile Gonadotropin-Releasing Hormone in Hypothalamic Amenorrhea: Effects of Dosage. J Clin Endocrinol Metab 1986;62:109—116.
14. Filicori M, Flamigni C, Meriggiola MC, Cognigni G, Valdiserri A, Ferrari P, Campaniello E. Fertil Steril 1991;56:1—13.
15. Hopkins CC, Hall JE, Santoro NF et al. Obstet Gynecol 1989;74:267—270.
16. Leyendecker G, Struve T, Plotz EJ. Arch Gynecol 1980;229:177—190.
17. Crowley WF Jr, McArthur JW. J Clin Endocrinol Metab 1980;51:173—175.
18. Filicori M, Santoro N, Merriam GR, Crowley WF Jr. J Clin Endocrinol Metab 1986;62:1136—1144.
19. Filicori M, Flamigni C, Campaniello E et al. Am J Physiol 1989;257:E930—E936.
20. Brown JB, Evans JH, Adey FS, Taft HP, Townsend SL. J Obstet Gynaec Br Cmwlth 1969;76:289—306.
21. Rabau E, David A, Serr DM et al. Am J Obstet Gynecol 1967;96:92—98.
22. Gemzell C, Roos P. Am J Obstet Gynecol 1966;94:490—496.
23. Callahan T, Hall J, Ettner S, Greene M, Crowley WF Jr. Clin Res 1993;41:234A.

Pulsatile GnRH in multifollicular and polycystic ovary patients

Howard S. Jacobs*

Division of Endocrinology, Department of Medicine, University College London Medical School, London, UK

Use of pulsatile GnRH in women with multicystic ovaries

Multicystic ovaries is a term we coined some years ago to describe the ovarian ultrasound pattern we had observed in two situations: the first was in girls progressing normally through puberty and the second was in young women emerging from a period of amenorrhoea caused by suppression of gonadotrophin secretion.

The physiological appearance of multicystic ovaries, together with its background endocrinology, was developed by Stanhope and Adams in a series of publications in the 1980s [1,2]. The key ultrasound features are the presence of six or more follicular structures of 4 mm or more in diameter, scattered at random throughout ovaries which have a normal stromal echo [3] (Fig. 1). It is salutary to note that this ultrasound appearance corresponds very closely to the actual appearance of the pubertal ovary, as described by Peters in postmortem examinations of young women killed in road traffic accidents [4]. Stanhope and his colleagues were able to reproduce this appearance in patients with delayed puberty caused by hypogonadotrophic hypogonadism by administering pulsatile GnRH therapy [1]. If the GnRH was applied only during the night (thus mimicking the physiological pattern of gonadotrophin secretion that occurs during the early stages of puberty) the small ovaries that characterise the hypogonadotrophic state enlarged and the multicystic appearance developed. When GnRH treatment was extended throughout the 24 h, a single dominant follicle emerged and ovulated and the multicystic appearance regressed.

We have interpreted the above findings as indicating that the multicystic appearance represents the response of an essentially normal ovary to an abnormality of pulsatile gonadotrophin secretion. The experiments during induction of puberty suggested that one abnormality is a shortened duration of pulsatile gonadotrophin stimulation. We suspect, but have not yet had the opportunity to prove, that in the pathological situation (vide infra) the underlying endocrinopathy is a decrease in the amplitude of pulsatile gonadotrophin secretion. Whether, as in the pubertal situation, there is a specific reduction of daytime GnRH activity is not clear. A practical point

---

Address for correspondence: Howard S. Jacobs, Cobbold Laboratories, The Middlesex Hospital, Mortimer Street, London W1N 8AA, UK.

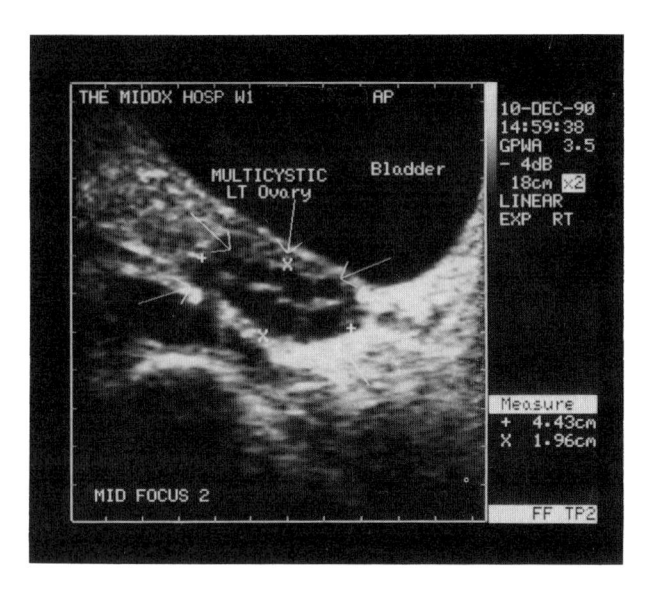

Fig. 1. Ultrasound appearance of multicystic ovary. Note the relative variability of the diameter of the cysts. There is no echodense stromal echo.

of clinical value is that if one detects a multicystic appearance in the ovary of a girl complaining of pubertal delay one can be reassuring about the status of gonadotrophin secretion and therefore about the prognosis, i.e., the appearance is not compatible with organic hypogonadotrophic hypogonadism. For the paediatric endocrinologist it implies therefore that the girl is experiencing the phenotypic consequence of early pubertal development of the hypothalamic — pituitary — ovarian axis.

Pathologically, multicystic ovaries occur in women who are emerging from a phase of suppression of gonadotrophin secretion. While I have seen this appearance in the very early phase of the response of hyperprolactinaemic women with amenorrhoea to treatment with bromocriptine, by far the most common association is with recovery from weight-loss-related amenorrhoea. The multicystic appearance typically occurs as the patient approaches a normal body mass index, a time parenthetically when pulsatile gonadotrophin secretion usually returns to its normal amplitude. Since for some years now we have declined to induce ovulation in women whose weight is subnormal because of the adverse effect of undernutrition on obstetric outcome [5], and perhaps on adult health too [6], my own experience of the outcome of pulsatile GnRH therapy in this situation is necessarily limited. Nonetheless, the experience we have had is that the treatment is seductively successful [7], as of course one would expect because one is offering it as a form of replacement therapy.

Use of pulsatile GnRH in women with polycystic ovaries

It is important at the outset to define terms: by polycystic ovaries I mean ovaries that by ultrasound are larger than normal with a highly echodense central stroma and 10 or more cysts (in a single plane) arranged around the circumference [3]. The cysts are usually from 2 to 8 mm in diameter although their exact size depends upon ambient gonadotrophin levels. Thus they are smaller in women with polycystic ovaries who are taking the combined birth control pill or using GnRH analogues; the stromal echo does not, however, change with these treatments. Figure 2 shows the typical appearance of a polycystic ovary.

Polycystic ovaries occur in about 20% of volunteer populations, as shown now in three large studies [8–10], although it must be accepted that each of them is subject to serious selection bias [11,12]. There is evidence that the phenotype runs in families [13] and one group has suggested it is inherited as a simple dominant [14]. The ultrasound appearance can be detected before puberty; its incidence rises with age from 6% at 6 years to the adult frequency at the age of 15 [15]. These are important observations because, as we shall see, they have provided an important stimulus for seeking the characteristic ultrasound features in women whose endocrine findings are unexpected, such as those with hypopituitarism [16].

Polycystic ovary syndrome is diagnosed when the characteristic ovarian ultrasound image is observed in association with a menstrual disturbance, clinical features of hyperandrogenisation (seborrhoea, acne, unwanted hair or male pattern baldness) and obesity. The prevalence of particular symptoms depends to a considerable extent on referral practice, more patients with disorders of androgenisation being referred to endocrinologists and more with fertility problems to gynaecologists. It is important

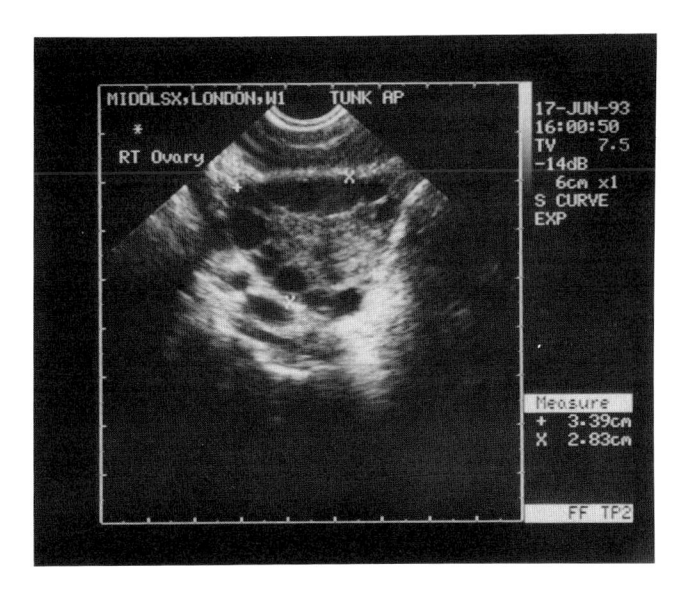

Fig. 2. Ultrasound appearance of a polycystic ovary. Note the arrangement of the cysts, their relative uniformity of size and the highly echodense central stroma.

to bear this referral bias in mind when interpreting the literature of this field.

There are two mechanisms of infertility in women with polycystic ovary syndrome. The first is failure to ovulate. Recent work has indicated that an important determinant of the rate of ovulation is the circulating serum insulin concentration [17]. Thus as insulin levels rise the interval between menstrual periods increases [18]. The fall in the ovulation rate is expressed clinically in the complaint of infertility. Since there is also a positive association between body weight and insulin secretion, development of obesity is typically associated with a fall in the rate of ovulation, both spontaneous and in response to GnRH therapy [19]. Conversely, a fall in insulin secretion, as induced by weight loss [20] or exercise is associated with a return of ovulation cycles and therefore a return of fertility. Hypersecretion of insulin also provokes hypersecretion of androgens in women with polycystic ovaries [21]. Excess insulin secretion is probably the explanation for the anovulation experienced by hirsute women with polycystic ovary syndrome; it seems unlikely to be caused by the androgens themselves, for reasons fully discussed elsewhere [22]. These observations are important when trying to interpret the published literature in this field because the success rates of all forms of treatment are clearly linked to body weight and therefore to insulin secretion.

The second mechanism of infertility in women with polycystic ovary syndrome is hypersecretion of LH. This subject is discussed elsewhere in this volume and has been the subject of two recent and complementary reviews from my group [23,24]. Suffice it to say here that, through mechanisms that frankly remain uncertain, women with high follicular phase LH concentrations have impaired fertility (both in vitro and in vivo) and a high rate of miscarriage. Hypersecretion of LH proves to be the only endocrine disturbance that exerts such adverse effects on fecundity despite a rate of ovulation, either spontaneous or induced, that may be normal. In terms of induction of ovulation it is therefore important to ensure that conception is attempted in an optimal endocrine milieu. Treatment with pulsatile GnRH tends to raise the serum levels of LH in women with amenorrhoea caused by polycystic ovary syndrome [25] and so, on a priori grounds, is unlikely to prove suitable.

Results of pulsatile GnRH treatment in women with polycystic ovary syndrome

The clinical implication of the above studies is that obese hyperadrogenaemic women with polycystic ovary syndrome and high LH concentrations are predicted to be unsuitable for treatment with pulsatile GnRH. Surveying the literature, we found that the ovulation rate per treated cycle was 50.7%, the pregnancy rate per ovulatory cycle was 28.7% but the pregnancy rate per treated cycle was only 14.6% [26]. These figures are compared with those obtained in women with hypogonadotrophic hypogonadism in Table 1, from which it can be seen that the major differences are that in the women with polycystic ovary syndrome the overall ovulation rate and the pregnancy rate per treatment cycle are about half of those in women with hypogonadotrophic hypogonadism.

Table 1. Results of treatment with GnRH in women with polycystic ovary syndrome compared with those with hypogonadotrophic hypogonadism. Data from the literature, reviewed by Shoham, Homburg and Jacobs, 1990 [26]

Diagnosis	No. of cycles	No. of patients	Ovulation rate (%)	Pregnancy per cycle (%)	Pregnancy per ovulation (%)
Hypogonadotrophic hypogonadism	464	150	90.1	28.6	32
Polycystic ovary syndrome	384	120	50.7	14.6	28.7

The rate of miscarriage was 22 out of a total of 56 pregnancies in the women with polycystic ovary syndrome compared with 30 out of 133 pregnancies in the women with hypogonadotrophic hypogonadism. The 17% difference between these two rates is statistically significant (Fisher's exact probability = 0.0321). These results were replicated in our own work [27] but with the additional observation that the miscarriages were significantly associated with hypersecretion of LH.

In contrast to these disappointing results, Filicori and colleagues [28] have reported that pretreatment of women with polycystic ovary syndrome with a superactive agonist of GnRH results in a considerable improvement in ovulation and pregnancy rates obtained with treatment with pulsatile GnRH. Presumably the major benefit of this pretreatment is mediated through sustained suppression of excessive LH secretion.

Pulsatile GnRH treatment in women with hypogonadotrophic hypogonadism and polycystic ovaries

The observations referred to earlier that polycystic ovaries can be detected in about one fifth of apparently normal women, as well as in children before puberty, prompted us to investigate whether the same might be true in women with hypogonadotrophic hypogonadism. The point of this study was the possibility that such a finding might provide us with a model in which we could investigate the role of spontaneous and induced gonadotrophin secretion in the development of the polycystic ovary syndrome.

So far we have assessed the ovaries in 77 women with hypogonadotrophic hypogonadism and found a polycystic appearance in 15, that is to say, in exactly the predicted number (Kaltzas, Conway, Patel and Jacobs, in preparation). The clinical and endocrine findings and the response to gonadotrophin therapy of a sample of these patients have been reported by Shoham et al. [29]. Briefly, we found that the women with ovaries that were polycystic but whose endocrine findings were those of patients with hypogonadotrophic hypogonadism made an ovarian response (in terms of the number of follicles that developed after a standard dose and duration of gonadotrophin treatment) that was indistinguishable from the patients in the same study who had fully developed polycystic ovary syndrome. There was thus a much more exuberant response in the women with polycystic ovaries than in the women with ovaries that were normal by ultrasound.

More recently we have analysed the response of these patients to treatment with pulsatile GnRH [30]. When we compared the results in the women with hypogonadotrophic hypogonadism with normal ovaries with those with polycystic ovaries, we found that while in the follicular phase serum FSH concentrations rose equally in the two groups, the ovarian follicular response was again much more striking in the women with polycystic ovaries. This result therefore confirmed the sensitive response of the polycystic ovary to endogenous FSH that we had observed with exogenous gonadotrophins. When we assessed the follicular phase serum LH concentrations we found that they rose to a higher level in the women with polycystic ovaries than in those with normal ovaries. Moreover, the statistically significant increase in LH concentrations was observed before any increase in serum oestradiol could be detected, suggesting that whatever was responsible for this exaggerated pituitary response to GnRH, it was unlikely to be an ovarian steroid. For these and other reasons we have postulated that the characteristic hypersecretion of LH that occurs in some 40% of women with polycystic ovaries is caused by a disturbance of a nonsteroidal ovarian pituitary feedback system [31]. It has led us to postulate a deficiency of a peptidergic ovarian factor (gonadotrophin surge attenuating factor, perhaps) as the cause of the unrestrained secretion of LH in this syndrome.

Finally, it should be mentioned that when we assessed the cumulative conception rate in the hypogonadotrophic patients with polycystic ovaries, we found that those treated with GnRH had a better response than those treated with gonadotrophin injections. We interpret this finding to indicate that although LH concentrations were higher in those receiving treatment with GnRH than with gonadotrophins, the level of LH was probably not high enough to cause all the adverse effects to which attention has earlier been drawn. In these patients the more important determinant of clinical outcome was probably the excessive follicular response of the polycystic ovary to gonadotrophin therapy.

Conclusions

The clinical problems presented by patients with multicystic ovaries only rarely need solving by application of pulsatile GnRH because they most commonly occur in the context of partially recovered weight-loss related amenorrhoea. This condition is appropriately managed by further weight increase with the evolution of spontaneous cycles, rather than by the application of "high tech" equipment. The management not infrequently involves psychiatric help. In my experience most patients readily understand the need for an improvement in their nutrition, particularly when the information about the impact of maternal malnutrition on fetal development is discussed.

The clinical problems presented by patients with polycystic ovary syndrome are among the most common that occur. The role of pulsatile GnRH therapy is limited in these patients because it does not really address the fundamental problems of hypersecretion of insulin being a major contributor to anovulation and hypersecretion of LH being a major contributor to infertility and miscarriage. While multiple pregnancy and ovarian hyperstimulation are major complications of gonadotrophin therapy that are avoided with pulsatile GnRH treatment, it should be possible with modern methods of surveillance and the judicious use of treatments like ovarian diathermy [32] to reduce the rate of these problems to normal or very close to normal.

References

1. Brook CGD, Jacobs HS, Stanhope R, Adams J, Hindmarsh P. Ballliere's Clin Endocrinol Metab 1987;1:23–41.
2. Stanhope R, Adams J, Jacobs HS, Brook CGD. Arch Dis Child 1985;60:116–119.
3. Adams J, Franks S, Polson DW, Mason HD, Abdulwahid N, Tucker M, Morris DV, Price J, Jacobs HS. Lancet 1985;2:1375–1379.
4. Peters H, Himelstein-Braw R, Faber M. Acta Endocrinol (Copenhagen) 1976;82:6127–6130.
5. van der Spuy ZM, Steer PJ, McCusker M, Steele SJ, Jacobs HS. Br Med J Clin Res 1988;296:962–965.
6. Barker DJP. Fetal and infant origins of adult disease. Br Med J 1992.
7. Homburg R, Eshel A, Armar NA, Tucker M, Mason PW, Adams J, Kilborn J, Sutherland IA, Jacobs HS. Br Med J 1989;298:809–812.
8. Polson DW, Adams J, Wadsworth J, Franks S. Lancet 1988;1:870–872.
9. Clayton RN, Ogden V, Hodgkinson J, Worswick L, Rodin DA, Dyer S, Meade TW. Clin Endocrinol 1992;37:127–134.
10. Farquharson CM, Birdsall M, Manning PJ, Mitchell JM. Prevalence and significance of polycystic ovaries. Ultrasound Obstet Gynaecol 1994 (in press).
11. Jacobs HS. Clin Endocrinol 1993;38:553.
12. Jacobs HS. Commentary. Ultrasound Obstet Gynaecol 1994 (in press).
13. Hague WM, Adams J, Reeders ST, Peto TEA, Jacobs HS. Clin Endocrinol 1988;29:593–606.
14. Carey AH, Chan KL, Short F, White D, Williamson R, Franks S. Clin Endocrinol 1993;38:653–681.
15. Bridges NA, Cooke A, Healy MJR, Hindmarsh PC, Brook CGD. Fertil Steril 1993;60:456–460.
16. Stanhope R, Adams J, Pringle JP, Jacobs HS, Brook CGD. Fertil Steril 1987;47:872–875.
17. Conway GS, Honour JW, Jacobs HS. Clin Endocrinol 1989;30:459–470.
18. Conway GS, Jacobs HS, Holly JMP, Wass JAS. Clin Endocrinol 1990;33:593–603.
19. Eshel A, Abdulwahid NA, Armar NA, Adams JM, Jacobs HS. Fertil Steril 1988;49:956–960.
20. Kiddy DS, Hamilton-Fairley D, Seppala M, Koistinen R, James VHT, Reed MJ, Franks S. Clin Endocrinol 1989;31:757–763.
21. Nestler JE, Barlascini CO, Matt DW, Steingold KA, Plymate SR, Clore JN, Blackgard WG. J Clin Endocrinol Metab 1989;68:1027–1032.
22. Conway GS, Jacobs HS. Clin Endocrinol 1993;39:623–632.
23. Shoham Z, Jacobs HS, Insler V. Fertil Steril 1993;59:1153–1161.
24. Balen AH, Tan S-L, Jacobs HS. Br J Obstet Gynaecol 1993;100:1082–1089.
25. Abdulwahid NA, Adams J, van der Spuy ZM, Jacobs HS. Clin Endocrinol 1985;23:613–626.
26. Shoham Z, Homburg R, Jacobs HS. Balliere's Clin Obstet Gynaecol 1990;4:589–608.
27. Homburg R, Armar NA, Eshel A, Adams J, Jacobs HS. Br Med J 1988;297:1024–1026.
28. Filicori M, Companiello E, Michelacci L, Pareschi A, Ferrari P, Bolelli G, Flamigni C. J Clin Endocrinol Metab 1988;66:327–333.

29. Shoham Z, Conway GS, Patel A, Jacobs HS. Fertil Steril 1992;58:37—47.
30. Schachter M, Balen AH, Patel A, Jacobs HS. Hypogonadotropic patients with ultrasonographically detected polycystic ovaries have aberrant gonadotropin secretion when treated with pulsatile gonadotropin releasing hormone — a new insight to the pathophysiology of polycystic ovary syndrome. Fertil Steril 1994 (in press).
31. Balen AH, Jacobs HS. Clin Endocrinol 1991;35:399—402.
32. Armar NA, McGarrigle HHG, Honour JW, Holownia P, Jacobs HS, Lachelin GCL. Fertil Steril 1990; 53:45—49.

Add-on regimens

Long-term GnRH agonist suppression and gonadotropins

David R. Meldrum

Department of Obstetrics and Gynecology, South Bay Hospital, Redondo Beach CA 90277, USA

Abstract. GnRH agonists are useful for preparation of the ovary for oocyte retrieval by decreasing the chance of a cancelled stimulation for poor response or a spontaneous LH surge. In addition, the number of eggs is increased and the number and quality of embryos is improved. These benefits result in an increased chance of pregnancy with both fresh and frozen embryo transfer. Use of this combination of GnRH-a and gonadotropins may also improve fecundity with ovulation induction in women with polycystic ovarian disease, but no benefit has been shown for women receiving gonadotropins and intrauterine insemination.

Following a period of marked stimulation of gonadotropins by a GnRH agonist, the pituitary becomes desensitized. Through primarily a postreceptor mechanism, the secretion of bioactive gonadotropins falls to low levels and the ovary becomes quiescent [1]. The combination of GnRH agonist suppression with stimulation of the ovary with exogenous gonadotropins has been used in an attempt to improve the response of the ovary to stimulation, the quality of developed oocytes, and to prevent premature release of luteinizing hormone (LH) [2]. This approach has been helpful in the induction of ovulation in women with polycystic ovarian disease (PCO) [3] and in preparation of the ovary for oocyte retrieval [2,4]. It is often referred to as a "long protocol" or downregulation protocol to distinguish it from protocols which add exogenous stimulation during the agonist phase of pituitary stimulation (the "short" protocol or "flare" technique).

Benefits of adjunctive use of GnRH agonists

Poor responders

Use of the long protocol for poor responders was predicated on the assumption that ovarian stimulation prior to the selection and dominance of a leading follicle could encourage development of secondary follicles. With the notable exception of women with an elevated level of follicle-stimulating hormone (FSH), this does appear to be the case, since poor responders appear to produce about twice as many follicles [4], and the number of oocytes retrieved is routinely greater than with gonadotropins given alone [2]. Since endogenous gonadotropins are suppressed, but the average daily requirement for gonadotropins is not increased [2], the ovary does indeed appear to be more sensitive. Since androgens are implicated in atresia of secondary follicles, the suppression of bioactive LH and testosterone during stimulation [5] may explain this improved response. The apparent increased incidence of ovarian hyperstimulation with combination therapy [6] is also consistent with increased ovarian sensitivity to gonadotropins.

Improved oocyte quality

A higher level of LH during the latter part of follicular maturation has been associated with a lower rate of pregnancy in women having oocyte retrieval and embryo transfer [7] and lower cycle fecundity in women attempting natural conception [8]. Embryo morphology has been reported to be significantly improved [6] and calculated embryo viability is increased [9] with combination therapy. Since bioactive LH is effectively suppressed by adjunctive use of a GnRH agonist [5], this lower exposure of LH to the developing oocyte may improve its quality, and that of the resulting embryo. The association of miscarriage with higher follicular phase LH levels [8], the increased rate of fetal loss in women with PCO, and the reduction of fetal loss in these women with GnRH agonist cycles [10] would also be consistent with a beneficial effect of LH suppression on embryo quality.

Improved oocyte quality should also be reflected in an improved pregnancy rate with IVF-ET. Because of the low statistical power of randomized studies, this has been difficult to ascertain in spite of strong trends in a number of investigations [6,11,12]. Meta-analysis has recently been used to combine these studies to improve statistical power [13]. A 2-fold higher odds ratio for pregnancy was found with the use of GnRH agonist. This finding could also result from improved implantation, but taken with the above, the bulk of evidence suggests improved oocyte and embryo quality.

Improved outcome with cryopreservation

Studies using the long protocol have consistently shown an increase in the number of oocytes retrieved, often with an increased rate of fertilization [2,4,6,11,12]. The resulting higher number of embryos available for cryopreservation should lead to a higher pregnancy rate with later transfer of thawed embryos if the survival rate and implantation rate per embryo are reasonably similar to non-GnRH-a cycles. In one study with cleaved embryos the survival rate was reduced, possibly due to a higher rate of embryo cleavage [14], whereas in another comparison, the survival rate and implantation rate were not significantly lower with cryopreservation at the pronuclear stage than without use of GnRH-a [15]. In this latter study, the pregnancy rate was significantly higher due to the transfer of more embryos. These apparent differences between outcome with pronuclear versus cleaving embryos may be specific to the use of propanediol as a cryoprotectant since actively dividing cells may be more sensitive to that agent. The short or flare GnRH-a procotol may not result in an increased number of pregnancies with cryopreservation, since significantly fewer oocytes are retrieved compared with the long protocol [16].

Use of GnRH-a in women not having oocyte retrieval

Women with PCO have particularly high levels of LH and a much lower cycle fecundity with use of human menopausal gonadotropins (hMG) than hypogonadotropic women with low LH levels [17]. The use of adjunctive leuprolide acetate in a long protocol has resulted in a strong trend towards increased fecundity (0.16 to 0.27 per cycle) [3]. Larger studies are warranted to examine the relative pregnancy rate and particularly the delivery rate using this approach, since a lower rate of miscarriage has been found with combination therapy of women with PCO having IVF [10]. The disadvantage of a 3- to 4-week pretreatment phase and the cost of the agonist may well be counterbalanced by the higher delivery rate achieved. However, newer approaches to hMG therapy in PCO using lower doses and more gradual increases in dose have also suggested trends toward higher cycle fecundity and result in lower hMG dose and total cost [18].

Women having hMG for intrauterine insemination could also benefit from LH suppression. However, results have been conflicting, with one study suggesting a benefit [19] and one suggesting a lower pregnancy rate with combination therapy [20]. Until further studies are carried out, the increased cost and inconvenience of this approach do not seem to be warranted.

Factors involved in the use of GnRH-a in a long protocol

Phase of menstrual cycle to begin the GnRH-a

The agonist phase of treatment can be troublesome, stimulating the ovary to develop follicular cysts. This requires an extended period of observation before hMG can be started. Estrogen secretion by the cysts generally resolves before the cyst disappears. The effect of cysts on the response of the ovary to stimulation has been controversial. The agonist phase is more prolonged when GnRH-a is started in the follicular phase. Suppression is more prompt and consistent when GnRH-a is started in the early follicular phase [21], and even more prompt when started in the midluteal phase [22]. Use of a split-dose regimen also significantly enhances suppression [22]. We routinely start GnRH-a in the luteal phase; if a follicular phase start is chosen for scheduling purposes, we give the GnRH-a each morning and evening. With PCO, the agonist can be started any time the ovary is in a resting state with follicles under 1.0 cm. The agonist phase is blunted and is consistently suppressed by 4 weeks [21]. The longer suppression may help to reduce hyperstimulation [23].

In one study the number of oocytes retrieved was significantly greater when the agonist was started in the mid to late luteal phase compared to the early luteal phase [24]. We therefore monitor ovulation and start GnRH-a about 8 days after the LH surge or temperature rise.

In one investigation there was a trend towards improved embryo morphology when the long protocol was begun in the early follicular rather than midluteal phase, and the required dose of GnRH-a was lower [25]. Further study of pregnancy outcome with varying times of GnRH-a initiation is warranted.

Dose and schedule of hMG

Because of the propensity toward hyperstimulation, caution must be exercised with the amount of exogenous gonadotropin administered. The dose can either be started low and increased as necessary [26] or started high (300 IU/day) and decreased when the follicles reach a certain stage and the level of estradiol (E2) reaches a given level [27]. No comparison has been made between these two approaches and both appear to be satisfactory.

Timing of hCG

A number of studies have noted a reduced pregnancy outcome with higher levels of circulating progesterone (P) on the day of hCG administration [28–30]. It is important to use a P assay which has sufficient accuracy and specificity for measuring levels in the subnanogram range [31]. Since high P levels in oocyte donors are associated with an increased pregnancy rate in recipients [32], the primary detrimental effect of progesterone appears to be on the endometrium. In other studies, the pregnancy rate was unchanged by arbitrarily delaying hCG by 1 or 2 days [33,34]. This finding, however, could indicate that further oocyte maturation is beneficial in some cases, counterbalancing the adverse effect of further P rises in other cases. The flexibility of hCG timing however, does appear to be much greater than with the short protocol, with which a dramatic fall in the pregnancy rate was found with a delay of only a single day [35].

Timing of ooycte retrieval

The accepted time for oocyte harvest of 34 to 36 h after hCG injection was based on protocols not using GnRH-a, with which substantial rises of bioactive LH have already occured before hCG is given [5]. In a recent study, an improved rate of oocyte maturity and cleavage was observed by increasing this interval to 36 to 38 h [36]. No ovulations were noted. This gives improved flexibility when delays occur in the timing of oocyte retrieval. Since the study was not large, there may be ovulations before 38 h in some individual patients.

Luteal support

Early luteal progesterone secretion was found to be significantly higher in GnRH-a/hMG cycles than with hMG only [37], probably due to the greater level of oocyte maturity generally allowed. However, E_2 and P levels fell dramatically about 8 days after hCG injection [38], probably due to the declining level of hCG and the continuing low level of endogenous LH. Randomized controlled trials (RCT) of supplementary hCG have shown significantly higher pregnancy rates [39,40] and luteal hormones. RCTs of intramuscular P [41] or intramuscular P plus oral E_2 valerate [42] have shown pregnancy rates similar to those using hCG. Vaginal micronized P also appears to be effective [43]. It is not clear whether luteal E_2 support is helpful [42], but in one report, a dramatic lowering of biochemical pregnancies was noted when high doses of E_2 and P were started at initial hCG detection [44]. Since luteal hCG support increases the chance of ovarian hyperstimulation [45], most programs use intramuscular P.

Ultralong GnRH-a

In women with endometriosis, pretreatment with 4 to 6 months of GnRH-a, then immediately proceeding to ovarian stimulation with hMG has been associated with particularly high pregnancy rates [46]. Endometrial defects have been found in women with endometriosis [47] and a lower implantation rate per transferred embryo has been reported when endometriosis is severe [48]. The level of CA-125 may be a practical way of following suppressive therapy, proceeding to stimulation when it is normal [46]. RTCs are needed to assess whether higher pregnancy rates can be achieved in women with endometriosis by such pretreatment. An alternative is to surgically ablate significant active endometriosis before doing IVF.

Summary

In preparation for oocyte retrieval, pituitary suppression with a GnRH agonist prior to ovarian stimulation with gonadotropins increases the number and quality of oocytes, the pregnancy rate, and the rate of additional pregnancies from cryopreservation because of the higher number of extra embryos available for freezing. Luteal support is necessary and may be provided by exogenous progesterone. Use of combined GnRH-a/hMG may also increase cycle fecundity in women with PCO having induction of ovulation, but benefits of combined therapy for superovulation/intrauterine insemination have been uncertain.

References

1. Meldrum DR, Tsao Z, Monroe SE, Braunstein GD, Sladek J, Lu JKH, Vale W, Rivier J, Judd HL, Chang RJ. J Clin Endocrinol Metab 1984;58:755—757.
2. Meldrum DR. Obstet Gynecol Surv 1989;44:314—318.
3. Dodson WC, Hughes CL, Yancy SE, Haney AF. Fertil Steril 1989;52:915—918.
4. Smitz I, Ron-El R, Terlatzis BC. Hum Reprod 1992;7:49—66.
5. Cedars MI, Surey E, Hamilton F, Lapolt P, Meldrum DR. Fertil Steril 1990;53:627—631.

6. Ron-El R, Herman A, Golan A, Nachum H, Soffer Y, Caspo E. Fertil Steril 1991;55:574−578.
7. Howles CM, Macnamee MC, Edwards RG. Hum Reprod 1987;2:17−21.
8. Regan L, Owen EJ, Jacobs HS. Lancet 1990;336:1141−1144.
9. Chetkowski RJ, Rode RA, Burruel V, Nass TE. Fertil Steril 1991;56:1095−1103.
10. Balen AH, Tan S-L, MacDougall J, Jacobs HS. Hum Reprod 1993;8:959−964.
11. Kingsland C, Tan S-L, Bickerton N, Mason B, Campbell S. Fertil Steril 1992;57:804−809.
12. Antoine JM, Salat-Baroux J, Alvarez S, Sornet D, Tibi CL, Mandelbaum J, Plachot M. Hum Reprod 1990;5:565−569.
13. Hughes EG, Fedorkow DM, Daya S, Sagle MA, Van de Koppel P, Collins JA. Fertil Steril 1992;58:888−896.
14. Keenan D, Cohen J, Suzman M, Wright G, Kort H, Massey J. Fertil Steril 1991;55:792−796.
15. Oehninger S, Toner JP, Veeck LL et al. Fertil Steril 1992;57:620−624.
16. Tan S-L, Kingsland C, Campbell S et al. Fertil Steril 1992;57:810−814.
17. Dor J, Itzkorvic DJ, Mashiach S, Lunenfeld B, Serr DM. Am J Obstet Gynecol 1980;136:102−105.
18. Meldrum DR. Fertil Steril 1991;55:1039−1040.
19. Gagliardi CL, Emmi AM, Weiss G, Schmidt CL. Fertil Steril 1991;55:939−944.
20. Dodson WC, Walmer DK, Hughes CL, Yancy SE, Haney AF. Obstet Gynecol 1991;78:187−190.
21. De Fazio J, Meldrum DR, Lu JKH et al. Fertil Steril 1985;44:453−459.
22. Meldrum DR, Wisot A, Hamilton F, Gutlay AL, Huynh D, Kempton W. Fertil Steril 1988;50:400−402.
23. Salat-Baroux J, Alvarez S, Antoine JM et al. Hum Reprod 1988;3:535−539.
24. Pellicer A, Simon C, Miro F et al. Hum Reprod 1989;4:285−289.
25. Ron-El R, Herman A, Golan A, Van der Ven H, Caspi E, Diedrich K. Fertil Steril 1990;54:233−237.
26. Meldrum DR, Wisot A, Hamilton F, Gutlay AL, Kempton W, Huynh D. Fertil Steril 1989;51:455−459.
27. Brzyski RG, Jones GS, Oehninger S, Acosta AA, Kruithoff CH, Muasher SJ. J In Vitro Fert Embryo Transfer 1989;6:290−293.
28. Schoolcraft W, Sinton E, Schlenker T, Huynh D, Hamilton F, Meldrum DR. Fertil Steril 1991;55:563−566.
29. Silverberg KM, Burns WN, Olive DL, Riehl RM, Schlenken RS. J Clin Endocrinol Metab 1991;73:797−803.
30. Franchin R, de Ziegler D, Taieb J, Hazout A, Frydman R. Fertil Steril 1993;59:1090−1094.
31. Meldrum DR. Fertil Steril 1991;56:154−155.
32. Legro RS, Ary BA, Paulson RJ, Stanczyk FZ, Sauer MV. Hum Reprod 1993;8:1506−1511.
33. Dimitry ES, Oskarsson T, Conaghan J, Margara R, Winston RML. Hum Reprod 1991;6:944−946.
34. Tan S-L, Balen A, El Hussein E et al. Fertil Steril 1992;57:1259−1264.
35. Clark L, Stanger J, Brinsmead M. Fertil Steril 1991;55:1192−1194.
36. Gudmundsson J, Fleming R, Jamieson ME, McQueen D, Coutts JRT. Fertil Steril 1990;53:735−737.
37. Brzyski RG, Jones GSS, Jones HW, Oehninger S, Muasher SJ. Fertil Steril 1991;55:119−124.
38. Smitz J, Devroey P, Braeckmans P et al. Hum Reprod 1987;2:309−314.
39. Smith EM, Anthony FW, Gadd SC, Masson GM. Br Med J 1989;298:1482−1485.
40. Belaisch-Allart J, De Mouzon J, Lapousterle C, Mayer M. Hum Reprod 1990;5:163−166.
41. Clamen P, Domingo M, Leader A. Hum Reprod 1992;7:487−489.
42. Smitz J, Devroey P, Camus M et al. Hum Reprod 1988;5:585−590.
43. Smitz J, Devroey P, Faguer B, Bourgain C, Camus M, Van Steirteghem AC. Hum Reprod 1992;7:168−175.
44. Prietl G, Diedrich K, van der Ven HH, Luckhaus J, Krebs D. Hum Reprod 1992;7:1−5.
45. Herman A, Ron-El R, Golan A, Raziel A, Soffer Y, Caspi E. Fertil Steril 1990;53:92−96.
46. Nakamura K, Oosawa M, Kondou M et al. J Assist Reprod Genet 1992;9:113−117.
47. Fedele L, Marchini M, Bianchi S, Dorta M, Arcaine L, Fontana PE. Fertil Steril 1990;53:989−993.
48. Yovich JL, Matson PL, Richardson PA, Hilliard C. Fertil Steril 1988;50:308−313.

Flare-up protocols in assisted reproductive technologies (ART): a re-evaluation

René Frydman* and Renato Fanchin

Department of Obstetrics and Gynecology, Hôpital Antoine Béclère, Clamart, France

Abstract. Flare-up GnRH-a protocols have been used as available alternatives to the classical long protocols for controlled ovarian hyperstimulation by many ART centers, worldwide. The objective of this outline is to overview the advantages and drawbacks of these protocols. Special interest will be given either to the use of flare protocols as diagnostic tools for the evaluation of the ovarian reserve, as well as to the possible adverse impact on the oocyte quality of the high LH levels induced by the flare-up effect in the early follicular phase. Finally, a number of comparative studies aiming at evaluating the relative efficacy of short and long protocols will be discussed.

Introduction

Gonadotropin-releasing hormone agonists (GnRH-a) have been routinely adopted as adjunct players in controlled ovarian hyperstimulation (COH) by the majority of ART centers, worldwide. GnRH-a are characterized by the selective substitution of amino acids at positions 6 and 10 of the native GnRH. These modifications allow a higher binding affinity to the GnRH receptor and decrease the susceptibility to degradation by pituitary endopeptidases, inducing a stable and durable pituitary desensitization. It is now generally accepted that the use of GnRH-a in COH provides a more comfortable monitoring of follicular growing and ovulation (no spontaneous LH surge), and leads to an overall improvement in pregnancy rates [1,2] likely due to an enhanced number of viable oocytes and embryos obtained [3]. Moreover, initially used exclusively in long regimens [1], GnRH-a have been applied successfully, during the last 5 years, concomitantly to the exogenous gonadotropin administration in ultrashort [4,5] and short [6,7] regimens. The putative rationale for choosing short rather than long protocols is based on the fact that the 4–5-day agonistic flare of gonadotropins may constitute a powerful synergistic add-back to the exogenous gonadotropin treatment. This leads to a significant reduction of the amount of exogenous gonadotropins required to achieve COH which renders the short protocols less expensive than the long regimens.

Although controversial results have been reported on the relative efficacy of short

---

Address for correspondence: René Frydman MD, Department of Obstetrics and Gynecology, Hôpital Antoine Béclère, 157, rue de la Porte de Trivaux, 92141 Clamart, France.

in comparison to long COH protocols concerning in vitro fertilization and embryo transfer (IVF-ET) results, the flare GnRH-a associations may provide, accessorily, useful diagnostic information about the ovarian responsiveness to gonadotropin stimulation (ovarian reserve). This double therapeutic/diagnostic application of the flare protocols will be the central issue of this article. Furthermore, the advantages and drawbacks of this type of GnRH-a regimen will also be overviewed.

The flare-up effect: an asymmetric LH/FSH release

Following GnRH-a administration and before installation of the complete suppression of endogenous gonadotropins, a significant and transient releasing of LH and FSH is observed for approximately 3 to 5 days. Both intensity and duration of this flare-up effect are directly related to the dose of GnRH-a administered. Marked differences concerning the kinetics of plasma LH- and FSH-release have, however, been reported. The post-GnRH-a releasing of LH has been recognized as being 2-fold higher than that observed for FSH [8–10]. In addition, complete suppression of plasma FSH levels occurs significantly more rapidly than that of plasma LH [8]. As discussed later, these abnormally high circulating LH levels during the early follicular phase seem to play a detrimental role on the pregnancy outcome presumably by hampering the oocyte quality.

Flare protocols: what has been proposed

Short or flare COH protocols combine characteristically the effects of endogenous (GnRH-a flare-up effect) and exogenous (hMG and/or hFSH) gonadotropins. Moreover, a number of models varying either the doses or the relative timing of this association have been proposed.

Classically, short COH protocols associate a daily administration of GnRH-a subcutaneously or intranasally, from the early follicular phase (cycle-days 2 or 3) until the day of hCG administration, with the administration of exogenous gonadotropins (hMG and/or hFSH). The doses of GnRH-a may be adapted according to the biological activity of GnRH-a preparations [6].

More recently, an abbreviated version of the short GnRH-a protocols (ultrashort) have been reported [4,5]. These consist of the daily administration of GnRH-a for only 3 [4] or 7 [5] days during the early follicular phase. GnRH-a treatment is, thereafter, overlapped by the exogenous gonadotropin administration until the day of hCG. No endogenous LH secretion has been detected for at least 9 days after the withdrawal of the GnRH-a administration [4] with satisfactory overall IVF-ET results. Therefore, others studies indicate that ultrashort protocol did not always prevent LH surge [11]. Ho and Co-workers [12] demonstrate that 6% of the 160 ultrashort protocol using buserelin nasal spray (500 µg/day) had an endogenous LH surge.

A recent study of our team [5] comparing the efficacy in IVF-ET of an ultrashort protocol in which a GnRH-a was administered from days 2 to 8 of the cycle with a classical time-release GnRH-a protocol revealed that the "7-day" regimen could safely prevent premature LH surges until hCG administration in all 86 cases (LH ≤2 mIU/ml). This study confirmed that the hypothalamus-pituitary axis does not immediately recover the positive feedback of estradiol (E2) after GnRH-a discontinuation. Furthermore, the IVF-ET results were similar between both protocols which was reassuring concerning the routine use of "7-day" ultrashort regimens.

Flare protocols: a diagnostic tool

Ovarian responsiveness to controlled ovarian hyperstimulation (COH) plays a major role in IVF-ET results [13]. Indeed, a suboptimal IVF-ET outcome is observed in cases of poor ovarian response to COH [14], likely due to a decreased oocyte/embryo quality. Moreover, poor responses to COH could represent an indirect sign of ovarian aging and early evidence of a reduction in the women's fertility potential. Hence, to avoid inadequate prescription of COH to women whose ovarian responsiveness to stimulation is definitely hindered, some approaches aiming to predict the performance of the ovaries under COH have been proposed.

Plasma FSH measurement on cycle-day 3 [15,16] has been routinely used to screen ovarian responsiveness to COH by a number of IVF-ET centers. Correlation of this test with COH results are, however, often disappointing. In fact, FSH levels during the early follicular phase can show marked intercycle fluctuations. To overcome this contingency of basal FSH measurements, some "dynamic" approaches for the evaluation of the ovarian reserve have been proposed, as the clomiphene citrate challenge test (CCCT) and the GnRH-a stimulation test.

The CCCT [17,18] analyses the FSH profiles before and after the administration of 100 mg of clomiphene citrate from day 5 to 9 of the menstrual cycle but monitoring of the E2 response during the CC challenge test did not predict ovarian responsiveness of pregnancy rates [19]. More recently, another approach based on the E2 response to the endogenous flare-up of gonadotropins induced by the administration of a GnRH-a was proposed by Padilla et al. [20,21] (Lupron test). This test aims at evaluating the increase in plasma E2 levels after the administration of a GnRH agonist (leuprolide acetate, 1 mg s.c.) on days 2, 3 and 4 of the menstrual cycle. The authors have found a good correlation between the E2 response and the ovarian response to COH: four distinct patterns of serum E2 response to the leuprolide acetate were identified, a lack of response of a sustained rise in peripheral E2 levels prognosticates a diminished pregnancy rate, whereas E2 levels elevation followed by a drop on the 3rd day of GnRH-a therapy bodes well.

Padilla conclude that E2 pattern is a better indicator than the baseline or stimulated serum FSH and LH levels. Winslow et al. [22] argue that these E2 patterns were unable to detect significant differences in any ovarian response outcomes. These authors have studied 228 patients who were stimulated with 1 mg of leuprolide acetate. The value of the agonist stimulation test was defined as the increase in E2 level from day 2 to day 3 (ΔE2). In contrast to Padilla et al., Winslow et al. observed no correlation of this test with pregnancy rates. Only ΔE2 is considered as a functional test of ovarian reserve and seems to be a sensitive predictor of ovarian response to stimulation. Hugues et al. [23] using a pretreatment with norethisterone demonstrate that the pattern of hormonal E2 flare-up can be modified by a progestogen pretreatment and specially the serum E2 cut-off value, but the relationship between the early events of the follicular phase and the subsequent pregnancy rate still exists. It was interesting to evaluate whether an early addition of pure FSH in patients without significant E2 flare-up is able to improve IVF. Unfortunately, early FSH supplementation does not improve IVF outcome in the preliminary data of those authors [24].

Flare protocols for poor responders

No consensus is available in the literature about the definition of poor responders. Moreover, patients who have presented E2 levels <1000 pg/ml at the end of COH with a daily dose of exogenous gonadotropins of at least 300 IU, whose total amount of exogenous gonadotropins exceeded 60, and who have produced <5 oocytes may be included in this group of patients.

Based on the theoretical benefits of the gonadotropin flare effect on the improvement of the follicular recruitment, short GnRH-a protocols have been proposed for the treatment of poor responders. Katayama et al. [25] have reported encouraging results using GnRH-a-hFSH-hMG in short association for COH in seven patients who had not previously developed a follicle larger than 15 mm or a peak E2 level >300 pg/ml in response to hFSH or hMG alone. Further publications, however, failed to confirm these preliminary results [26,27].

Flare protocols: what about premature elevation of plasma progesterone (P)?

Despite suppression of endogenous gonadotropins by GnRH-a, some cases (up to 20%) of premature elevation of plasma P (>0.9 ng/ml) have been reported during COH for IVF-ET [28–30]. These authors concurred to observe poorer IVF-ET results in such cases likely due to an adverse effect of prematurely high P levels on the endometrial receptivity [30]. The etiology of this phenomenon remains, however, unclear. One of the plausible hypotheses is a pituitary escape from the GnRH-a action with a consequent impact of endogenous LH on the follicular cells. As in ultrashort protocols GnRH-a treatment is discontinued several days before hCG administration, pituitary LH secretion should recover theoretically more rapidly in these protocols than in the long GnRH-a regimens. Surprisingly, not only plasma LH levels remained low until hCG administration (≤2 mIU/ml) [5] but also the incidence of premature elevation of plasma P was similar in ultrashort and long protocols. These observations concur to disclaim the hypothesis that the pre-hCG elevations of P observed during

COH are due to an action of endogenous gonadotropins on the ovarian steroidogenic cells.

Flare protocols: what about oocyte quality?

As described above, the 3—5-day releasing of pituitary gonadotropins (FSH and LH) into the circulation following the administration of a GnRH-a is biologically asymmetric: higher plasma LH in comparison to FSH levels have been observed after GnRH-a [8—10]. In addition, plasma P levels also display a significant increase during the gonadotropin flare [9] as a result of the action of the endogenous gonadotropins on the ovarian granulosa/thecal cells. These two phenomena (altered LH/FSH ratios and increased P — and androgen? — levels during the early follicular phase) have been pointed out as possible clues responsible for suboptimal IVF-ET outcome. Putative mechanisms center around direct oocyte effects, decreasing clinical and ongoing pregnancy rates [31,32]. These hormonal disarrangements observed on the early follicular phase with flare protocols seem to constitute a serious drawback against their use in ART.

Flare protocols: lower pregnancy rates?

The relative results between short and long protocols concerning the IVF-ET outcome are controversial. Some recent studies concurred to demonstrate poorer IVF-ET results with short in comparison to long protocols. Ron-El et al. [33] compare a 3-day GnRH-a administration in 92 cases to 92 long protocols. They conclude that the ultrashort group needed significantly less amount of hMG ampoules than the long regimen but the same numbers of oocytes. They obtained less embryos and concluded that the ultrashort protocol, despite its convenience, is inferior in outcome compared with the long protocol in term of embryos per retrieval and pregnancies rate.

Tarlatzis and co-workers [34] randomly allocated 527 cycles in short and long protocols obtained a 19 vs. 25% pregnancy rate but the difference was not significant. Tan and colleagues [35] also found a 25.7 vs. 17% in favour of long protocols but still the difference was not significant.

The French Registry of 1992 [36], analysing approximately 18,000 IVF-ET cycles, reported significantly lower overall pregnancy rates with short (15% per cycle) in comparison to long (19.2% per cycle) GnRH-a regimens ($p < 0.001$). On the other hand, results of an extensive meta-analysis failed to show a significant difference in either cycle cancellation or pregnancy rates when comparing flare (n = 368) and long protocols (n = 476) [37]. Our group compare classical short protocols and long protocols [38] or 7-day protocols against long protocols [5]. We observed a remarkably lower hMG amount requiring 24 vs. 42 vials but the number of embryos and pregnancy rate were similar in the two treatment groups.

Conclusion

Flare-up protocols may be useful as therapeutic options for COH in ART with these comments:
– All short protocol are very well tolerated without any side effects.
– Three days of GnRH-a administration seems to be too short and 14 days too long.
– Results in term of pregnancies are still controversial comparing short to long protocols.
– Specific indication has to be defined and proved.
– Prognostic value can be one of the interest in the flare-up protocol if it:
  – individualises the risk of hyperstimulation syndrome by measurement of LH,
  – identifies poor responders by measurement of FSH,
  – predicts the success or cancels the cycle by measurement of E2.

References

1. Frydman R, Parneix I, Belaish-Allart J, Hazout A, Fernandez H, Testart J. Hum Reprod 1988;3:559–561.
2. Meldrum DR, Wisot A, Hamilton F. Fertil Steril 1989;51:455.
3. Liu HC, Lai YM, Davis O, Berkeley AS, Graf M, Grifo J, Cohen J, Rosenwaks Z. J Assit Reprod Genet 1992;9:338–344.
4. Macnamee MC, Howles CM, Edwards RG, Taylor PJ, Elder KT. Fertil Steril 1989;52:264–269.
5. Hazout A, de Ziegler D, Cornel C, Fernandez H, Lelaidier C, Frydman R. Fertil Steril 1993;59:596–600.
6. Barrière P, Lopes P, Borffand JP, Pousset C, Quentin M, Sagot P, Lhermitte A, Lerat MF, Charbonnel B. J Assist Reprod Genet 1987;4:64–65.
7. Garcia JE, Padilla SL, Bayati J, Baramki TA. Fertil Steril 1990;53:302–305.
8. Crowley WF Jr, Beitins IZ, Vale W, Kliman B, Rivier J, Rivier C, McArthur JW. N Engl J Med 1980;302:1052–1057.
9. Brzyski R, Muasher SJ, Droesch K, Simonetti S, Jones GS, Rosenwaks Z. Fertil Steril 1988;50:917–921.
10. Loumaye E, Vankrieken L, Depreester S, Psalti I, De Coonana S, Thomas K. Fertil Steril 1989;51:105–111.
11. Acharya U, Irvine S, Hamilton M, Templeton A. Fertil Steril 1992;58:1169–1173.
12. Ho PC, Chan YF, So WK, Yeung WS, Chan ST. Asia Oceania J Obstet Gynaecol 1993;19:159–163.
13. Jones HW Jr, Acosta A, Andrews MC, Garcia JE, Jones GS, Mantzavinos T, McDowell J, Sandow B, Veeck L, Whibley T, Wilkes C, Wright G. Fertil Steril 1983;40:317.
14. Pellicer A, Lightman A, Diamond MP, Russell JB, Decherney AH. Fertil Steril 1987;47:812–815.
15. Muasher SJ, Oehninger S, Simonnetti S, Matta J, Ellis LM, Liu HC et al. Fertil Steril 1988;50:298–307.
16. Scott RT, Toner JF, Muasher SJ, Oehninger SC, Robinson S, Rosenwaks Z. Fertil Steril 1989;51:651–654.
17. Navot D, Rosenwaks Z, Margalioth EJ. Lancet 1987;2:645–647.
18. Loumaye E, Billion JM, Mine JM, Psalti I, Pensis M, Thomas K. Fertil Steril 1990;53:295–301.
19. Scott RT, Illions EH, Host ER, Dellinger C, Hoffmann GE, Navot D. Fertil Steril 1993;60:242–246.
20. Padilla SL, Bayati J, Garcia JE. Fertil Steril 1990;53:288.
21. Padilla SL, Smith RD, Garcia JE. Fertil Steril 1991;56:79–83.

22. Winslow KL, Toner JP, Brzyski RG, Oehninger SC, Acosta AA, Muasher SJ. Fertil Steril 1991;56:711–717.
23. Hugues JN, Attalah M, Herve F, Martin-Pont B, Kohler LM, Santarelli J. Hum Reprod 1992;7:1079–1084.
24. Cernin-Durnerin I, Hugues JN, Attalah M, Hervé F, Huet L, Kottler ML. Réf Gyn Obst 1993;1:277–286.
25. Katayama KP, Roesler M, Gunnarson C, Stehlik E, Jagusch S. J In Vitro Fert Embryo Transf 1988;5:332–334.
26. Matthews CD, Warnes GM, Norman RJ, Phillipson G, Kirby CA, Wang X. Hum Reprod 1991;6:817–821.
27. Regan L, Owen EJ, Jacobs HS. Lancet 1990;336:1141–1144.
28. Schoolcraft W, Sinton E, Schlenker T, Huynh D, Hamilton F, Meldrum DR. Fertil Steril 1991;55:563–566.
29. Silverberg KM, Burns WN, Olive DL, Riehl RM, Schenken RS. J Clin Endocrinol Metab 1991;73:797–803.
30. Fanchin R, de Ziegler D, Taieb J, Hazout A, Frydman R. Fertil Steril 1993;59:1090–1094.
31. Stanger JD, Yovitch JL. Br J Obstet Gynecol 1985;92:385–393.
32. Shoham Z, Jacobs HS, Insler V. Fertil Steril 1993;59:1153–1161.
33. Ron-El R, Herman A, Golan A, Soffer Y, Nachum H, Caspi E. Fertil Steril 1992;58:1164–1168.
34. Tarlatzis BC, Pados G, Bontis J, Lagos S, Grimbizis G, Spanos E, Mantalenakis S. Hum Reprod 1993;8:807–812.
35. Tan S-L, Kingsland C, Campbell S, Mills C, Bradfield J, Alexander N, Yovich J, Jacobs HS. Fertil Steril 1992;57:810–814.
36. Dossier FIVNAT 1992. Association FIVNAT, Ed. ORGANON 1992, Laboratoire Organon S.A., 93204 St Denis Cedex 01, France.
37. Hughes EG, Fedorkow DM, Daya S et al. Fertil Steril 1992;58:888.
38. Frydman R, Belaisch-Allart J, Parneix I, Forman RG, Hazout A, Testart J. Fertil Steril 1988;50:471–475.

The role of GnRH during the periovulatory period: a basis for the use of GnRH antagonists in ovulation induction

P. Bouchard[1], B. Charbonnel[2], A. Caraty[3], H.M. Fraser[4], S. Dubourdieu[1], I. Leroy[1], F. Olivennes[1] and R. Frydman[5]

[1]Departments of Endocrinology, Hôpital Saint Antoine, 184 rue du Faubourg Saint Antoine, 75012 Paris, France; [2]Hotel Dieu, Place Alexis Ricordeau, 44000 Nantes, France; [3]INRA, 37380 Nouzilly, France; [4]MRC Reproductive Biology Unit, 37 Chalmers Street, Edinburgh EH9 3EW, UK; and [5]Department of Obstetrics and Gynecology, Hôpital Antoine Béclère, 92141 Clamart Cedex, France

The menstrual cycle is controlled by the gonadotropins LH and FSH released by the pituitary [1,2]. This pituitary-ovarian axis is driven by the hypothalamic GnRH pulse generator which releases GnRH in the hypothalamic-pituitary portal circulation in a pulsatile manner [1]. In primates, the midcycle LH surge which triggers ovulation is induced by an increase in circulating estradiol (E_2) levels [1,2]. Administration of estrogens to oophorectomized nonhuman primates or postmenopausal women during the early follicular phase of the menstrual cycle can mimic the LH surge [3–6]. Although several studies suggest that E_2 acts on the pituitary, it is still not clear if GnRH is involved. Indeed, E_2 administration to monkeys with hypothalamic lesions elicited the LH surge if carried out within 48 h of the last administration of GnRH [7]. Moreover, administration of a weak GnRH antagonist reduced or slightly delayed the E_2-induced LH surge [8]; also, electrophysiological recordings of the hypothalamic multiunit activity, a marker of the pulse generator activity, show a significant decrease of activity at the time of the surge [9]. Although these findings do not provide strong evidence that GnRH is needed to trigger the LH surge, more recent studies in ewes have shown that the LH surge is accompanied by a 50-fold increase in secretion of GnRH in the portal circulation [10]. This has been confirmed in the monkey [11]. In the ewe, using two different antibodies with different specificity against the C- and N-terminal portions of the GnRH molecule respectively, we could demonstrate that mainly one form of GnRH is released at the time of the surge: native GnRH [12]. In order to suppress the effect of the first part of the surge, we administered i.v. a potent GnRH antagonist ([Ac-D2Nal^1, D4-ClPhe^2, D3Pal^3, Arg^5, DGlu^6 (AA), DAla^{10}]GnRH) (Nal-Glu) [12]. The antagonist administration postponed the LH surge which occurred during the latter part of the GnRH surge. This indicates that the GnRH released at the end of the surge is biologically active [12].

We then attempted to clarify the role of GnRH during the periovulatory period by using the same GnRH antagonist (Nal-Glu) in normal women [13,14]. To suppress GnRH action over various periods, we administered various regimens of antagonists (1–5 injections) when plasma E_2 levels were sufficient to elicit LH surges.

Administration of Nal-Glu antagonist (for 1—5 consecutive days) to normal women during the periovulatory period blocked the LH surge during the entire course of treatment; an LH surge occurred in most subjects after the effects of Nal-Glu had worn off. No LH surge occurred as long as the antagonist was circulating in the plasma.

In order to study whether or not the effect of the antagonist was related to the dramatic decrease in plasma E_2 observed after antagonist administration, we coadministered estradiol benzoate (EB) together with Nal-Glu [14]. This coadministration of Nal-Glu and EB did not trigger the LH surge. These findings suggest that the positive feedback effect of E_2 is abolished during the periovulatory period in normal women by the blockade of GnRH receptors by GnRH antagonist, and support the hypothesis that endogenous GnRH is required for the E_2-induced LH surge. In contrast, the data do not support the hypothesis that E_2 can act directly as a gonadotropin-releasing hormone and induce the gonadotropin surge in the absence of GnRH. Our findings are consistent with those of a recent study [15] which showed that progesterone administration, following 72 h of priming with ethinyl-estradiol, resulted in a surge-like release of LH and FSH in all subjects treated (estrogen-primed postmenopausal women); concomitant administration of the GnRH antagonist abolished this progesterone-induced surge-like release of both gonadotropins in all subjects. In a last experiment, to further demonstrate the direct role of GnRH, we treated, with pulsatile GnRH, women that had received Nal-Glu in the periovulatory period as described before [14]. The occurrence of an LH surge in the woman cotreated with GnRH antagonist and pulsatile GnRH therapy during the late follicular phase confirmed that GnRH plays an important role in the induction of the LH surge.

If it is clear that GnRH is required to initiate the estrogen-induced LH surge in women, the amount of GnRH needed, and its modalities of secretion, remain to be established. Our data also suggest that treatment with GnRH antagonists during the late follicular phase could be used to block premature LH surges in women undergoing ovarian hyperstimulation.

In order to try to solve the question whether or not the LH surge needs GnRH support to be maintained we went back to the same experimental paradigm, and this time we looked at the 6 women in whom the antagonist was administered when the surge had already started. We observed that the surge was interrupted in all women and LH dropped immediately and reached a nadir 24 h following antagonist administration (unpublished data). The surge was interrupted transiently in three women with a follicular rest. The surge was interrupted for 12—15 days in three women. Surprisingly, on the day of Nal-Glu administration, no criteria could allow us to predict the pattern of response. These data suggest that GnRH is also necessary to maintain the LH surge in addition to its role on the initiation of the surge. One possible application is that it is possible to block the surge even after LH has already started to rise. This is not only a theoretical consideration but is actually the base of a new practical approach to prevent endogenous rise in LH in controlled ovarian hyperstimulation.

Even under those circumstances, if the antagonist is administered after the surge has started, the LH rise is interrupted and ovulation can be triggered by hCG when it is suitable. The follicular maturation can thus be resumed after antagonist treatment.

While the approach of using agonist desensitisation for controlled ovarian stimulation and induction of multiple follicular development is widely used clinically, its full potential has not been realised with respect to its use as a key to understanding the normal process of follicular development. This is because the agonist analogues lack precision as scientific tools in suppressing LH and FSH secretion. We are now on the verge of improvements in the way pituitary-ovarian function can be precisely controlled in the human and further advances in our understanding of the requirements for follicular growth and luteal function. These advances should be brought about by the introduction of the new antagonists into clinical practice and the availability of FSH preparations, produced by means of recombinant DNA technology, which have half-lives similar to that of FSH produced during the normal cycle.

In patients undergoing IVF, premature LH surges are certainly unwarranted since they occur when follicular develoment is inadequate. This can have a deleterious effect on the oocytes and in addition, the subsequent rise in progesterone has a negative effect on the endometrium [16–18]. In the superovulation protocols used in IVF, the use of GnRH agonist is now generalized in order to prevent this rise in LH [18]. However, a period of 3 weeks is necessary for the desensitization to occur. This alters the luteal phase P secretion and requires large doses of hMG/FSH which increase the risks of ovarian hyperstimulation. Pilot studies using GnRH antagonists have confirmed the interest of GnRH antagonists in controlled ovarian superovulation in IVF [16,17,19–21].

Such a treatment does not require support of the luteal phase, and in addition would allow the triggering of ovulation with a GnRH agonist or GnRH itself if a hyperstimulation is feared.

The first pilot studies of the use of GnRH antagonist for prevention of a premature LH rise in controlled ovarian hyperstimulation have been described recently. In a simplified protocol for in vitro fertilisation cycles, GnRH antagonist was administered daily for 3 days beginning during the early follicular phase to achieve suppression of pituitary-ovarian function. Daily human menopausal gonadotropin (hMG) was given alone to obtain follicular development, followed by resumption of antagonist treatment when follicles reached 14–16 mm in diameter and was continued until the day of hCG administration to prevent the induction of premature surges of LH [20]. In an alternative approach, patients were treated with clomiphene citrate and hMG [17]. When serum concentrations of oestradiol exceeded 600 pg/ml 5 mg Nal-Glu antagonist was administered that evening and repeated 48 h later. hMG injections were maintained to stimulate follicle growth. The antagonist treatment prevented untimely LH surges. In a second group of women, hCG was administered 48 h after the last injection of antagonist. Resulting luteal function was normal, indicating that the antagonist treatment was without deleterious effect.

A third approach has been examined in monkeys in which follicular growth was induced by hFSH (Metrodin) beginning on day 2 of the cycle and continuing through to cycle day 10. GnRH antagonist was administered daily starting either from day 2, 5 or 8 of the cycle [22]. In the latter groups advantage was taken of endogenous gonadtropin stimulation. hCG was administered on cycle day 10. Of 33 monkeys treated, all but 4 responded moderately well or very well, irrespective of the treatment protocol and spontaneous LH surges were blocked in all but one. Ovarian stimulation was also performed on a flexible protocol based on delaying antagonist administration until serum oestradiol had reached 400 pg/ml.

All three regimens described were notable in that only with short-term GnRH antagonist administration was the positive feedback action of oestradiol blocked, at least during exogenous gonadotropin-induced multiple follicular development cycles.

The antagonists which are now entering clinical trials have 100 times less the histamine-releasing activity than the previous compounds, with a 2—10-fold increase in biological potency and high water solubility. The question of effects of exposure of the oocyte to antagonist needs to be addressed and prolonged action resulting in a carry-over to the developing embryo raises the issue of potential toxic or teratogenic effects.

In a recent study including 17 healthy women undergoing superovulation using 225 IU of hMG every day starting on day 2 of the cycle, the GnRH antagonist cetrorelix (SB-75; Ac-D-Nal(2)^1·D-Phe(4Cl)^2,D-Pal(3)^3,D-Cit^6,D-Ala^{10}) (Asta-Medica AG, Frankfurt, Germany) was administered s.c. at a dose of 5 mg when E_2 levels were between 550—730 pmol/l per follicle of at least 14 mm [23]. A second dose was injected 48 h later if the triggering of ovulation was not achieved in the mean time. In all the patients treated, LH levels remained low for at least 5 days following treatment. The total number of ampules of hMG was 28 ± 4, the number of mature oocytes was 7 ± 3 and the number of embryos was 6 ± 4. A mean of 2.6 embryos were transferred. Five pregnancies were observed.

In conclusion, our results clearly indicate that in women, continued ongoing GnRH action is required to initiate the estrogen-induced LH surge. It remains to be demonstrated whether or not a continuous secretion of GnRH is necessary to sustain the estrogen-induced LH surge. In addition, these findings support the use of GnRH antagonists during the late follicular phase for blocking premature LH surges in women undergoing ovarian hyperstimulation regimens. If these results are confirmed by larger, randomised studies, the good tolerance and efficacy that we observed suggest a bright future for this product in assisted reproductive technologies.

References

1. Knobil E. Recent Prog Horm Res 1980;36:53—88.
2. Crowley WF Jr, Filicori M, Spratt DI, Santoro NF. Rec Progr Horm Res 1985;41:473—531.
3. Yen SSC, Tsai CC. J Clin Endocrinol Metab 1971;33:882—890.
4. Liu JH, Yen SSC. J Clin Endocrinol Metab 1983;57:797—802.
5. Keye WR, Jaffe RB. J Clin Endocrinol Metab 1974;38:805—810.
6. Nakaï Y, Plant TM, Hess DL, Hoegh EJ, Knobil E. Endocrinology 1978;102:1008—1014.
7. Wildt L, Hausler A, Hutchison JS, Marshall G, Knobil E. Endocrinology 1981;108:2011—2013.

8. Wilks JW, Folkers K, Humphries J, Bowers CY. Biol Reprod 1980;23:1—9.
9. O'Byrne KT, Thalabard JC, Grosser PM, Wilson RC, Williams CL, Chen MD, Ladendorf D, Hotchkiss J, Knobil E. Endocrinology 1991;129:1207—1214.
10. Moenter SM, Caraty A, Locatelli A, Karsch FJ. Endocrinology 1991;129:1175—1182.
11. Xia L, Van Vugt D, Alston EJ, Lucklaus J, Ferin M. Endocrinology 1992;131:2812—2820.
12. Caraty A, Antoine C, Delaleu B, Locatelli A, Bouchard P, Gautron JP, Evans NP, Moenter SM, Karsch F. In: Bouchard Ph, Caraty A, Coelingh Bennink HJT, Pavlou SN (eds) Recent Progress on GnRH, GnRH analogs, Gonadotropins and Gonadal Peptides. Cambridge UK: Parthenon Press, 1993:113—124.
13. Bouchard P, Dubourdieu S, Hajri S, Le Nestour E, d'Acremont MF, Leroy I, Spitz IM, Frydman R, Charbonnel B. In: Bouchard Ph, Caraty A, Coelingh Bennink HJT, Pavlou SN (eds) Recent Progress on GnRH, GnRH analogs, Gonadotropins and Gonadal Peptides. Cambridge UK: Parthenon Press, 1993:265—284.
14. Dubourdieu S, Charbonnel B, d'Acremont MF, Carreau S, Spitz IM, Bouchard P. Effect of administration of a GnRH antagonist (Nal-Glu) during the preovulatory period: the LH surge requires the secretion of GnRH. J Clin Endocrinol Metab 1994 (in press).
15. Kolp LA, Pavlou SN, Urban RJ, Riviers FC, Vale WW, Veldhuis JD. J Clin Endocrinol Metab 1992;75:993—997.
16. Frydman R, Cornel C, De Ziegler D, Taïeb J, Spitz IM, Bouchard P. Hum Reprod 1992;7:930—933.
17. Frydman R, Cornel C, De Ziegler D, Taïeb J, Spitz IM, Bouchard P. Fertil Steril 1991;56:923—927.
18. Loumaye E. Hum Reprod 1990;5:357—376.
19. Ditkoff EC, Cassidenti DL, Paulson RJ. Am J Obstet Gynecol 1991;165:1811—1817.
20. Cassidenti DL, Sauer MV, Paulson RJ, Ditkoff EC, Rivier J, Yen SSC, Lobo RA. Am J Obstet Gynecol 1991;165:1806—1810.
21 Diedrich K, Diedrich E, Santos E, Zoll C, Al-Hasani Reissmann T et al. Supression of the endogenous LH-surge by the GnRH-antagonist Cetrorelix during ovarian stimulation. Hum Reprod 1994 (in press).
22. Byrd SB, Itskovitz J, Chillik C, Hodgen GD. Fertil Steril 1992;57:209—214.
23. Olivennes F, Fanchin R, Bouchard Ph, de Ziegler D, Taieb J, Frydman R. The single or dual administration of the GnRH antagonist cetrorelix prevents premature LH surges in an IVF-ET program. Fertil Steril 1994 (in press).

Potential for embryo damage by GnRH analogs

T.M. Siler-Khodr[1*], I.S. Kang[2], T.J. Kuehl[3] and G.S. Khodr[4]
[1]*University of Texas, Health Science Center at San Antonio, Texas, USA;* [2]*Yonsei University, Seoul, Korea;* [3]*Scott & White Clinic and Texas A&M University, College of Medicine; and* [4]*Southwest Genetics, San Antonio, Texas, USA*

Abstract. The utilization of gonadotropin-releasing hormone (GnRH) or an analog of this decapeptide in assisted reproductive protocols, such as in vitro fertilization, is now a common practice. However, the question of safety of treatment for the pregnancy resulting during that cycle or mistaken administration during pregnancy must be considered. The action of GnRH and its analogs in the intrauterine tissues, factors known to regulate GnRH production and metabolic degradation within the intrauterine tissues, and our current experience with GnRH analogs in these protocols is reviewed. In assisted reproductive protocols where exposure to GnRH analogs may occur, analogs without sustained delivery systems, that have limited binding to ovarian or intrauterine receptors and that can be degraded by the chorionic tissues, should be best suited for this use.

Introduction

The utilization of gonadotropin-releasing hormone (GnRH) or an analog of this decapeptide in assisted reproductive protocols, such as in vitro fertilization, is now a common practice. However, the question of safety of treatment for the pregnancy resulting during that cycle or mistaken administration during pregnancy must be considered, especially for an agent, such as GnRH, which has been shown to be produced by the intrauterine tissues and to regulate intrauterine functions during pregnancy.

To address this question, a review of what is known about GnRH in the intrauterine tissues, especially in early pregnancy, will be given. The factors known to regulate GnRH production will be described, as well as its metabolic degradation within the intrauterine tissues. The actions and metabolism of exogenous GnRH or its analogs during pregnancy will be discussed. Finally, how this information relates to the use of GnRH analogs for in vitro fertilization protocols and our current experience with GnRH analogs in these protocol will be discussed.

Address for correspondence: T.M. Siler-Khodr, Department of Obstetrics and Gynecology, University of Texas Health Science Center at San Antonio, 7703 Floyd Curl Drive, San Antonio, TX 78284, USA.

GnRH in pregnancy

The capability of an intrauterine tissue to synthesize a physicochemically, biologically and immunologically active GnRH-like molecule was first described by ourselves in 1980 [1]. Prior data by ourselves [2–5] and others [6] had indicated both its presence and activity within the intrauterine tissues. The concentration of GnRH in the placenta [2] as well as in the maternal circulation [7] varies throughout pregnancy with highest levels in the first trimester of pregnancy.

Subsequent studies established the presence of a mRNA for GnRH in human placenta tissue which was thought to be identical to that found in the hypothalamus [8,9]. However, later studies have shown that the placental mRNA contains the first exon which is not transcribed in the hypothalamus [10]. This mRNA appears to code for a peptide very similar to that of the pro-GnRH-GAP molecule of the hypothalamus. However, immunologic studies of both ours [11] and Gautron [12] indicate that a difference at the N-terminal of chorionic GnRH (cGnRH) may exist. Recent studies have demonstrated the presence of a pro-GnRH-GAP molecule that is immunologically indistinguishable from the hypothalamic species at the 6–16th amino acid. A hydroxyproline GnRH has also been isolated from human placenta [13].

Our immunofluorescent studies using an antiserum directed to the 3–10 amino acids of GnRH in human placental tissues of 10–12-week gestation localized GnRH immunoactivity primarily to the cytotrophoblast with uptake along the outer syncytial border and patchy uptake in the stroma of the villous [3]. Other investigators have localized GnRH to the syncytiotrophoblast [14] or the cytotrophoblast [15] and one group to both cells [16]. Other studies have shown production of cGnRH from cytotrophoblast only [17]. These apparently conflicting results may be related to the gestational age of the tissues studied and/or the antisera used. However, recent studies utilizing in situ localization have found the message for pro-GnRH in the syncytio- and cytotrophoblast but not the stroma of early human placenta [18].

Characterization of a placental receptor for GnRH has been completed [19–24]. Its interaction with numerous analogs of GnRH or GnRHs from different species indicate a specific placental receptor that differs from that of the pituitary; however, it does exhibit a high affinity for GnRH the decapeptide, buserelin and numerous other analogs of GnRH. Clearly these existing data establish the synthesis of a cGnRH in the peri-implantation embryo [25] throughout gestation, and indicate a paracrine and/or autocrine role for it during pregnancy.

GnRH production and action during pregnancy

Studies in vitro

GnRH activity within the intrauterine tissues throughout pregnancy has been established through numerous studies in vitro. Initially we demonstrated that GnRH could stimulate hCG production from the 10-week placenta [5] and subsequently demonstrated that this action was dose-related [26]. However, the pattern and duration of response was dependent on the gestational age of the placental tissue studied [27]. Multiple studies have expanded and refined this observation [19,28—31]. In early gestation, the amplitude and frequency of the pulsatile release of hCG is increased by physiologic concentrations of GnRH and by an agonist of GnRH [32,33]. Chronic high levels of GnRH inhibited hCG release similar to downregulation observed at the pituitary level. Further studies of ours [34,35] demonstrated that GnRH antagonist can inhibit the production of hCG. GnRH antagonist can also reverse the stimulation of hCG by exogenous GnRH or GnRH agonist [32,33].

The action of GnRH on steroid production is biphasic and is mediated by hCG as well as other mechanisms. At high doses of GnRH, placental progesterone is inhibited [36—39]. At physiologic concentrations of GnRH, stimulated hCG leads to increased progesterone and estrogen production [30,38—40]. The progesterone in turn has a negative feedback on the production of hCG in the placenta [41—44]. Estrogens appear to have a biphasic action on hCG and thus progesterone. At lower doses estrogens can stimulate GnRH-induced hCG production [44—46], while at high concentration they inhibit the GnRH stimulation of hCG and progesterone [30,37,41,43] as well as inhibit GnRH production itself [43].

One mechanism by which estrogen and progesterone affect their actions appears to be via modulation of a second messenger such as cAMP [43], which in turn leads to release of cGnRH [47] and hCG production [48]. Progesterone inhibits the dibutryl cAMP-stimulated release of cGnRH, while estradiol augments the dibutryl cAMP stimulation of hCG [43]. When given concomitantly, the inhibitory action of progesterone overrides.

A stimulatory role for calcium in the GnRH-induced hCG release has been demonstrated [49,50], while other investigators have also shown an effect of protein kinase C [51,52]. We [53—55] and Haning [48,56] have demonstrated a biphasic action of GnRH on placental prostaglandin E (PGE) and prostaglandin F (PGF) production. In first trimester placentas, increasing concentrations of GnRH led to a dose-related inhibition of PGE and PGF, while in term placentas, over long-term static incubation with GnRH, an increase was observed. Recent studies using a short-term perfusion system have also demonstrated an inhibition of thromboxane production by GnRH [55]. A stimulatory feedback by PGE and PGF on GnRH secretion has been reported [47].

Neurotransmitters may also regulate GnRH production. Epinephrine stimulates the secretion of GnRH [47]. Opiates have been shown to inhibit the cAMP-induced release of cGnRH without altering its basal release and thus reduces hCG production [57]. Other factors have also been shown to affect hCG production via GnRH, such as activin and inhibin, which stimulate and inhibit hCG, respectively [58—60]. Inhibin has been shown to both modulate the GnRH stimulation of hCG as well as inhibit the actual production of GnRH. Growth factors such as EGF stimulate GnRH production, and is at least one of the mechanisms by which hCG production is increased by growth factors [61].

Studies in vivo

In addition to the studies in vitro, numerous investigations on the in vivo effect of GnRH and its analogs in pregnant animals and humans have been completed. As early as in the mid-70s, an antipregnancy effect of GnRH analogs [62,63] was observed. Initially this activity was ascribed to a luteolytic action of GnRH via downregulation of pituitary LH [64]. The extrapituitary actions of GnRH were not appreciated at that time. However, further studies in rats at midgestation [65,66] or in hypophysectomized pregnant rats [67—70] led to the recognition of direct ovarian and uterine action of GnRH. In the ovarian-dependent pregnant rat suppression of ovarian steroid is effected by GnRH [71,72]. Administration of a GnRH analog to hCG-stimulated baboons or humans resulted in a suppression of progesterone production [41,73]. A direct action of GnRH on ovarian progesterone is now well recognized.

Concomitant with these studies was our demonstration of a cGnRH and our proposal of its regulation of hCG, and thus its role in the maintenance of pregnancy. Initially studies using GnRH antagonist or antiserum were used to establish this hypothesis. GnRH antiserum given to pregnant bonnet monkeys [22], the wallaby [74], the marmoset [75] and the baboon [76] supported the hypothesis that GnRH plays a critical role in the maintenance of CG and progesterone during pregnancy. Studies with antagonists of GnRH given to pregnant bonnet monkeys [77] and baboons [78] after the ovarian luteal shift also supported this conclusion. Thus, a direct action on the intrauterine tissues was demonstrated. In early pregnant humans a GnRH bolus at appropriate doses can evoke a stimulation of hCG [79].

However, other studies administering GnRH pituitary agonists to early pregnant baboons resulted in reduction of CG and progesterone and abortions [80]. Das and Talwar [81] observed similar findings but noted that the same dose in the early luteal phase reduced progesterone without leading to abortion. Further studies of ours [82] administering either Zoladex pellets (day 14) or an antagonist of GnRH to pregnant baboons (day 14—21) resulted in increased abortions or jeopardized fetal outcomes (Fig. 1). These data all support the conclusion that GnRH or its analogs can jeopardize the outcome of pregnancy.

We also observed that of 162 cycles, 72 resulted in implanted pregnancies, a rate of 44% [83]. This may seem high but it must be realized this is the count at the time of implantation even prior to the next expected menses. Of these pregnancies we then observed a 60% loss, all of which could be retrospectively predicted due to their abnormal CG and/or progesterone patterns during the peri-implantation period. In one anecdotal observation, one animal aborted 3 times (Fig. 2), each time having a similar abnormal endocrine pattern, i.e., low CG and progesterone. However, one pregnancy in this animal was maintained, the one treated with Zoladex. This pregnancy continued to term and resulted in a normal fetal outcome.

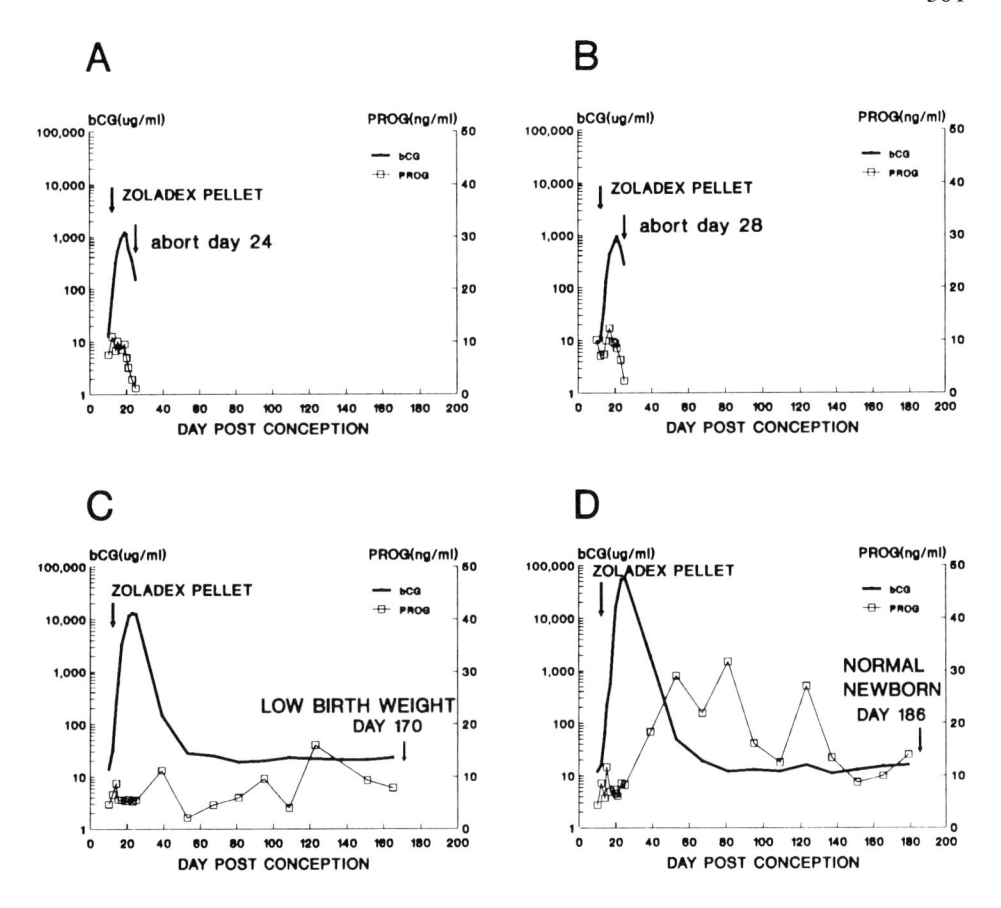

Fig. 1. The maternal circulating bCG and progesterone concentrations and their pregnancy outcome in four baboons receiving Zoladex implants on day 10 postconception. Reprinted with permission from Kang IS, Kuehl TJ, Siler-Khodr TM. Fertil Steril 1989;52:846–853.

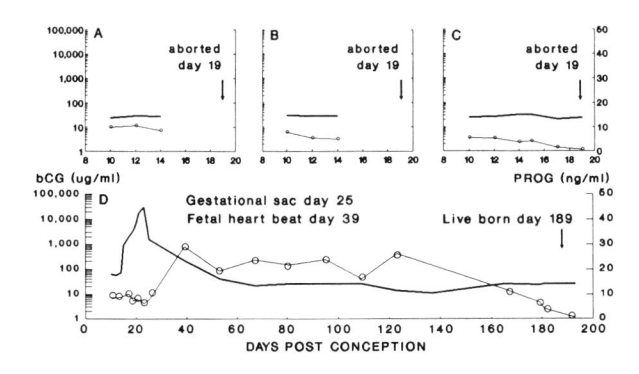

Fig. 2. The bCG and progesterone concentrations in a baboon having consecutive repeated spontaneous abortions (top graphs) was treated with Zoladex and that pregnancy continued to term (bottom graph). Reprinted with permission from Kuehl TJ, Kang IS, Siler-Khodr TM. Am J Primatol 1992;28:41–48.

Metabolism of cGnRH in the intrauterine tissues

A very important factor in the regulation of the concentration of any hormone, and one which is frequently overlooked, is its metabolism. In the development of appropriate analogs of a factor, metabolism is a crucial issue. We have isolated from human placenta a chorionic peptidase, which we have named chorionic peptidase-1 (C-ase-1), that actively degrades GnRH [84]. Interestingly and probably fortunately, as we will expand on below, C-ase-1 degrades GnRH at the 9—10 amino acids [85], a site different from the primary pituitary and serum enzymes that degrade GnRH [86]. C-ase-1 is a postproline peptidase that is present in high concentrations in the term placenta, and will actively degrade proline-containing peptides such as GnRH, angiotensin II or thyrotropin-releasing hormone. However, it appears that C-ase-1 has the greatest activity for the degradation of GnRH and angiotensin. Analogs of GnRH which are not altered at the ninth amino acid are also degraded by C-ase-1. Peptides without proline or with a cyclic structure prior to the proline, such as oxytocin, are not degraded by the enzyme. Therefore, alteration of the proline in GnRH analogs may lead to major changes in the metabolism of that analog in the intrauterine tissues, and thus affect its activity in the intrauterine tissues.

Effect of GnRH or its analogs on the outcome of pregnancy

The data clearly demonstrate that GnRH or its analogs can act directly on the ovary, the uterus and the placenta. Thus, the potential action of GnRH analogs administered prior to or during a pregnancy cycle are real. However, the effect of GnRH analogs administered prior to fertilization and implantation will present a different set of potential interactions than GnRH analogs accidentally administered in early pregnancy.

Considering the first and most common situation, i.e., the use of GnRH analogs to better regulate the timing of ovulation prior to pregnancy, a vast experience of these protocols now exist. A teratogenic action of GnRH on the embryos conceived in these cycles has not been observed [87]. There does seem to be a decreased production of progesterone, and thus, there is an increased need for luteal support [41]. Most commonly this luteal support is given progesterone supplements; however, a few studies report that hCG supplementation is superior to oral progesterone [88]. An important consideration in the need for and type of support may be related to the type of GnRH analog used, i.e., is it a short- or long-acting GnRH analog. Further investigation is needed to clearly determined the best protocol for each particular analog.

Another effect of GnRH analogs may be an increase in ectopic pregnancies [89,90]; this may be due to decreased progesterone production and/or a direct action on tubal motility, neither of which have been thoroughly investigated; whereas IVF patients with hypothalamic amenorrhea had an increased abortion rate, this was associated with increased twinning [91]. On the other hand, a decreased abortion rate in patients having endometriosis following long-term GnRH therapy has been reported [92]. Once again the action of GnRH is clearly indicated but which may be the best analog to overcome and produce the positive and negative actions needs to be determined. One study found that use of a shorter-acting analog resulted in a lower miscarriage rate. Yet neither analog studied utilized progesterone supplementation [93].

The second situation, the accidental administration of GnRH analogs during early pregnancy, is one with limited experience. A literature review yields four cases treated with decapeptyl [94–97]; six with buserelin [98,99] and seven with leuprolide [100,101]. In general, pregnancy continued and the fetal outcome was good. The decapeptyl was administered from the time of implantation to two patients, and beginning at the 5th week of pregnancy to two others. In each case normal term pregnancy with normal fetal outcome resulted. In the patients receiving buserelin exposure was from the time of fertilization in one case (900 µg/day for 14 days), or for 5 days (100 µg/day) starting on the 7th day of fetal age (n = 6). In five of the latter cases, hCG was supplemented at the time of missed menses and normal pregnancies ensued. In the one patient not supplemented with hCG a first trimester spontaneous abortion occurred. Leuprolide was accidentally administered beginning at 3 weeks from the last menstrual period (LMP) for 14–21 days in six pregnancies. In four cases the pregnancies progressed to term without complication, in one a missed abortion occurred and one elected termination of a trisomy 18 fetus. Thus, in the reported case where early exposure to a GnRH analog occurred 14 of 16 pregnancies bearing chromosomally normal fetuses continued to term with an apparently normal fetal outcome.

Prior to drawing conclusions from these findings, we should consider the structure of these analogs, their potency and their half-lives. Each molecule contains the proline at the ninth position, and thus can still be metabolized by the C-ase-1. Their potency, if related to its receptor-binding in the chorionic tissues [23,24] both buserelin and decapeptyl, is equal to GnRH for buserelin and decapeptyl. Thus, in pregnancies these are not superagonist in the intrauterine tissues as at the pituitary, probably due to their rapid degradation by C-ase-1, although a direct measurement of their half-lives during pregnancy has not been done. From our studies in pregnant baboons Zoladex implants may be active as long as 60 days.

Conclusion

GnRH is a primary hormone in both the regulation of the corpus luteal function during the luteal phase of early pregnancy and intrauterine paracrine and endocrine function throughout pregnancy. Interruption of its normal production and feedback interactions during pregnancy can lead to deleterious effects on the pregnancy. However, the placenta contains a very active enzymatic system which may protect it from exogenous GnRH by degrading the incoming molecules. The most active enzyme, C-ase-1, is a postproline peptidase and thus depends on a peptide bond following the proline to degrade GnRH or the GnRH analog. GnRH analogs are frequently administrated to women in assisted reproductive protocols who may become pregnant. Thus, their action must be considered. Analogs without sustained delivery systems and that can be degraded by the chorionic tissues should be best suited for this use. In addition, since the chorionic receptor may differ from that at the pituitary, it may be possible to design analogs having little activity within the intrauterine tissue yet maintaining activity at the pituitary. Should the ovarian receptor or its metabolic degradation differ from that at the pituitary, similar designs to overcome luteal suppression may be possible. Future development of GnRH analogs for use in assisted reproduction or in women who may become pregnant while using GnRH analogs should be developed with these points in mind.

Acknowledgements

These studies were supported by the WHO grant No. 85058A, NIH Center for the Study of Reproductive Biology, RIA Core — HD 10202.

References

1. Khodr GS, Siler-Khodr TM. Science 1980;207:315–317.
2. Siler-Khodr TM, Khodr GS. Am J Obstet Gynecol 1978;130:216–219.
3. Khodr GS, Siler-Khodr TM. Fertil Steril 1978;29:523–526.
4. Siler-Khodr TM, Khodr GS. Fertil Steril 1979;22:294–296.
5. Khodr GS, Siler-Khodr TM. Fertil Steril 1979;30:301–304.
6. Gibbons JM, Mitnick M, Chieffo V. Am J Obstet Gynecol 1975;121:127–131.
7. Siler-Khodr TM, Khodr GS, Valenzuela G. Am J Obstet Gynecol 1984;150:376–379.
8. Seeburg PH, Adelman JP. Nature 1984;311:666–668.
9. Adelman JP, Mason AJ, Hayflick JS, Seeburg PH. Proc Natl Acad Sci USA 1986;83:179–183.
10. Radovick S, Wondisford FE, Nakayama Y, Yamada M, Cutler GB Jr, Weintraub BD. Mol Endocrinol 1990;4:476–480.
11. Siler-Khodr TM, Kang IS, Kuehl TJ, Khodr GS, Harper MJK. In: Bouchard P, Haour F, Franchimont P, Schatz B (eds) Recent Progress on GnRH and Gonadal Peptides. New York: Elsevier, 1990; 101–112.
12. Lundin-Schiller S, Mitchell MD. Placenta 1991;12:353–363 (abstract).
13. Currie WD, Steele GL, Yuen BH, Dordon C, Gautron JP, Leung PC. Endocrinology 1992;130(5):2871–2876.
14. Seppala M, Wahlstrom P, Lehtovirta P, Lee JN, Leppalouto J. Clin Endocrinol 1980;12:441–451.
15. Miyake A, Sakumoto T, Aono T, Kawamura Y, Maeda T, Kurachi K. Obstet Gynecol 1982;60:444–449.
16. Petraglia F, Woodruff TK, Wotticelli G, Botticelli A, Genazzani AR, Mayo KE, Vale W. J. Clin Endocrinol 1992;74(5):1184–1188.
17. Zhuang LZ, Li RH. Sciences in China — Series B, Chemistry, Life Sciences & Earth Sciences 1991; 34(9):1092–1097.
18. Duello TM, Tsai SJ, Van Ess PJ. Endocrinology 1993;133:2617–2623.
19. Belisle S, Bellabarba D, Gallo-Payet N, Lehoux J-G, Guevin J-F. Can J Physio Pharmacol 1986; 64:1229–1235.
20. Kliman HJ, Nestler JE, Sermasi E, Sanger JM, Strauss III JF. Endocrinology 1986;118:1567–1582.

21. Escher E, Mackiewicz Z, Lagace G et al. J Recept Res 1988;8:391–405.
22. Rao AJ, Moudgal NR. Obstet Gynecol 1984;12:1105–1106.
23. Bramley TA, McPhie CA, Menzies GS. Placenta 1992;13(6):555–581.
24. Menzies GS, Bramley TA. Placenta 1992;13(6):583–595.
25. Seshagin PB, Terasawa E, Hearn JP. The 26th Annual Meeting of the Society for the Study of Reproduction (Fort Collins), 1993;Abstract#342:144.
26. Siler-Khodr TM, Khodr GS. Biol Reprod 1981;25:353–358.
27. Siler-Khodr TM, Khodr GS, Valenzuela G, Rhode J. Biol Reprod 1986;34:245–254.
28. Butzow R. Int J Cancer 1982;29:9–11.
29. Mathialagan N, Rao AJ. Biochem Int 1986;13:757–765.
30. Haning RV Jr, Choi L, Kiggens AJ, Kuzma DL, Summerville JW. J Clin Endocrinol Metabol 1982;55:213–218.
31. Kim SJ, Namkoong SE, Lee JW, Jung JK, Kang BC, Park JS. Placenta 1987;8:257–264.
32. Barnea ER, Kaplan M, Naor Z. Hum Reprod 1991;6(8):1063–1069.
33. Szilagyi A, Benz R, Rossmanith WG. Gynecol Endocrinol 1992;6(4):293–300.
34. Siler-Khodr TM, Khodr GS, Vickery BH, Nestor JJ Jr. Life Sci 1983;32:2741–2745.
35. Siler-Khodr TM, Khodr GS, Rhode J, Vickery BH, Nestor JJ Jr. Placenta 1987;8:1–14.
36. Wilson EA, Jawad MJ. Fertil Steril 1980;33:91–93.
37. Branchaud CL, Goodyer CG, Lipowski LS. J Clin Endocrinol Metabol 1983;56:761–766.
38. Shi CZ, Zhang ZY, Zhuang LZ. Science in China – Series B, Chemistry, Life Sciences & Earth Sciences 1991;34(9):1098–1104.
39. Zhu BT, Chu YH. Yao Hsueh Hsueh Pao-Acta Pharm Sinica 1990;25(6):469–472.
40. Siler-Khodr TM, Khodr GS, Valenzuela G, Rhode J. Biol Reprod 1986;34:255–264.
41. Casper RF, Yen SSC. Science 1979;205:408–410.
42. Barnea ER, Kaplan M. J Clin Endocrinol Metabol 1989;69:215–217.
43. Petraglia F, Vaughan J, Vale W. J Clin Endocrinol Metabol 1990;70:1173–1178.
44. Barnea ER, Feldman D, Kaplan M. Hum Reprod 1991;6(7):905–909.
45. Bhattacharya S, Chaudhary J, Das C. Biochem Int 1992;28(2):363–371.
46. Zhou MH, Han GZ, Chu YH. Yao Hsueh Hsueh Pao-Acta Pharm Sinica 1991;26(11):801–804.
47. Petraglia F, Lim AT, Vale W. J Clin Endocrinol Metabol 1987;65:1020–1025.
48. Haning RV Jr, Choi L, Kiggens AJ, Kuzma DL. Prostaglandins 1982;24:495–506.
49. Mathialagan N, Rao AJ. Placenta 1989;10:61–70.
50. Belisle S, Petit A, Bellabarba D, Escher E, Lehoux J-G, Gallo-Payet N. J Clin Endocrinol Metabol 1989;69:117–121.
51. Iwashita M, Watanabe M, Setoyama M et al. Placenta 1992;13:213–221.
52. Tertrin-Clary C, Dela Llosa-Hermier MP, Roy M, Chenut MO, Hermier C, Dela Llosa P. Cellular Signalling 1992;4(6):727–736.
53. Siler-Khodr TM, Khodr GS, Valenzuela G, Harper MJ, Rhode J. Biol Reprod 1986;35:312–319.
54. Siler-Khodr TM, Khodr GS, Harper MJ, Rhode J, Vickery BH, Nestor JJ Jr. Prostaglandins 1986;31:1003–1010.
55. Kang IS, Koong MK, Forman J, Siler-Khodr TM. Am J Obstet Gynecol 1991;165:1771–1776.
56. Haning RV Jr, Choi L, Kiggens AJ, Kuzma DL, Summerville JW. Prostaglandins 1982;23:29–40.
57. Cemerikic B, Maulik D, Ahmed MS. Placenta 1992; Abstract #9.
58. Petraglia F, Sawchenko P, Lim ATW, Rivier J, Vale W. Science 1987;237:187–189.
59. Musah AI, Schwabe C, Willham RL, Anderson LL. Biol Reprod 1987;37:797–803.
60. Steele GL, Currie WD, Yuen BH, Jia XC, Perlas E, Leung PC. Endocrinology 1991;133(1):297–303.
61. Zhuang L-Z, Li R-H. The 23rd Annual Meeting of the Society for the Study of Reproduction (Vancouver) 1990; Abstract #362:161.
62. Beattie CW, Corbin A, Foell TJ, Garsky V, Rees RWA, Yardley J. Contraception 1976;13:341–353.
63. Hilliard J, Pang C-N, Sawyer CH. Fertil Steril 1976;27:421–425.
64. Beattie CW, Corbin A, Cole G et al. Biol Reprod 1977;16:322–332.
65. Humphrey RR, Windsor BL, Reel JR, Edgren RA. Biol Reprod 1977;16:614–621.

66. Corbin A, Beattie CW, Rees R et al. Fertil Steril 1977;28:471–475.
67. MacDonald GJ, Beattie CW. Life Sci 1979;24:1103–1110.
68. MacDonald GJ, Greeley LK, Beattie CW. Int J Fertil 1980;25:198–202.
69. Bex FJ, Corbin A. Endocrinology 1981;108:273–280.
70. Rivier C, Vale W. Endocrinology 1982;110:347–351.
71. Sridaran R. Proc Soc Exp Biol Med 1986;182:120–126.
72. Sridaran R, Mahesh VB. Biol Reprod 1989;40:276–282.
73. Vickery BH, McRae GI. Life Sci 1980;27:1409.
74. Wilcox AJ, Weinberg CR, O'Connor JF et al. N Engl J Med 1988;319:189–194.
75. Hodges JK, Hearn JP. Nature 1977;265:746–748.
76. Das C, Gupta SK, Talwar GP. J Steroid Biochem 1985;23:803–806.
77. Rao AJ, Chakraborti R, Kotagi SG, Ravindranath N, Moudgal NR. J Steroid Biochem 1985;23:807–809.
78. Siler-Khodr TM, Kuehl TJ, Vickery BH. Fertil Steril 1984;41:448–454.
79. Egyed J, Gati I. Endocrinol Exp 1985;19:11–15.
80. Vickery BH, McRae GI, Stevens VC. Fertil Steril 1981;36:664–668.
81. Das C, Talwar GP. Fertil Steril 1983;39:218–223.
82. Kang IS, Kuehl TJ, Siler-Khodr TM. Fertil Steril 1989;52:846–853.
83. Kuehl TJ, Kang IS, Siler-Khodr TM. Am J Primatol 1992;28:41–48.
84. Siler-Khodr TM, Kang IS, Jones MA, Harper MJK, Khodr GS, Rhode J. Placenta 1989;10:283–296.
85. Kang IS, Siler-Khodr TM. Placenta 1992;13:81–87.
86. Griffiths EC, Kelly JA. Mol Cell Endocrinol 1979;14:3–17.
87. De Sutter P, Dhont M, Vandekerckhove D. J Assist Reprod Genet 1991;9(3):254–258.
88. Bovat J, Malcoffer G, Guittard C, Herbaut JC, Louvet AL, Dehaene JL. Fertil Steril 1990;53(3):490–494.
89. Al-Hussaini T, Mettler L. Hum Reprod 1992;7(10):1479–1480.
90. Forman R, Robinson J, Egan D, Ross C, Gosden B, Barlow D. Fertil Steril 1990;54(1):169–170.
91. Braat DD, Ayalon D, Blunt SM, Bogchelman D, Coelingh Bennink HJ, Handelsman DJ et al. Gynecol Endocrinol 1989;3(1):35–44.
92. Dicker D, Goldman JA, Levy T, Feldberg D, Ashkenazi J. Fertil Steril 1992;57(3):597–600.
93. Gonen Y, Dirnfeld M, Goldman S, Koifman M, Abramovici H. J In Vitro Fertil Embryo Transf 1991;8(5):254–259.
94. Ronel R, Golan A, Herman A, Raziel A, Soffer Y, Caspi E. Fertil Steril 1990;53(3):572–574.
95. Rocco V. Minerva Ginecologica 1992;44(11):585–586.
96. Har-Toov J, Brenner SH, Jaffa A, Yavetz H, Peyser Mr, Lessing JB. Fertil Steril 1993;59(2):446–447.
97. Weissman A, Shoham Z. Hum Reprod 1993;8(3):496–497.
98. Dicker D, Goldman JA, Vagman I, Eckstein N, Ayalon D. Hum Reprod 1989;4(3):250–251.
99. Jackson AE, Curtis P, Amso N, Shaw RW. Hum Reprod 1992;7(9):1222–1224.
100. Ghazi DM, Kemmann E, Hammond JM. J Reprod Med 1991;36(3):173–174.
101. Young DC, Snabes MC, Poindexter AN. Obstet Gynecol 1993;81(4)587–589.

Gonadotropins and growth hormone regimens for ovarian stimulation

Roy Homburg[1*] and Hanne Østergaard[2]
[1]*Infertility Unit, Golda Medical Center, Petah Tikva, Israel (Affiliated to Sackler Medical School, Tel Aviv University); and [2]Novo Nordisk A/S, Gentofte, Denmark*

Abstract. The use of growth hormone (GH) as an adjuvant for ovarian stimulation with human menopausal gonadotropin is critically reviewed. A select group of infertile patients may benefit from this cotreatment, particularly those who have a surgical, pathological or medically-induced dysfunction of GH kinetics. The mechanism of this action, the effective dose needed and the implications regarding the interface of GH, insulin-like growth factor I and ovarian physiology and pathology are now becoming clearer. A greater understanding of GH action on the ovary may in future benefit patients afflicted by anovulatory infertility.

Introduction

The role of growth hormone (GH) in adult life remains uncertain. However, the reality of GH and growth factor interaction with gonadotropins in the ovary are now established. Several observations initially suggested this possibility. The lowering of GH levels in female rats led to delayed puberty and decreased ovarian steroidogenesis in response to stimulation by gonadotropins [1]. Puberty is delayed and prolonged in children with Laron-type dwarfism (i.e., resistance to the action of GH) [2] whereas puberty and gonadal maturation could be induced by administration of GH to hypophysectomised animals [3].

The realization of the existence of an intraovarian regulating mechanism involving growth factors and, in particular, the ability of insulin-like growth factor-I (IGF-I) to augment the responses of granulosa cells (GC) to follicle-stimulating hormone (FSH) [4] suggests a role for GH in the reproductive process. There is now clear evidence of the existence of functional GH receptors in human GC which mediate the stimulation of basal and FSH-induced steroid production [5]. This action may be direct and/or produced by an intermediary growth factor. IGF-I receptors are found in abundance in the ovary and the actions of IGF-I have been well elucidated in in vitro experiments. Lately, growth hormone-releasing hormone (GHRH) has been found in thecal cells, GC and the oocyte [6]. These facts collectively suggest that the ovary is a target of growth hormone action and a hive of growth factor activity.

Address for correspondence: Prof. Roy Homburg, Infertility Unit, Golda Medical Center, (Hasharon Hospital), Petah Tikva 49372, Israel.

Although these actions appear mainly to be permissive and regulatory, the exploration of possible clinical applications of cotreatment with GH and gonadotropins was inevitable. It is the purpose of this presentation to review briefly the in vitro studies that prompted the resulting human clinical trials which are analysed more fully. One of the sequelae of the numerous clinical studies involving cotreatment with GH is that we now have a much clearer idea of those patients who may benefit from such treatment, the mechanism of action, and some indication of the dose required. The time is thus ripe for a prospective insight into the possible clinical applications of GH therapy in the field of infertility.

Physiological basis

A direct stimulatory effect of low levels of GH on estradiol (E_2) production by human GC independent of the effect of FSH and without an increase in IGF-I have been shown by Mason et al. [7] in addition to its additive effect with FSH. In support of the hypothesis that GH alone may augment ovarian steroid production, Lanzone et al. [8] demonstrated the ability of human thecal cells incubated with GH (albeit in supraphysiological concentrations) to augment progesterone production in a dose-dependent manner in addition to its synergism with human chorionic gonadotropin in more physiological amounts. However, rather than being regarded as a gonadotropin per se, in the context of normal ovarian physiology, GH can be more accurately seen as a cogonadotropin, synergising with FSH and LH in promoting ovarian function.

There is now a great deal of evidence demonstrating the existence of a complex intraovarian regulatory system involving IGFs, complete with ligands, receptors and binding proteins [4]. Whether the system is mediated by GH through its receptor, indirectly stimulating ovarian IGF gene expression, is not yet clear. Whatever the case, IGFs do seem to have a meaningful role in the regulation of ovarian function, particularly in the amplification of gonadotropin hormonal action. IGF-I amplifies the action of FSH on the proliferation and differentiation of GC and stimulates aromatase activity, enhances proteoglycan biosynthesis, induces LH receptors and potentiates LH action, increasing progesterone production [4]. These actions of IGF-I in the rat have been confirmed in human GC regarding aromatase activity [9,10] and progesterone production [11]. In addition to its direct action on the ovary, GH administration distinctly increases circulatory concentrations of IGF-I by inducing hepatic production [12] and IGF-I binding sites exist on human GC [13]. On the basis of these in vitro studies and with the advent and availability of administration of recombinant human GH, we initiated clinical studies to explore the possible use of recombinant hGH as an adjuvant for induction of ovulation and superovulation.

Clinical trials

Using the hypothesis that it might be possible to increase endogenous IGF-I concentrations and thereby sensitize the ovaries to the action of gonadotropins, the obvious group of patients on whom to experiment consisted of those who were undergoing induction of ovulation or superovulation for IVF and who were resistant to treatment with human menopausal gonadotropins (hMG) [14]. All seven patients recruited had a chronic anovulatory hypogonadotropic state. They were treated concurrently with a combination of hMG and GH (Norditropin, Novo Nordisk A/S, Gentofte, Denmark), 20 IU on alternate days to a total of 120 IU. This cotreatment significantly augmented the ovarian response to hMG in four patients undergoing conventional ovulation induction and in three others undergoing IVF when a total of 33 gonadotropin cycles was compared with 19 cycles featuring the combined regimen. The amount, duration of treatment with, and daily effective dose of hMG were reduced by the concurrent provision of GH. In the IVF cycles, the number of oocytes obtained rose from a mean of 3 to 7.5 per cycle and the fertilization rate improved enormously. The three patients who conceived with GH therapy all delivered normal healthy babies.

The positive results of this open study encouraged us to perform a large, randomized, prospective, placebo-controlled trial to examine the role of GH in the treatment of poor responders to conventional induction of ovulation with hMG [12]. A total of 16 such women, all afflicted with chronic hypogonadotropic anovulation, were randomly allocated to treatment with hMG and GH (24 IU on alternate days, total dose 144 IU) or hMG and placebo. Seven patients receiving placebo were offered a second cycle of treatment with combined hMG and GH for ethical considerations. The cotreatment with GH was again associated with a 36% reduction in the required dose of hMG and a significant reduction in the duration of treatment and daily effective dose. There was no significant difference in the number of large or cohort follicles induced. Three patients conceived in their first study cycle, one in the placebo and two in the GH group and delivered healthy babies. Serum IGF-I concentrations rose during GH treatment and peaked at more than twice the upper limit of normal, falling back into the normal range within 1 week of the last GH injection. Serum IGF-I concentrations remained unchanged during placebo cycles. No change was seen in serum IGF-II concentrations in either GH or placebo cycles. Using a broad range of "safety" screening tests, other than a transient rise in serum alanine transferase and a mild dip in serum urea concentrations in those receiving GH therapy, no changes were noted.

In a single case report [15] a similar potentiating effect using just four injections of 4 IU of GH was demonstrated in a panhypopituitary patient. Burger et al. [16] in an open study, commented on by Fowler and Templeton [17], also examined the utility of adjunctive GH therapy in three patients with chronic hypogonadotropic anovulation using three different doses of GH. A very striking benefit was obtained from GH therapy, reducing the dose of hMG required to achieve ovulation from a mean of eight to 11 ampules per day to three to six ampules per day. This effect of GH given in one cycle of treatment appeared to carry over and persist for four further cycles in one patient without further GH therapy. It is possible that this was due to GH itself but this point is debatable as other factors such as the initial induction of ovulation itself may have set off a chain reaction.

A further report by our group [18] included two more patients who had hypogonadotropic hypogonadism and who displayed a dramatic response within 7 days of cotreatment with GH and hMG. One of these patients had previously shown no response in two cycles of treatment with large amounts of hMG. Following cotreatment with GH (96 IU over 7 days) ovulation was successfully induced.

From the above studies it now seems clear that additive GH can dramatically sensitize the ovaries of patients afflicted by chronic hypogonadotropic hypogonadism to stimulation by gonadotropins. As the majority of these patients were probably also suffering from a relative deficiency of GH and possibly IGF-I, the adding on of GH may be regarded as successful substitution therapy. This potential utility of adjunctive GH therapy was hinted at by two early studies [19,20] which both described the inordinately high amounts of hMG required to induce ovulation in patients with blatant GH deficiency. In addition, a thought-provoking study by Ovesen et al. [21] demonstrated intriguingly that women with primary anovulatory infertility and regular menses had a relative GH insufficiency as illustrated by a blunted response to GH stimulation tests in these patients compared with controls.

Several studies have examined the effect of adjuvant GH added to a regimen of GnRH agonist (GnRH-a) and hMG for superovulation in the context of an IVF program. It is important to note that, in contrast to the studies just described, the vast majority of the patients involved were normally cycling and therefore normogonadotropic. Ibrahim et al. [22] gave GH to 10 women who had responded poorly in their previous cycle of GnRH-a/hMG. Growth hormone was given concurrently with hMG in a dose of 144 IU over 6 or 12 days. Results were pooled and revealed that GH had reduced the total number of hMG ampules required per cycle from 94 to 59 and the duration of treatment per cycle by 6 days. The rate of follicular growth, the number of oocytes collected and embryos replaced were all increased by GH. Of most significance was that 6 out of 10 women conceived in their GH cycle in this open trial.

Using a similar treatment regimen, Owen et al. [23] performed a randomized, double-blind, placebo-controlled trial in similar patients. Cotreatment with GH was associated with a significant reduction in gonadotropin requirement. Of the 25 patients assessed, 18 had ultrasonically diagnosed polycystic ovaries and it was in this particular subgroup of patients that more follicles developed and more oocytes were collected, fertilized and cleaved in those receiving GH compared to placebo.

A recent report by Tzeng et al. [24] employed 19 patients who had previously failed to conceive with IVF on a regimen of GnRH-a and FSH. They were given GH, 4 IU on day 2, 4 and 6 of the next cycle. Results were compared with their previous cycles and with those of a matched control group of 38 women without GH cotreatment. The pregnancy rate in GH-treated patients was 58% (11 of 19) compared with 21% (8 of 38) in the control group. The number of gestational sacs per embryo transferred was 19% in the GH-treated cycles, compared with 5% in controls. The authors concluded that cotreatment with GH may improve the embryo quality and endometrial maturation and enhance embryo implantation.

Shaker et al. [25] in contrast found that GH had no effect at all when GH was added to GnRH-a/hMG cycles in 10 poor responders. However, it appeared that the reason for the previous poor response in at least half of these patients was approaching incipient failure as witnessed by elevated FSH levels at entry to the study. As we have already indicated [18] no effect of adjuvant GH treatment can be expected in patients who are poor responders with elevated FSH levels.

A recent randomized double-blind and placebo-controlled study from Bergh et al. [6] on 40 women undergoing IVF with GnRH-a/hMG has shown no beneficial effect of adjuvant GH other than a significantly improved fertilization rate. The authors comment that this may be clinically important in a group of patients from which very few oocytes are retrieved.

When GnRH-a was not involved in the standard treatment protocol for IVF, the results of adjunctive GH therapy have been less encouraging. Owen et al. [26] reported that in a controlled trial on a group of 20 poor responders on a protocol of clomiphene and hMG no significant improvement in ovarian response was noted from the addition of GH. Again, a subgroup of women with ultrasonically diagnosed polycystic ovaries did respond to GH with an increased number of oocytes collected but, on the whole, results were disappointing. Volpe et al. [27] examined the effect of GH on 11 patients deemed resistant to therapy with FSH/hMG for IVF. Whereas all previous cycles had been cancelled for lack of response, the addition of GH to the same dose of FSH/hMG employed in previous cycles, induced a considerable improvement in ovarian responsiveness in the younger patients (<36 years) but no improvement whatsoever in the older age group (>39 years).

Several groups have tested the utility of adjuvant GH therapy to standard GnRH-a/hMG protocols in patients who respond normally [25,28,29]. Results were uniformly negative in that the addition of GH to standard protocols of GnRH-a/hMG did not affect dose of hMG, oocytes recovered or pregnancy rates.

Employing the principle that GHRH will activate the somatotropic axis to increase endogenous GH secretion, three studies have employed this agent in an attempt to promote follicular responsiveness in IVF programs [30–32]. Hugues et al. [30] gave 500 μg of GHRH twice daily from day 2 of hMG treatment and a flare-up protocol of GnRH-a while Volpe et al. [31] used GHRH with a standard GnRH-a regimen. Both studies showed minor benefits from additive GH of borderline clinical significance. Tulandi et al. [32] improved the pregnancy rate in 13 women with hMG and GHRH compared with hMG and placebo.

Indications for GH adjuvant therapy

The summary of the clinical trials described here provides a clearer idea of which patients may benefit from cotreatment with GH and hMG. In general, patients suffering from a blatant or more subtle disturbance of GH kinetics causing a dysfunction of the putative GH/IGF-I intraovarian regulatory system are a small but select group who may benefit. This disturbance may have been induced by surgical (e.g., hypophysectomy), pathological (e.g., idiopathic hypothalamic hypogonadism) or medical (e.g., the use of GnRH-a) reasons. Thus, clear evidence of an adjuvant effect of GH in increasing ovarian response to gonadotropins has been obtained in women with hypopituitarism [12,14—18]. The positive effect of GH in these series may be regarded as successful substitution therapy for GH insufficiency.

Poor responders to conventional GnRH-a/hMG therapy for IVF have been reported to have a mixed response to additive GH therapy. While some have shown a significant improvement in ovarian sensitivity and number of oocytes collected [22,23,27], fertilization rates [6,24], pregnancy rates [22,24] or a selective improvement in women with polycystic ovaries [23], others have shown no effect [25,26]. Without the use of GnRH-a, younger poor responders have accelerated ovarian response with additive GH but in older patients and in a further controlled series no significant effect was noted [26,27]. Older patients, those with incipient ovarian failure or normal responders have shown no improvement [18,25,27].

It was perhaps over optimistic to expect that additive GH to hMG in normal responders would improve ovarian responsiveness to gonadotropins. These patients have a balanced pituitary-ovarian axis with normal GH kinetics. Follicular development is already maximal in patients with a normal response to hMG and the system is already saturated.

However, in poor responders for whom GnRH-a was employed, a relative GH deficiency may have been created, thus explaining the benefit achieved in a number of these patients from GH cotreatment. In addition to the induced hypoestrogenic state, despite the fact that GnRH-a does not affect IGF-I or GH peripheral circulating levels, the pituitary GH response to GHRH is reduced [33]. In addition, GnRH-a has been shown to reduce the number of IGF-I receptors induced by FSH in granulosa cells [4].

Prediction of patients who may benefit from additive GH therapy

It would, of course, be a singular advantage to be able to predict those patients who would benefit from cotreatment with GH and hMG. Clinically, it is obvious that patients displaying overt GH deficiency or severe hypoestrogenic states will do so. Several studies have attempted to utilize tests of GH reserve as predictors of relative GH deficiency which may, putatively, affect ovarian function. Ovesen et al. [21] employing arginine and heat exposure as stimulation tests, found that the GH response was significantly lower in eight anovulatory women compared with a group of healthy women controlled for age, body weight and E_2 levels. Menashe et al. [34] employed clonidine, a stimulator of GHRH and observed a very low or absent response of GH in 17 of 25 anovulatory patients with cyclic spontaneous bleeding. Seven of these 17 responded very poorly to hMG stimulation. All clonidine-positive patients produced a good response to hMG. Blumenfeld [35] had a similar experience. Nine of 12 poor responders were clonidine negative and all responded favourably to additive GH and five conceived. Three patients who responded to clonidine derived no benefit from GH. It is tempting to suggest that clinically inevident subtle GH insufficiency may play a role in the anovulatory infertility of some women.

Dose required

In our original studies [12,14] we had clearly used a pharmacological dose of GH so we then proceeded to explore the utility of a single intramuscular injection of GH (24 IU) administered on the first day of hMG therapy in seven patients [36] who had participated in the controlled study [12]. This allowed a comparison of a placebo, single dose and six dose added GH cycle in the same woman. Whereas there was a very significant difference between the placebo and six dose cycles, the single dose and six dose GH regimens produced almost identical results. The six dose cycles required slightly, but not significantly, less ampules of hMG, daily effective dose and duration of treatment than the single dose regimen. The single dose regimen was clearly superior to the placebo cycles using these criteria as a guide. More prolonged increments in the circulating levels of IGF-I were noted in the six dose regimen compared to the one dose. The results of this study suggest that a single sharp rise in IGF-I concentration sensitizes the ovary to gonadotropin stimulation, that this effect is dose dependent and that a single injection of 24 IU GH may well suffice to enhance ovarian sensitivity to gonadotropins.

Utilizing three hypogonadotropic patients Burger et al. [16] tested the effect of 4, 12 and 24 IU of GH with gonadotropins for 5 to 7 doses on alternate days and found that these doses were equally effective in terms of gonadotropin requirements. This despite the fact that the increase in circulating IGF-I levels was less in the patient given 4 IU. In a single case report of a woman with panhypopituitarism, a total of 16 IU of additive GH given in 4 doses was sufficient to produce a dramatic change in ovarian response to gonadotropins [15]. The minimum dose of GH required to synergize with gonadotropins may thus be quite low in these patients although it has proved difficult to pinpoint an exact effective dose. A multicenter trial organized by the Novo Nordisk company is now in progress to elucidate this point and its preliminary findings are that a definite dose-dependent effect has been established.

Mechanism of action

There are several possible mechanisms by which GH may produce its effect in sensitizing the ovary to gonadotropin stimulation. Treatment with GH causes a distinct increase in serum IGF-I concentrations by stimulating hepatic production and exerting an endocrine effect [12]. This is borne out by the fact that in women receiving GH (but not in controls) serum IGF-I concentrations correlated with, but were always higher than, follicular fluid levels [23]. This suggests that the follicular fluid IGF-I diffuses from the serum. However, the action of GH on the ovary may be mediated through an increase in the local production of IGF-I activating a paracrine effect on the GC [37] although following a study on IVF patients, Owen et al. [23] failed to support this hypothesis. Following the results of a study by Mason et al. [7] a third possibility exists and that GH exerts a direct stimulatory effect on E_2 biosynthesis by the human ovary without any concomitant increase in IGF-I concentration. This may even occur without the presence of FSH [7].

Summary

The reality of the interaction of GH and its mediator IGF-I with gonadotropins is now established. Much has been learnt about the physiological implications. Clinically, a select group of patients may benefit from cotreatment with GH and hMG, namely, those with hypoestrogenic, hypopituitary amenorrheic states and some poor responders receiving GnRH-a, particularly those with polycystic ovaries. This cotreatment serves no purpose in normal responders or perimenopausal patients. While the induced increase in ovarian sensitivity may be highly desirable, particularly in obstinate poor responders, the cost benefit index will only be appreciated when an accurate estimate of the dose of GH required will be completed. Further research into the possibility of improving pregnancy rates, the most ardently desired end point is needed and this may well involve examination of the effect of GH/IGF-I on the endometrium, follicle and oocyte.

References

1. Advis JPS, White S, Ojeda SR. Endocrinology 1981;108:1343–1352.
2. Laron Z, Sarel R, Pertzelan A. Eur J Pediatr 1980;134:79–83.
3. Sheikholislam BM, Stempfel RS. Pediatrics 1972;49:362–374.
4. Adashi EY, Resnick CE, D'Ercole AJ, Svoboda ME, Van Wyk JJ. Endocr Rev 1985;6:400–420.
5. Carlsson B, Bergh C, Bentham J, Olsson JH, Norman MR, Billig H, Roos P, Hillensjo T. Hum Reprod 1992;7:1205–1209.
6. Bergh C, Hillensjo T, Wikland M, Nilsson L, Borg G, Hamberger L. Adjuvant growth hormone treatment during IVF; a randomized, placebo-controlled study. Fertil Steril (in press).
7. Mason HD, Martikainen H, Beard RW, Anyaoku V, Franks S. J Endocrinol 1990;126:R1–R4.
8. Lanzone A, Di Simone N, Castellani R, Fulghesu AM, Caruso A, Mancuso S. Fertil Steril 1990; 57:92–96.
9. Erickson GF, Garzo VG, Magoffin DA. J Clin Endocrinol Metab 1989;69:716–724.
10. Christman GM, Randolph JF, Peegel H, Menon KM. Fertil Steril 1991;55:1099–1105.
11. Bergh C, Olsson JH, Hillensjo T. Acta Endocrinol (Copenh) 1991;125:177–185.
12. Homburg R, West C, Toressani T, Jacobs HS. Fertil Steril 1990;53:254–260.
13. Gates GS, Bayer S, Siebel M, Poretsky L, Flier JS, Moses AC. J Recept Res 1987;7:885–890.
14. Homburg R, West C, Toressani T, Jacobs HS. Clin Endocrinol 1988;29:113–117.
15. Blumenfeld Z, Lunenfeld B. Fertil Steril 1989;52:328–331.
16. Burger HG, Kovacs GT, Polson DM, McDonald J, McCloud PI, Harrop M. Clin Endocrinol 1991; 35:119–122.
17. Fowler PA, Templeton A. Clin Endocrinol 1991;35:117–118.
18. Homburg R, West C, Ostergaard H, Jacobs HS. Gynecol Endocrinol 1991;5:33–36.
19. Cassar J, Verco CG, Joplin GF. Br J Obstet Gynaecol 1980;87:337–339.

20. Dawood MY, Jarrett JC, Choe JK. Fertil Steril 1982;38:415–418.
21. Ovesen P, Moller J, Moller N, Christiansen JS, Jorgenson JOL, Orskov H. Fertil Steril 1992;57:97–101.
22. Ibrahim ZHZ, Matson PL, Buck P, Lieberman BA. Fertil Steril 1991;55:202–204.
23. Owen EJ, Shoham Z, Mason BA, Ostergaard H, Jacobs HS. Fertil Steril 1991;56:1104–1110.
24. Tzeng CR, Chien LW, Cheng YF, Chang SR, Chen AC. J Assist Reprod Genet 1993;10(suppl):111 (abstract).
25. Shaker AG, Fleming R, Jamieson ME, Yates RWS, Coutts JRT. Fertil Steril 1992;58:919–923.
26. Owen EJ, West C, Mason BA, Jacobs HS. Hum Reprod 1991;6:524–528.
27. Volpe A, Coukos G, Barreca A, Artini PG, Minuto F, Giordano G. Gynecol Endocrinol 1989;3:125–133.
28. Hughes SM, Huang ZH, Matson PL, Buck P, Lieberman BA, Morris ID. Hum Reprod 1992;7:770–775.
29. Younis JS, Dorembus D, Simon A, Schenker JG, Koren R, Laufer N. Fertil Steril 1992;58:575–580.
30. Hugues JN, Torresani T, Herve F, Martin-Point B, Tamboise A, Santarelli J. Fertil Steril 1991;55:945–951.
31. Volpe A, Coukos G, Barreca A, Giordano G, Artini PG, Gennazzani AR. Hum Reprod 1991;6:1228–1232.
32. Tulandi T, Falcone T, Guyda H, Hemmings R, Billiar R, Morris D. Hum Reprod 1993;8:525–527.
33. Word RA, Odom MJ, Byrd W, Carr BR. Fertil Steril 1990;54:73–78.
34. Menashe Y, Lunenfeld B, Pariente C, Frenkel Y, Mashiach S. Fertil Steril 1990;53:432–435.
35. Blumenfeld Z. J In Vitro Fertil 1991;8:127–136.
36. Homburg R, West C, Torresani T, Jacobs HS. Clin Endocrinol 1990;32:781–785.
37. Barreca A, Minuto F, Volpe A, Cecchelli E, Cella F, Del Monte P. Clin Endocrinol 1990;32:497–505.

Ovarian hyperstimulation

Pathophysiology and clinical management of ovarian hyperstimulation

Daniel Navot[1*], Paul A. Bergh[2] and Roberto Palermo[3]

[1]Department of Obstetrics and Gynecology, Division of Reproductive Endocrinology, New York Medical College, Valhalla, NY 10595, USA; [2]Department of Obstetrics and Gynecology, Division of Reproductive Endocrinology St. Barnabas Medical Center, Livingston, NJ 07039, USA; and [3]Istituto Materna Infantile, Palermo, Italy

Abstract. Ovarian hyperstimulation is the consequence of pharmacological intervention into the ovulatory or anovulatory menstrual cycle. In general terms there are two types of intervention; the so-called controlled ovarian hyperstimulation (COH) for the novel reproductive technologies, and the much less aggressive ovulation induction (OI) practised for anovulatory infertility. Controlled ovarian hyperstimulation is an intentional effort to exert positive selection on the recruited cohort of follicles. In contrast to conventional ovulation induction, COH poses several theoretical and practical differences. The oocyte is not allowed to be extruded, rather the follicle is aspirated with its contents, including the oocyte-corona-cumulus complex and a large supplement of granulosa cells. Thus, the iatrogenic intrafollicular hemorrhage and reduction in granulosa cell mass may significantly impact on the quality of the ensuing luteal phase and on the prospect of ovarian hyperstimulation syndrome (OHSS). Lastly, in ART, complete control can be exercised over the number of ova reaching the female reproductive tract (including completely deferring ovum transfer with the use of cryopreservation) without severely compromising the chances for an eventual pregnancy. Ovulation induction is typically applied in anovulatory women, with an attempt to closely simulate the phases characteristic of a natural ovulatory cycle. Although theoretically a single dominant follicle represents an optimal cycle of OI, in practice codominance of 2–3 follicles yield the best pregnancy results. Ovarian enlargement and accumulation of extravascular exudate are the hallmarks of OHSS. The underlying mechanism responsible for the clinical manifestation of OHSS appears to be an increase in capillary permeability of mesothelial surfaces, and intense neovascularization (angiogenesis) which is a prerequisite for the rapidly enlarging ovary. Although currently the ovarian renin-angiotensin cascade provides the most attractive and comprehensive explanation for the pathophysiological processes comprising the OHSS, alternate mediators may also play a role in the genesis of this syndrome. In addition to the classical description of OHSS, we have redefined severe OHSS and added a critical, life-threatening form of the syndrome. In this classification, generalized edema (anasarca) and liver dysfunction are considered additional signs of severe OHSS, while adult respiratory distress syndrome (ARDS), a tense ascites, severe hemoconcentration (hct >55%), and profound leukocytosis (>25,000) are signs of the severest life-threatening form. The severe and life-threatening forms of the syndrome call for aggressive medical and surgical intervention; significant hemoconcentration and stress (hct >45%, leukocytosis >20,000), subjective or objective oliguria, massive ascites and rising serum creatinine (≥ 1.0 ng/ml) indicate immediate hospitalization and initiation of fluid therapy. NaCl with or without glucose is the crystalloid of choice. The daily volume infused may vary from 1.5 to >3.0 l. Whenever adequate fluid balance cannot be restored by crystalloids alone, plasma expanders (albumin) should be utilized. If OHSS cannot be controlled by medical therapy, paracentesis becomes an alternate

---

Address for correspondence: Daniel Navot MD, Department of Obstetrics and Gynecology, Division of Reproductive Endocrinology, New York Medical College, Valhalla, NY 10595, USA.

option. Although severe OHSS should be largely preventable, the significant overlap between target values leading to successful outcome and criteria conducive of severe OHSS means that at least occasionally this iatrogenic syndrome will continue to haunt clinicians.

The pathophysiology of ovarian hyperstimulation syndrome (OHSS) is best understood through the principles of the ovulatory cycle as laid down by Hodgen and co-workers [1] and the new insights provided by Geugon et al. [2]. The classical view of the menstrual cycle describes five distinct periods: a period of follicular recruitment and subsequent periods of follicular selection and follicular dominance which culminate in ovulation of the dominant follicle [1]. After extrusion of the mature oocyte, the dominant follicle transforms into the corpus luteum dominating the luteal phase of the cycle. Geugon's supposition [2] adds a new dimension to the above concept, namely that "recruitment" is a predetermined process which most probably starts about a year prior to the index ovulatory cycle. A personal interpretation of Geugon's contribution implies a genetic programming, which initiates the growth of primordial follicles and conversion of these to primary follicles. This step is assumed to take upward of 150 days. Additional follicular development creates the secondary and preantral follicles (120 days). Acquisition of an antrum is the next step, a phase which marks the beginning of the gonadotropin-dependent "growth period" (65 days) which is divided into 5 classes. The transition between classes 4 and 5 marks the beginning of the "selection" phase which spans a 10-day period overlapping the late luteal phase of the previous and the early to midfollicular phase of the index ovulatory cycle. Class 4 and 5 follicles range between 2–5 mm in size corresponding to the necklace of follicles often observed on transvaginal ultrasonography in PCO-like patients [3]. From this point on, selection and dominance proceed in succession. However, the cohort of follicles which is amenable for selection has been destined to proceed on the trajectory of follicular growth some 340 days prior [2]. Thus all of the follicles which may be saved from atresia by high dose gonadotropins and driven towards codominance already exist in the ovary as class 5 small antral follicles. Figure 1 illustrates this concept clearly; on cycle day 3 a palisade of follicles 2–8 mm in size (panel A) are launched into rapid growth by exogenous gonadotropin stimulation. It is obvious that all of the larger follicles depicted on cycle day 11 (panel B) have already been there and thus were not recruited as much as saved from atresia. In a clinical sense the above explains the predisposition of some patients to develop ovarian hyperstimulation even with minute doses of gonadotropins. In these high responders all of the existing follicles are driven into codominance and thus significantly enhance the prospects of hyperstimulation. Indeed the patient whose ovary is depicted in Fig. 1 had 72 oocytes aspirated from a corresponding number of follicles.

Pharmacological intervention

Ovarian hyperstimulation is the consequence of pharmacological intervention into the

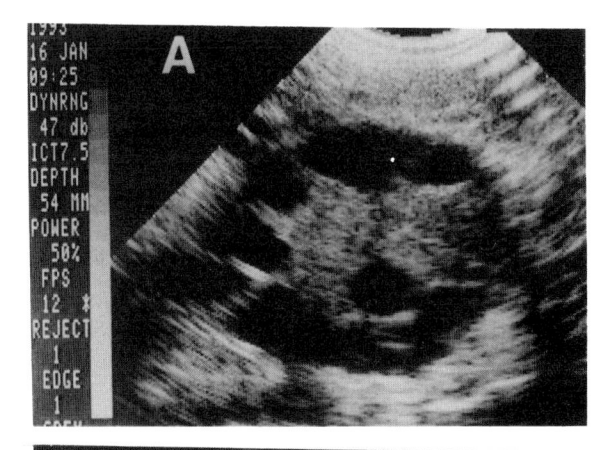

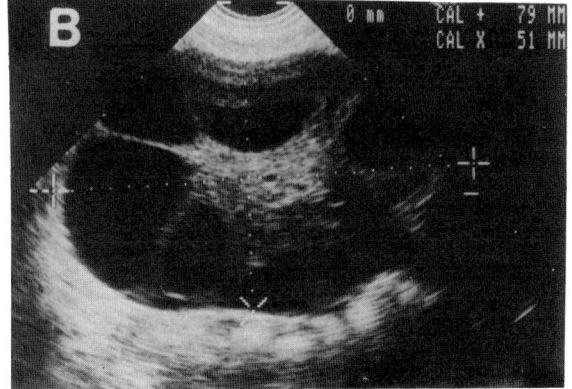

Fig. 1.

ovulatory or anovulatory menstrual cycles. In general terms there are two types of intervention; the so-called controlled ovarian hyperstimulation (COH) for the novel reproductive technologies, and the much less aggressive ovulation induction (OI) practiced for anovulatory infertility.

Controlled ovarian hyperstimulation

This is an intentional effort to exert positive selection on the recruited cohort of follicles. Through continuous application of moderate to high doses of exogenous gonadotropins, multiple follicles will be saved from atresia and launched towards maturation and codominance. This is feasible since all of the selected follicles have acquired at least a minimal content of FSH receptors to sustain maturation in a milieu rich in FSH and LH. In order to exert complete control over a COH cycle, a GnRH agonist (GnRH-a) is continuously administered to prevent an ill-timed endogenous LH surge. The indications for COH include in vitro fertilization (IVF), gamete intrafallopian transfer (GIFT) and zygote intrafallopian transfer (ZIFT). In contrast to conventional ovulation induction, COH poses several theoretical and practical differences. The oocyte is not allowed to be extruded, rather the follicle is aspirated with its contents, including the oocyte-corona-cumulus complex and a large supplement of granulosa cells. Thus, the iatrogenic intrafollicular hemorrhage and reduction in granulosa cell mass may significantly impact on the quality of the ensuing luteal phase and on the prospect of OHSS. Lastly, in ART, complete control can be exercised over the number of ova reaching the female reproductive tract (including completely deferring ovum transfer with the use of cryopreservation) without severely compromising the chances for an eventual pregnancy.

Ovulation induction

This is typically applied in anovulatory women, with an attempt to closely simulate the phases characteristic of a natural ovulatory cycle. Although theoretically a single dominant follicle represents an optimal cycle of OI, in practice codominance of 2—3 follicles yields the best pregnancy results. Simulation of such a cycle is either achieved by relatively small doses of follicle-stimulating hormone (FSH) and luteinizing hormone (LH), or alternately by a stepwise reduction of the dose of gonadotropins. This step-down approach will exert a strong negative selection by allowing maturation and dominance solely to a few selected follicle(s). These follicles would have accumulated enough FSH receptors to be able to respond to a reduced stimulus of exogenous FSH. Although theoretically an OI cycle is less prone to severe OHSS, the inherently inadequate control over the actual number of maturing follicles and the complete lack of control over the number of ova reaching the female reproductive tract poses a significant risk for both OHSS and multiple gestations.

Pathophysiology of OHSS

Ovarian enlargement and accumulation of extravascular exudate are the hallmarks of OHSS. The underlying mechanism responsible for the clinical manifestation of OHSS appears to be an increase in capillary permeability of mesothelial surfaces, and intense neovascularization (angiogenesis) which is a prerequisite for the rapidly enlarging ovary.

Angiogenesis

The process of follicular maturation, ovulation, and corpus luteum formation are associated with a significant increase in capillary permeability which, at least in part, is believed to be secondary to angiogenesis [4,5]. The work of diZerega and Hodgen [4] as well as Zeleznick et al. [6] established the presence of an increased density of blood vessels in the infrastructure of the dominant follicle in primates. Subsequently, the presence of angiogenic activity in follicular fluid of various species including humans was demonstrated [4,5]. Angiotensin II (A-II), the active end-product of the renin-angiotensin cascade was the prime substance implicated in ovarian angiogenesis

[7]. Indeed, A-II has been shown to have a wide range of actions including vasoconstriction, aldosterone biosynthesis, prostaglandin formation enhanced steroidogenesis, increased vascular permeability and angiogenesis [8].

The ovarian-renin-angiotensin system

Renin and its high molecular weight precursor, prorenin, circulate in plasma. While the juxtaglomerular cells in the walls of the afferent arterioles of the kidney are the richest source of active renin, prorenin originates from a variety of other tissues including the placenta and the ovary. Irrespective of the production site, the main steps of the renin-angiotensinogen cascade are uniform; renin, an acid protease, specifically cleaves the substrate, angiotensinogen, at the leucine-leucine bond. This cleavage of angiotensin results in the formation of the decapeptide angiotensin I (A-I), which is further cleaved by the zinc-containing exopeptidase (angiotensin-converting enzyme (ACE) or peptidyl dipeptidase) into the potent A-II. While the converting enzyme is found in most tissues in the body, the very rapid conversion of A-I to A-II is due to the activity of the tissue-bound enzyme present on the luminal aspect of the vascular endothelial cells.

Sealey and co-workers described plasma prorenin to be at a baseline level throughout the follicular phase. There is a 2—4-fold rise near the midcycle LH peak, starting 8—16 h after the initiation of the LH surge and returning to baseline approximately 16 h after LH. A second, smaller midluteal rise in prorenin was noted coinciding with the time of the luteal phase progesterone peak. This second, midluteal peak in plasma prorenin was related to a similar rise in plasma levels of active renin, peaking in the midluteal phase. The temporal relationship of prorenin to LH suggests that LH may stimulate its production. Fernandez and co-workers as well as Glorioso et al. demonstrated preovulatory follicular fluid levels of prorenin up to 12 times higher than plasma prorenin after gonadotropin stimulation [7,9]. Navot et al. established the link between the renin-angiotensin cascade and OHSS by the demonstration of a direct correlation between the plasma renin levels and the severity of the OHSS [10]. They speculated that through the elaboration of A-II, the ovarian-renin-angiotensin system may play a crucial role in the pathophysiology of the OHSS as well as in normal ovarian physiology. A confirmatory report to the above speculation came from Ong et al. who found in patients with OHSS pronounced elevations in plasma renin activity and plasma aldosterone concentrations [11]. Although A-II is best known for its pressor effect, its ability to enhance vascular permeability and initiate angiogenesis would account for a pivotal role in the dramatic fluid shifts seen in the OHSS. In addition to the increase in capillary permeability seen in relation to A-II's ability to induce angiogenesis, it also acts to increase capillary filtration pressure by constricting postcapillary venules. Additional increases in vascular permeability in larger arterioles are caused by the separation of endothelial cells by a possible contractile response. The overall effect is a marked decrease in blood volume and an increase in extravascular fluid and flow of lymph (Fig. 2).

Although currently the ovarian renin-angiotensin cascade provides the most attrac-

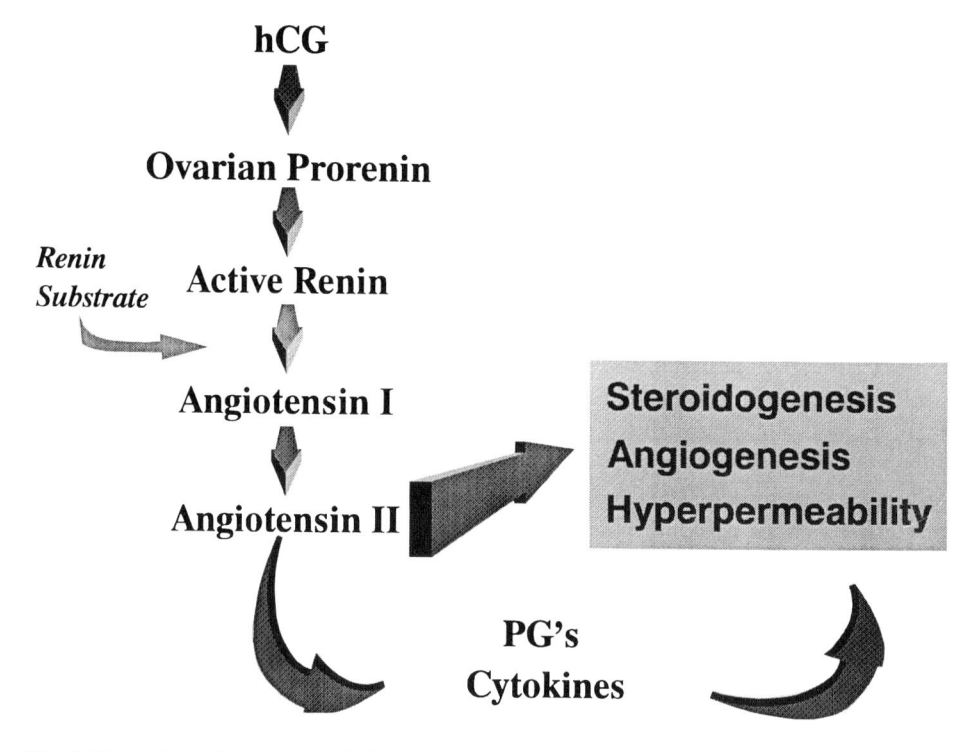

```
                    hCG
                     ↓
              Ovarian Prorenin
                     ↓
  Renin       Active Renin
Substrate ⟶         ↓
              Angiotensin I         ┌─────────────────┐
                     ↓              │ Steroidogenesis │
              Angiotensin II ──────▶│ Angiogenesis    │
                     ↓              │ Hyperpermeability│
                                    └─────────────────┘
                   PG's
                 Cytokines
```

Fig. 2. The renin-angiotensin cascade in OHSS (from reference [12], with permission).

tive and comprehensive explanation for the pathophysiological processes comprising the OHSS, alternate mediators may also play a role in the genesis of this syndrome. Notable amongst these are histamine, prostaglandins and cytokines. Histamine has been implicated as a possible mediator of the OHSS. Although early animal studies yielded promising results in reduction of ascites and ovarian size in OHSS, more recent reports have been less promising [12]. Prostaglandins have also been proposed as key mediators in the pathogenesis of OHSS [13]. Prostaglandins, directly or through their enhanced production by A-II, may account for the induction of OHSS. However, indomethacin in pharmacologic doses failed to prevent ascites and ovarian enlargement in rabbits despite its ability to suppress ovarian prostaglandin formation [14]. Similarly, human trials of indomethacin for the treatment of the OHSS have been disappointing [15].

Cytokines

Recent work regarding cytokine modulation of ovarian function has focused on the interleukin family. Analysis of follicular fluid aspirated from women undergoing in vitro fertilization reveals that macrophages and monocytes compromise 5–15% of the cell population found in preovulatory human follicular fluid [16]. This apparent acute inflammatory reaction is likely to be secondary to the increased periovulatory follicular neovascularization combined with the release of follicular chemotactic factors. The presence of cytokines within the ovary does not appear to depend solely on lymphocytic infiltration since the ovum was found to contribute to their production as well [17].

Interleukin-1 (IL-1) is an activated macrophage-derived cytokine, previously known as lymphocyte activating factor. While the macrophage is the principle source for this polypeptide, other tissues (vascular, epithelial, lymphoid, epidermal, and possibly granulosa cells) produce IL-1. Interleukin-1 exists in two structurally related but distinct forms, IL-1α and IL-1β; the latter form appears to be more potent. Both forms of IL-1 have been found to modulate luteinization, proliferation and progesterone production of granulosa cells [18–20]. Hurwitz et al. recently presented evidence that the intraovarian IL-1 system may modulate the intraovarian regulation of somatic ovarian cell differentiation and thus follicular maturation [21]. Although this cytokine appears to play primarily a paracrine role in ovarian physiology, the detection of IL-1 in the plasma of women after ovulation has led to the hypothesis for a possible endocrine function.

Another cytokine, interleukin-6 (IL-6), was first described as a type of interferon that was purified with hepatocyte and hybridoma growth factor. The mRNA of IL-6 has been reported to be produced in vivo in two self-limiting angiogenic processes: 1) the neovascularization accompanying ovarian follicular development; and 2) the formation of the capillary network in the maternal decidua following embryonic implantation [22]. This limited expression of IL-6 suggests a role for this cytokine in reproductive angiogenesis.

Although these cytokines have not been examined in the context of the OHSS, evidence continues to accumulate on their importance in the modulation of most aspects of ovarian physiology. It is not unreasonable to anticipate a significant role for these ovarian regulators in the pathophysiology of OHSS.

Clinical presentation of OHSS

The mildest form of OHSS is characterized by chemical hyperstimulation, namely, high serum estradiol and progesterone. The ovaries are mildly enlarged, up to 5 cm in diameter. Moderate OHSS features include, in addition to the chemical hyperstimulation, bloating, abdominal distension, and discomfort accompanied by nausea, vomiting, and/or diarrhea. The ovaries, in moderate hyperstimulation, range in size from 5 to 12 cm in diameter. Severe OHSS is comprised of massive ovarian enlargement (>12 cm) usually with ascites, less often with hydrothorax, or pericardial effusion. In addition to the above classical description of OHSS, we have redefined severe OHSS and added a critical, life-threatening form of the syndrome [23]. In this classification, generalized edema (anasarca) and liver dysfunction are considered additional signs of severe OHSS, while adult respiratory distress syndrome (ARDS), a tense ascites, severe hemoconcentration (hct >55%), and profound leukocytosis (>25,000) are signs of the severest life-threatening form [23].

Treatment of OHSS

Medical

Mild to moderate forms of OHSS require little more than reassurance that in the absence of pregnancy, symptoms should abate by 10–12 days after ovulation. However, if the cycle is conceptual symptoms may progress but as a rule no more than one degree in severity. In patients with moderate ascites and mild hemoconcentration (hematocrit (hct) <45%), bed rest and abundant liquid intake should be prescribed [23]. The tendency for intravascular volume depletion and hyponatremia may be treated by balanced salt solution. Gatorade, a popular drink among athletes, seems to be particularly suitable. The patient should be alerted to decrease in urine output, significant weight gain or bloating. These symptoms may be the first warning signs to accumulation of ascitic fluid. The rapidly amassing ascites, secondary to marked vascular and mesothelial permeability, brings about a dramatic reduction in intravascular plasma volume, and thus to hemoconcentration. This disturbance in normal hemodynamics has a wide range of serious consequences including: ascites and pleural effusion, electrolyte imbalance, liver and kidney damage and thromboembolic phenomena. This wide range of systemic effects resulting from the OHSS is ultimately derived from a rapid and relentless depletion of intravascular plasma volume.

Hyperpermeability leads to progressive depletion of intravascular volume and protein, with a reciprocal increase in third space fluid. The protein-rich fluid in third spaces draws more fluid out of the vascular tree through increased oncotic pressure. The formation of tense ascites increased blood viscosity and hypoperfusion of vital organs may follow unless this vicious cycle is interrupted (from reference [12] with permission). Thus, the single most important parameter that indicates the severity of the OHSS is hemoconcentration as reflected in the hematocrit. It is a common misconception that the magnitude of change in the hematocrit is directly proportional to the change in plasma volume; however, the true relationship between hematocrit and plasma is such that a relatively minor rise in hct (i.e., 2%) is 4 times smaller than the actual drop in plasma volume. Thus, even a small change in hematocrit may signify marked hemodynamic deterioration [24]. An additional useful measure for the severity of OHSS is the magnitude of leukocytosis, which may surpass 40,000/ml (Table 1). This massive neutrophilia may to some extent be attributed to a generalized stress reaction. Thus, the concurrent finding of an elevated WBC count (stress and hemoconcentration) becomes very helpful in the clinical assessment of OHSS. In addition to plasma electrolytes and kidney function tests, it is imperative to periodically assess the patient's coagulation profile and liver enzymes. A patient without clinically significant ascites and hemoconcentration may be observed as an outpatient. However, significant hemoconcentration and stress (hct >45%, leukocytosis >20,000), subjective or objective oliguria, massive ascites and rising serum creatinine (≥ 1.0 ng/ml) call for immediate hospitalization and initiation of fluid therapy. The profound vascular hyperpermeability coupled with the high protein content of the fluid accumulated in third spaces, account for the fact that crystalloids

Table 1. Clinical signs and laboratory criteria of ovarian hyperstimulation syndrome

	Mild to moderate	Severe	Critical
Ovarian enlargement	5–12 cm	>12 cm	Variable
Abdominal distention	Moderate	Severe	Tense
Clinical ascites	None	Yes	Tense
Hydrothorax	None	Possible	Yes
Pericardial effusion	None	Infrequent	Infrequent
Decreased renal function	None	Infrequent	Frequent
Renal failure	None	None	Possible
Thromboembolism	None	None	Possible
ARDS	None	None	Possible
Hemoconcentration	Hct < 45%	Hct ≥ 45%	Hct ≥ 55%
WBC/ml	<15,00	≥15,000	≥25,000
Liver enzymes	Normal	Elevated	Elevated
Creatinine (ng/ml)	<1.0	1.0–1.5	≥1.6
Creatinine clearance (ml/min)	>100	50–100	<50

alone, although seldom sufficient in restoring homeostasis, do remain the mainstay of therapy. Because of the tendency for hyponatremia, NaCl with or without glucose is the crystalloid of choice. The daily volume infused may vary from 1.5 to >3.0 l.

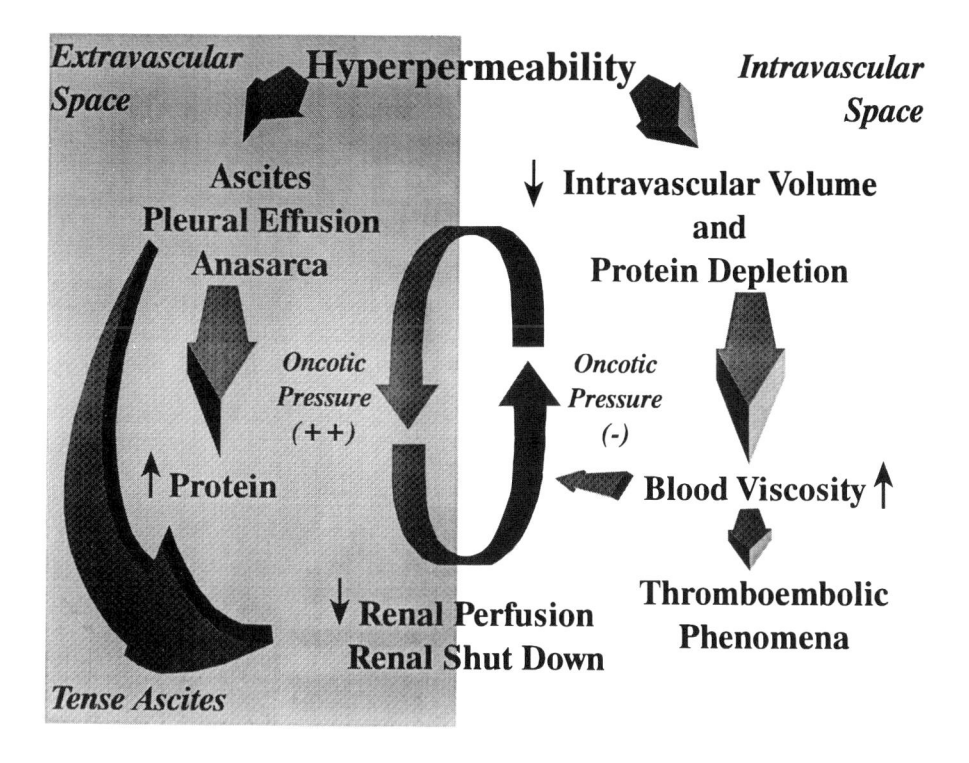

Fig. 3. Schematic layout of the complex hemodynamic changes in OHSS.

Whenever adequate fluid balance cannot be restored by crystalloids alone, plasma expanders should be utilized. Albumin is the protein which is lost in OHSS, and it is safe from viral contamination, thus low-salt human albumin is the preferred volume expander. Albumin at doses of 50 to 100 gm (50 to 100 cc i.v.), repeated every 2 to 12 h, is an extremely effective plasma expander in OHSS. Whenever the above regimen is successful in restoring plasma volume and hemoconcentration is alleviated, i.v. Lasix may be administered. The stage of relative hemodilution, however, may be at the expense of rapid accumulation of ascites and tightening of the abdominal wall. This creates a tense ascites which calls for surgical intervention [23].

Paracentesis

In severe and life-threatening OHSS, which cannot be controlled by medical therapy, paracentesis becomes an alternate option. Both abdominal or vaginal paracentesis are safe and exceptionally beneficial [25]. Dramatic improvements in the clinical symptoms of severe OHSS, with almost instantaneous diuresis are the rule. The indications for paracentesis include the need for symptomatic relief, tense ascites, oliguria, rising creatinine or falling creatinine clearance, and hemoconcentration unresponsive to medical therapy. Paracentesis should only be performed with ultrasound guidance, and it is contraindicated in the patient who is hemodynamically unstable.

In the critical form of OHSS, reduced organ perfusion may lead to multiple system failure. This gravest form of the disease requires management in an intensive care facility and expertise in monitoring and maintenance of the precarious hemodynamic balance inherent in critical OHSS. Impending renal failure, first signaled by minimal rise in serum creatinine and oliguria, should be intensely treated by volume expansion and paracentesis; however, if diuresis does not ensue, a dopamine drip (renal rescue protocol) may prove to be beneficial.

Surgical intervention in OHSS should be reserved solely for abdominal catastrophes and even those can as a rule be approached by laparoscopy. Rupture of ovarian cysts with hemorrhage, ovarian torsion and ectopic gestation, may all indicate surgical intervention. There should be a high index of suspicion for heterotopic gestation whenever a conceptual cycle with severe OHSS coexists with low or decreasing hematocrit. The low hematocrit may actually be secondary to intraperitoneal blood loss and should not be regarded as a reassuring sign of relative hemodilution.

Although severe OHSS should be largely preventable, the significant overlap between target values leading to successful outcome and criteria conducive of severe OHSS means that, at least occasionally, this iatrogenic syndrome will continue to haunt clinicians.

References

1. Goodman A, Hodgen GD. Rec Prog Horm Res 1983;39:1–73.
2. Gougeon A. Hum Reprod 1986;1:81–87.

3. Salat-Baroux J, Tibi L, Alvarez S, Gomez A, Antoine JM, Cornet D. In: Mashiach S, Ben-Rafael Z, Laufer N, Schenker JG (eds) Advances in Assisted Reproductive Technologies. New York: Plenum Publishing 1990:559–565.
4. diZerega GS. Hodgen GD. J Clin Endocrinol Metab 1980;51:903–907.
5. Gospodarowicz D, Thakral K. Proc Natl Acad Sci USA 1978;75:847–851.
6. Zeleznik A, Schuller H, Reichert L Jr. Endocrinology 1981;109:356–362.
7. Fernandez LA, Tarlatzis BC, Rzasa PJ et al. Fertil Steril 1985;44:219–223.
8. Paulson RJ, Hernadez MF, Do YS, Hsuesh WA. Society for Gynecologic Investigations, San Diego, CA 1991; abstract 197.
9. Glorioso M, Atlas SA, Laragh JH, Hewelewicz R, Sealey JE. Science 1986;233:1422–1424.
10. Navot D, Margalioth EJ, Laufer N et al. Fertil Steril 1987;48:57–61.
11. Ong ACM, Eisen V, Rennie DP et al. Clin Endocrinol 1991;34:43–49.
12. Bergh PA, Navot D. J Assist Repro Genet 1992;9:429–438.
13. Schenker JG, Polishuk W Z. Eur J Obstet Gynecol Reprod Biol 1976;6:47–50.
14. Pride SM, Yuen BH, Moon YS, Leyung PCS. Am J Obstet Gynecol 1986;154:1155–1160.
15. Borenstein R, Elhalah U, Lunenfeld B, Shoham-Schwartz Z. Fertil Steril 1989;51:791–795.
16. Loukides JA, Loy RA, Edwards R, Honig J, Visintin I, Polan ML. J Clin Endocrinol Metab 1990; 71:1363–1367.
17. Zolti M, Ben-Rafael Z, Meirom R et al. Fertil Steril 1991;56:265–272.
18. Fukuoka M, Mori T, Taii S, Yasuda K. Endocrinology 1987;122:367–369.
19. Fukoka M, Hasuda K, Taii S, Takakura K, Mori T. Endocrinology 1989;124:884–894.
20. Gottschall PE, Uehara A, Hoffmann ST, Arimura A. Biochem Biophys Res Commun 1987;149:502–509.
21. Hurwitz A, Ricciarelli E, Katz E et al. Annual meeting of the SGI 1991; abstract 5.
22. Motro B, Itin A, Sachs L, Keshet E. Cell Biol 1990;87:3092–3096.
23. Navot D, Bergh PA, Laufer N. Fertil Steril 1992;58:249–260.
24. van Beaumont W. J Appl Physiol 1972;5:712–713.
25. Rizk B, Aboulghar MA. Hum Reprod 1991;6:1082–1087.

Prevention of ovarian hyperstimulation

Josef Blankstein

Department of Obstetrics & Gynecology, Mount Sinai Hospital Medical Center, California Avenue at 15th Street, Chicago, IL 60608, USA

The ovarian hyperstimulation syndrome (OHSS) is one of the severest complications associated with the use of human menopausal gonadotropin (hMG) for ovulation induction. Death and severe morbidity have been reported with this syndrome [1]. The reaction occurs when ovaries respond with the formation of too many follicles and, after administration of human chorionic gonadotropin (hCG), develop ovarian follicular and corpus luteum cysts.

The clinical symptoms of OHSS usually appear 5 to 10 days following hCG administration. To provoke hyperstimulation, both hMG and hCG must be administered. The hCG alone, even in large doses, does not lead to severe side effects. On the other hand, therapy with hMG alone may still result in ovarian enlargement, sometimes with cyst formation and ovulation. Hyperstimulation in such cases, however, is extremely rare, because the endogenous feedback mechanism is usually able to prevent massive luteinization. In cases of severe hyperstimulation, abnormally high levels of ovarian steroids (that is, estradiol, estriol, progesterone, 17-hydroxy-progesterone, pregnanediol, pregnanetriol, testosterone, and Δ5 steroids) have been found. The abnormal hormonal secretion apparently leads to capillary damage and permeability, with loss of fluid from the intravascular compartment, leading to hypovolemia, hemoconcentration, and decreased renal perfusion, together with increased blood viscosity and coagulation abnormalities. Aldosterone production also increases salt retention.

The elevation of aldosterone and antidiuretic hormone can be considered as secondary to the intravascular volume deficit produced by the loss of fluid and protein into the peritoneal and pleural cavities [2].

If not promptly recognized and vigorously treated, the syndrome may be complicated by the occurrence of dangerous thromboembolic phenomena. Since OHSS is Iatrogenic and it may be life-threatening to otherwise healthy females careful measures should be employed to prevent its occurrence.

Classification of OHSS

A comprehensive classification of the OHSS into six grades has been suggested. This was later modified into three grades (Table 1) [3].

Table 1. Hyperstimulation classification

Laboratory and clinical findings	Adverse reaction					
	Mild				Severe	
	I		II		III	
	I	II	III	IV	V	VI
Excessive steroid production	+	+	+	+	+	+
Ovarian enlargement		+	+	+	+	+
Abdominal discomfort		+	+	+	+	+
Ovarian palpable cysts		?	+	+	+	+
Abdominal distension			+	+	+	+
Nausea			+	+	+	+
Vomiting				+	+	+
Diarrhea				?	+	+
Ascites					+	+
Hydrothorax						+
Severe hemoconcentration						+
Thromboembolic phenomena						?

Grade I includes patients with variable ovarian enlargement and sometime small cysts. Laboratory findings in grade I hyperstimulation cases include urinary estrogen levels over 200 μg per 24 h (or serum E_2 levels above 2,000 pg/ml) and pregnanediol excretion of over 10 mg per 24 h (or serum progesterone above 30 mg/ml). Although treatment is not necessary, it is important that patients report back immediately if additional symptoms appear, since severe complications may develop from initially innocent-looking disturbances.

Grade II (mild hyperstimulation) includes patient with distinct ovarian cysts, accompanied by various additional symptoms such as abdominal distension, nausea, vomiting, diarrhea, and weight gain. In cases of rapid weight gain associated with vomiting and diarrhea, hospitalization for symptomatic treatment may be advisable.

Grade III (severe hyperstimulation) includes patients with large ovarian cysts, ascites and sometimes hydrothorax.

Monitoring objectives

The treatment monitoring serves to assess the dose that is effective in evoking an ovarian response, the time required for follicular maturation, and the appropriate time for induction of ovulation with hCG. Furthermore, it should aim to prevent hyperstimulation or at least to detect it as early as possible. Ideally, for these purposes, a combination of estrogen determination and ultrasonography should be used.

Monitoring of E_2 levels

In case of multifollicular development, much higher levels of estrogens will be obtained. In this case, the decision to inject hCG should be carefully weighed against the risk of hyperstimulation or multiple pregnancies.

Although OHSS is associated with high preovulatory estrogen levels [4,5] many cases of OHSS occur with normal or low estrogens, whereas high estrogen levels do not always lead to hyperstimulation.

Since the higher the E_2 content around the assumed time of ovulation, the greater the chances of OHSS, many authors suggested withholding hCG when E_2 levels were higher than 1,000 to 2,000 pg/ml [6–8].

Jaffe et al. [9] have recently reported on a large number of patients who had preovulatory serum estradiol levels >3,000 pg/ml. For cycles with preovulatory E_2 levels of 3,000–3,999 pg/ml the incidence of severe OHSS was less than 1% while in cycles with preovulatory E_2 >4,000 pg/ml the incidence was 5.97%. Since OHSS is more common in young and lean women [10] the authors support withholding hCG whenever serum E_2 >4,000 pg/ml especially in young patients with primary ovarian failure.

In our experience the most important hint during treatment is the slope of ascent of blood estrogens. A steep increase of estrogens — that is, 2 or 3 consecutive days during which serum estrogen more than doubles — should be regarded as serious warning signs, especially with patients who are prone to develop HS, and who will have high levels of E_2 around the assumed time of hCG administration.

Ultrasonographic monitoring

The development of sophisticated ultrasonographic techniques enables us to monitor ovarian follicular growth. While some investigators [11,12], have demonstrated that there is a linear correlation between the follicular diameter and estradiol level in the plasma of normal ovulatory cycles, such correlation is poor in induced cycles where there are many intermediate and small follicles.

Many infertility clinics induce ovulation by means of ultrasonographic measurements of the leading follicle, disregarding the presence of other follicles or the level of ovarian estrogenic secretions. However, this management does not lead or has not led to a reduction in the rate of ovarian hyperstimulation. This is not surprising since it has been shown that the small and intermediate follicles around the assumed time of ovulation may have a crucial role in the later development of ovarian hyperstimulation.

Is it possible to predict OHSS by the number and size of preovulatory ovarian follicles? [13]

Sixty-five infertile patients were included in a prospective study to try and correlate the preovulatory ultrasonography findings and the later occurrence of hyperstimulation. All patients ovulated during clomiphene therapy but did not conceive following three treatment cycles. Patients were treated with hMG according to their daily response and the treatment was continued until urinary estrogen levels reached 80 to 180 µg per 24 h. Subsequently human chorionic gonadotropin hCG was administered intramuscularly on 3 consecutive days. All patients underwent pelvic ultrasound scanning. The results of the ultrasonographic examinations were unknown to the treating physicians, i.e., that did not influence the treatment regime. The number and diameter of the ovarian follicle larger than 5 mm were assessed in both ovaries on the day of assumed ovulation (Table 2). Ovarian follicles were classified according to their size into small follicles of 5 to 8 mm, intermediate follicles, 9 to 15 mm and large follicles greater than 15 mm. It was found that patients who later develop OHSS had significantly more follicles at the time of hCG compared to patients without OHSS. Mild OHSS was characterized by the presence of eight to nine follicles, 68.7% of which were of intermediate size (9 to 15 mm). In moderate to severe OHSS 95% of the preovulatory follicles were <16 mm, most of them (54.7%) <9 mm in diameter. Thus a decrease in the fraction of the mature follicles and an increase in the fraction of the very small follicles correlated with an augmented risk for the development of severe OHSS. From this study one can conclude that ultrasonography is of good predictive value in the occurrence of clinically moderate to severe OHSS in women treated by hMG and hCG. Even with estrogen levels within accepted normal limits, it is suggested that hMG/hCG administration should be interrupted in the presence of 11 or more preovulatory follicles especially if most of them are immature (<9 mm).

Imminent hyperstimulation: what are the options?

Withholding hCG
With very few exceptions it has been reported that withholding hCG prevents the development of OHSS [14,15]. Consequently the current concept is that when biochemical or ultrasonographic signs indicate imminent OHSS hCG should not be given and the cycle should be aborted. Kushnir's study [16] supports this view since none of his patients with excessive E_2 levels and multiple follicular development developed this syndrome. Furthermore, Kushnir et al. [16] evaluated hormonal profiles and follicular growth in cycles with imminent OHSS in which hCG was withheld. Following discontinuation of hMG three distinct periods were observed: 1) day 1 to 2, the level of estradiol testosterone and prolactin and the total number of

Table 2. Ovarian follicles

COE	Small (<9 mm)		Intermediate (9 to 15 mm)		Large (>15 mm)	
	No.	%	No.	%	No.	%
Grade 0	1.8 ± 0.3	30.0	2.8 ± 0.4	46.7	1.4 ± 0.2	23.3
Grade 1	0.8 ± 0.3	9.6	5.7 ± 0.8	68.7	1.8 ± 0.5	21.7
Grade 2	5.8 ± 1.4	54.7	4.3 ± 0.9	40.6	0.5 ± 0.5	4.7

follicles continued to rise; 2) day 3 to 6, the levels of estradiol testosterone and prolactin declined sharply and the total number of follicles was reduced significantly while the large and medium sized follicles continued to increase, levels of follicle-stimulating hormones (FSH) and luteinizing hormone (LH) gradually declined to reach their lowest levels by day 5 to 6 and then increased; 3) thereafter, the number of follicles and steroid output declined to early follicular phase levels.

Delay of hCG administration
Is it possible to rescue cycles prone to develop hyperstimulation?

Since the abortion of human menopausal gonadotropin cycles involve a substantial financial loss to the patient and since their repeated occurrences may ultimately have a negative effect on the physician/patient relationship it is desirable to find a way to prevent the loss of the induced cycle. One has to remember that during the menstrual cycle a secondary decrease in FSH induced by negative feedback causes atresia of all recruited follicles but one. If it was possible to imitate this spontaneous endocrinological behavior it may also be possible to rescue cycles prone to OHSS. Furthermore, if the intrinsic gonadotropin activity of the patient could maintain the growth of only one or two leading follicles after hMG administration has been stopped due to high estrogens or many premature follicles, then a controlled ovulation could be induced at a later stage of the cycle when few mature follicles secrete adequate preovulatory estrogen levels. Rabinovici et al. [17] studied 12 consecutive women with anovulatory cycles who were prone to develop hyperstimulation based on their E_2 and ultrasonographic configuration. hMG administration was stopped in these patients, but the cycle was not aborted. Daily blood E_2 levels and ovarian follicular development were assessed ultrasonographically. If E_2 levels became adequate (<1,700 pg/ml) and the diameter of the leading follicle was between 17 and 22 mm, hCG was administered. Despite the discontinuation of hMG one could observe growth of many follicles. E_2 plasma levels declined in nine of 12 patients from day 1 of the obligatory pause until hCG injection. In three women with rising E_2 levels in whom hMG was discontinued due to many small follicles, E_2 levels rose proportionately to ovarian follicular growth until the day of hCG administration. All three pregnancies recorded occurred in these three patients (Table 3).

Table 3. Duration of pause in menotropin administration and outcome [17]

Duration of pause (days)	No. of patients	Ovulation	Pregnancy
2	1	1	0
3	4	4	1
4	2	2	2
6	2	1	0
7	2	1	0
10	1	0	0
Total	12	9	3

One can conclude that the rescue of overstimulated hMG cycles prone to develop hyperstimulation is possible and appears to offer a satisfactory alternative to abortion and complete loss of the cycle. The successful management seems to depend on an early detection of the events leading to overstimulation i.e., rising estrogen levels accompanied by small leading follicles.

Reduce the dose of hCG
Ovulatory hCG dosages range from 5,000–25,000 IU. Uncontrolled studies indicate that the frequency of OHSS was lower in patients given 1,000–5,000 IU compared to patient treated with higher dosages.

Use of gonadotropin-releasing hormone (GnRH) agonist
Several studies have shown that the use of GnRH agonist can trigger LH and probably reduce the later occurrence of OHSS [18–20].

In a recent study by Levit [21] et al., a single dose of 0.2 mg D-trp-6-LHRH (Decapeptyl) was administered subcutaneously to 19 IVF patients in 24 treatment cycles stimulated by FSH/hMG. The women so-treated either reached estradiol level of >13,000 pmol/l or had a history of OHSS in previous cycles (median 23,600 pmol/l). In all cases oocytes were successfully retrieved. Luteal phase was supported with daily progesterone and estradiol valerate. It was interesting to see that no clinical or sonographic evidence of OHSS was recorded during the above cycles.

The data indicate that GnRH agonist is a probably a safe and efficient way to induce LH surge and prevent OHSS with superovulatory women.

Use of albumin
The potential development of OHSS can be prevented by the prophylactic administration of intravenous albumin. In a study of 36 high risk patients given albumin within 45 min after follicular aspiration the complications related to OHSS were completely avoided [22]. Apparently a pilot double-blind study using albumin also indicates that albumin may avert severe OHSS [23]. We have to await further studies to confirm these encouraging data.

Converting to in vitro fertilization (IVF) cycle
It is believed that aspiration of all follicles reduces the risk of OHSS. Rabinovitz et al. [24] have demonstrated such a protective effect which was associated with a decline in hormonal levels.

It is not surprising that some authors felt that IVF does not offer complete protection from the development of OHSS [25,26] since generally in IVF cycles E_2 levels around the assumed time of aspiration are several fold higher when compared to regular induction of ovulation cycles where the aim is to recruit only one to three mature follicles.

If a patient has multifollicular development associated with elevated E_2 levels, it makes sense to consider converting the cycle to an IVF cycle, and to aspirate all but one to three mature follicles. The aspirated oocytes should be fertilized in vitro for possible later use.

Summary

Before starting treatment with hMG/hCG for ovulation induction one has to identify the patients who are at risk of developing OHSS. The young and lean patients [10] who after relatively few ampules of hMG, develop high E_2 levels and multiple small follicles are at higher risk of developing this syndrome. Patients with polycystic ovarian disease and those with a previous history of hyperstimulation are also at a significant risk of OHSS.

It is again emphasized that prevention is the best way to manage OHSS. There is no doubt that proper monitoring will reduce OHSS; however, one has to remember that strict adherence to the "rules" may be overly conservative and cause a significant fall in pregnancy rates.

An individual approach for ovulation induction is definitely recommended. One has to try and rescue cycles prone to develop OHSS as described above. However, if the risk is very significant it is suggested that hMG/hCG administration should be interrupted.

References

1. Mozes M, Bogokowsky H, Anatebi E et al. Lancet 1965;11:1213.
2. Hanning RV, Strawn EY, Nolten WE. Obstet Gynecol 1985;66:220–224.
3. Lunenfeld B, Insler V, Rabau E. In: Moricard R, Ferin J (eds) L'Ovulation. Paris, Masson et Cie, 1969;291.
4. Oelsner G, Serr DM, Mashiach S, Blankstein J, Snyder M, Lunenfeld B. Fertil Steril 1978;30:538.
5. Yloestalo P, Lindgren PG, Nillius SJ. Acta Endocrinol (Copenhagen) 1981;98:592.
6. Schenker JG, Polishuk WZ. Obstet Gynecol 1975;46:23.
7. Blankstein J, Mashiach S, Lunenfeld B. In: Blankstein J, Mashiach S, Lunenfeld B (eds) Induction of Ovulation and In Vitro Fertilization. Chicago: Yearbook Medical Publishers, 1986.
8. Check JH, Wu CH, Gocial B, Adelson HG. Fertil Steril 1985;43:317.
9. Jaffe, SB, Jaffe, LH, Jewelowicz R. Gynecol Obstet Invest 1993;35:222–227.
10. Navot, D, Relou, A, Birkenfeld A, Rabinowitz R et al. Am J Obstet Gynecol 1988;159:210–215.
11. Hackeloer BJ, Nitschkes S, Daume E, Sturm G, Buchholz R. Geburtshilfe Frauenheilkd 1977;37: 185–190.
12. Schenker JG, Lewin A, Ben-David M. In: Kurjak A. (ed) Ultrasound and Infertility. Boca Raton, FL: CRC Press, 1989;23.
13. Blankstein J, Shalev J, Tova S, Kukiam E, Rabinovici J et al. Fertil Steril 1987;47:4.
14. McGarrigle HHG, Radwanska E, Lihe V, Swyer GIM. J Obstet Gynaecol Br Comm 1974;81:657–660.
15. Wu CH. Fertil Steril 1978;30:617–630.
16. Kushnir O, Ben-Rafael Z, Shalev J, Lipitz S, Bider D, Mashiach S, Blankstein J. Hum Reprod 1991; 6(4):665–669.
17. Rabinovici J, Kushir O, Shalev J, Goldenberg M, Blankstein J. Br J Obstet Gynecol 1987;99:1098–1102.

18. Gonen Y, Balakier H, Powell W, Casper F. J Clin Endocrinol Metab 1990;71:918–922.
19. Lanzone A, Fulghesu AM, Apa R, Caruso A, Mancuso S. Gynecol Endocrinol 1989;3:312–320.
20. Imoedemhe DAG, Sigue AB, Pacpaco ELA, Olazo AB. Fertil Steril 1991;55:328–332.
21. Levit N, Peretz BA, Manor J, Itskovitz E. Prevention of ovarian hyperstimulation by using GnRH agonist for the induction of LH surge in superovulated women (abstract). Ovulation Induction: Basic Science and Clinical Advances. Palm-Beach USA, January 1994.
22. Ascl HR. Albumin may avert severe ovarian hyperstimulation (abstract). The Annual Meeting of the Pacific Coast Fertility Society 1992.
23. Shoham-Schwartz Zeev: Personal Communication 1994.
24. Rabinowitz R, Laufer N, Lewin A, Schenker JG. Fifth Congress on IVF-ET. Norfolk, USA, 1987; abstract 500;111.
25. Friedman CI, Schmidt GE, Chang FE and Kim MJH Am J Obstet Gynecol 1984;150:436–437.
26. Golan A, Ron-El R, Herman A, Weinraub Z, Sofler Y, Caspi E. Fertil Steril 1988;50:912–916.

Pregnancy reduction in iatrogenic multifetal pregnancies

M. Dommergues[1*], Y. Dumez[1] and M.I. Evans[2]

[1]*Maternité Port Royal Baudelocque, 123 Boulevard Port Royal, 75014 Paris, France;* [2]*Department of Obstetrics and Gynecology, Molecular Biology and Genetic Pathology, Wayne State University, Detroit, Michigan, USA*

Abstract. The aim of multifetal pregnancy reduction (MFPR) is to improve perinatal outcome of multiple pregnancies by reducing their prematurity rate. MFPR can be achieved by several techniques including transcervical aspiration and intrathoracic KCl injection either transabdominally or transvaginally. The 10–15% miscarriage rate following MFPR should be compared to that of multiple pregnancies without MFPR. Prevention of prematurity is best achieved when a single embryo is left, but even in that case, prematurity rate following MFPR are higher than in natural singleton pregnancies. MFPR is efficient in improving the outcome of multifetal pregnancies, unambiguously for quadruplets, and arguably for triplets. However, after thorough counseling, parental autonomy should be given a high priority in the decision-making. To obviate the need for MFPR, infertility specialists must continue to be vigilant in the use of fertility drugs.

Introduction

Multiple pregnancies of high order usually result from infertility therapies, including ovulation induction by parenteral gonadotropins [1,2], GIFT, IVF, but also clomiphene citrate [3,4]. Perinatal mortality and morbidity are positively correlated to the number of fetuses [5], mainly due to a high rate of premature deliveries.

The aim of multifetal pregnancy reduction (MFPR) is to improve perinatal outcome of multiple pregnancies of high order by reducing the risk of premature delivery.

Techniques of MFPR

All MFPR techniques are ultrasound guided and can be performed under local anesthesia on an outpatient basis. MFPR can be done either by transcervical suction (before or at 10 menstrual weeks) or by transabdominal or transvaginal needling (8–12 weeks). Although there is no definitive consensus regarding the optimal gestational age for MFPR, our opinion is that it should be done at 10–11 weeks. At

---

Address for correspondence: M. Dommergues, Maternité Port Royal Baudelocque, 123 Boulevard Port Royal, 75014 Paris, France. Tel.: +33-14-234-1204. Fax: +33-14-234-1991.

this gestational age, the odds for spontaneous in utero death of one of the embryos are small, and some gross birth defects can be identified or suspected, which may contribute to the choice of which embryos should be terminated.

Ultrasound guidance

The aim of preoperative sonography is to assess the number of live embryos and their growth, to map their respective locations, and to check for interovular membranes (monochorial vs. multichorial type). The embryos not to be terminated should be precisely identified to avoid any trauma of their ovular cavities throughout the procedure. Careful mapping of the embryos to be reduced is also crucial since survival after a failed attempt of feticide can potentially result in survival with sequellae. Therefore any attempt should be thoroughly completed. If there are no fetal abnormalities, the choice of the embryos to be terminated is mainly based on topographic criteria, and the easiest to reach should be chosen. If a set of monochorial embryos is recognized within a multiple pregnancy, both monochorial fetuses should be terminated altogether.

Transcervical aspiration

This technique was developed by Martene-Duplan et al. [6] in the early 80s. Briefly, the patient is placed in the lithotomy position and ultrasound control is obtained using an abdominal probe. The uterine cervix is exposed by a single valve speculum, cleansed and gently grasped using a Pozzi tenaculum. Progressive cervical dilatation is achieved using Hegar dilators. A Karman cannula, connected to a 20 ml syringe is then inserted transcervically and brought in contact with the embryo located next to the internal cervical os. The embryo is aspirated by a brisk depression operated manually. The corresponding placenta is not aspirated. The operation can be repeated if more than one embryo is to be terminated [3,6–8].

Transabdominal needling

Under sonographic guidance by an abdominal probe, a 20 gauge needle is inserted through the mother's abdomen into the thorax of the embryo. Fetal demise can be achieved by mechanical trauma or the injection of air or potassium chloride (KCl). Nowadays, only the latter method is routinely in use, since mechanical trauma is not always effective and air injection alters sonographic images [9–12].

Transvaginal needling

This approach is similar to the latter technique, but the needle is inserted through the vagina and guided by a vaginal ultrasound probe connected to a needle guide. Although transvaginal needling can be done at earlier gestational ages, it is usually performed at 9–10 weeks [13,14].

Postoperative follow-up

Spotting is usually noticed following transcervical aspiration, but not after transvaginal or transabdominal MFPR. The usefulness of prophylactic antibiotics, tocolytic agents, or cervical suture is not demonstrated. Nevertheless, the major goal of subsequent obstetrical follow-up is to achieve prevention of prematurity, since the risks of premature delivery are decreased but not completely suppressed by MFPR.

Obstetrical and perinatal results

The main goal of MFPR is to decrease the risk of premature delivery associated with multiple pregnancies of high order. This can be at least partly achieved, but obstetrical benefits of MFPR should be weighed against potential drawbacks of the procedure including fetal loss and maternal morbidity.

Fetal loss

Following MFPR, spontaneous in utero death of one of the surviving embryos is infrequent. In contrast miscarriage of the whole pregnancy before 24 weeks occurs in a significant number of cases (10–15%) [11]; these miscarriages often take place 4 to 8 weeks postprocedure. However, this relatively high pregnancy loss rate must be compared with the incidence of miscarriages in multiple pregnancies of high order. For example, in our institution, pregnancy loss before 24 weeks occurs in up to 10% of triplet pregnancies without MFPR. An increased fetal loss rate has been reported with transcervical MFPR [3], but this has not been confirmed in all series [8]. Not surprisingly, the starting number of fetuses and the number of fetuses terminated are positively correlated to the fetal loss rate following MFPR [11].

Maternal morbidity

Apart from miscarriages, no significant maternal morbidity is associated with MFPR, while maternal complications are not infrequent in multiple pregnancies of high order. The use of local anesthesia is recommended to avoid the potential side effects of general anesthesia.

Neonatal morbidity and gestational age at birth

MFPR has not been found to be associated with an increase in the incidence of intrauterine growth retardation or malformations in surviving fetuses.

In multiple pregnancies, prematurity is the major factor of pediatric morbidity, and therefore gestational age at birth should be the prominent criteria to evaluate the efficacy of MFPR.

The obstetrical follow-up of 463 MFPRs performed since 1981 [11] has shown that among potentially viable deliveries (≥24 weeks), mean gestational age at birth was 36 menstrual weeks. However, nearly half of the patients delivered before 37 completed weeks, and before 34 weeks in one out four cases.

The finishing number of embryos left following MFPR was the major factor correlated with gestational age at birth. [3,11].

Following MFPR to a finishing number of three embryos, 89% of the patients delivered before 37 weeks, and 33% before 32 weeks. With a finishing number of two embryos, 52% of the MFPR patients delivered before 37 weeks, and 13% before 32 weeks. In contrast, with a finishing number of one embryo, 30% of the MFPR patients delivered before 37 weeks, and 10% before 32.

Indications and preoperative counseling

In the absence of MFPR, prematurity, as well as neonatal mortality and morbidity, are correlated to the number of fetuses [5]. Nearly all quadruplets are delivered before 37 weeks, and 30 to 40 % of them are born before 32 weeks [15]. In our institution, 78% of potentially viable triplets deliver before 37 weeks, and 21% before 32 weeks. Similar results have been found by others [1]. These data and the results presented above suggest that MFPR is likely to provide a major decrease in the risk of premature delivery in quadruplets, and that a more arguable benefit can be expected from MFPR in triplets. Therefore, we feel that MFPR should be proposed to patients with quadruplet pregnancies, and that in the case of triplets, parental autonomy should be given a high priority in the decision-making after thorough counseling on the potential risks and benefits of MFPR.

The final number of embryos to be left following MFPR is debatable. While leaving a single embryo is the most effective way of preventing prematurity, this approach is associated with a slightly higher risk of miscarriage. Moreover, some couples with a long history of infertility are wishing to keep a twin pregnancy despite an increased perinatal risk.

The choice of a particular technique cannot be based on objective criteria. While we and others had better results with transabdominal MFPR than with transcervical aspiration [3,9], this has not been universally confirmed [8]. Whatever technique is used, the experience of the operator is likely to be an important factor of safety and we believe MFPR should be performed in tertiary care centers.

The psychological distress of couples considering MFPR should never be underestimated. The pregnancy was extremely desired by parents who often underwent stressful infertility therapies, sometimes during many years. However, the birth of triplets or quadruplets is perceived negatively. Usually, the couple is considering MFPR mainly for "social" reasons, and do not realize that maternal or pediatric outcome may be significantly compromised in a multiple pregnancy of high order. The tremendous guilt experienced by these parents is at least partly amended by the information that perinatal outcome should be improved by MFPR.

Despite the relatively good results of MFPR, it must be stressed that this technique reduces but does not completely eliminate the increased risk of prematurity associated with multiple pregnancies of high order. Therefore, our major goal remains prevention of iatrogenic multiple fecundations. During IVF, this can be easily achieved by limiting the number of embryos transferred. However, despite careful monitoring, induction of ovulation can result in the recruitment of multiple follicles. In such cases, follicle aspiration is probably the best alternative. It is clear that to obviate the need for MFPR, infertility specialists must continue to be vigilant in the use of fertility drugs.

References

1. Holcberg G, Biale Y, Lewenthal H, Insler V. Obstet Gynecol 1982;59:472–479.
2. Schenker JG, Yarkoni S, Granat M. Fertil Steril 1981;35:105–123.
3. Dommergues M, Nisand I, Mandelbrot L, Isfer E, Radunovic N, Dumez Y. Fertil Steril 1991;55:801–811.
4. Evans MI, Fletcher JC, Zador IE. Obstet Gynecol 1988;71:289–296.
5. Botting BH, Mc Donald Davies I, Mc Farlane AJ. Arch Dis Child 1987;62:941–950.
6. Martene-Duplan J, Aknin AJ, Alamowitch R. Contraception Fertilité Sexualité 1983;11:745–748.
7. Dumez Y, Oury JF. Contr Gynaecol Obstet 1986;15:50–53.
8. Salat-Baroux J, Aknin J, Antoine JM, Alamowitch R. Hum Reprod 1988;3:399–401.
9. Berkowitz R, Lynch L, Chitkara U. N Engl J Med 1988;318:1043–1047.
10. Bessis R, Milanese C, Frydman R. Partial termination of pregnancy. 2nd Congress "Fetus as a Patient". Jérusalem, Mai 1985.
11. Evans MI, Dommergues M, Wapner RJ, Lynch L, Dumez Y, Goldberg JD et al. Obstet Gynecol 1993;82:61–66.
12. Jeny R, Leroy B. Ann Radiol 1983;26:446.
13. Itskovitz J, Boldes R, Thaler I, Bronstein M, Erlik Y, Brandes J. Am J Obstet Gynecol 1989;160:215–217.
14. Timortritsch IE, Peisner DB, Monteagudo A, Lerner JP, Sharma S. Am J Obstet Gynecol 1993;168:799–804.
15. Pons JC, Le Moal S, Dephot N, Papernik E. In: Papiernik (ed) Les Grossesses Multiples. Paris: Doin, 1991;319–328.

Pregnancy complications

© 1994 Elsevier Science B.V. All rights reserved.
Ovulation Induction: Basic Science and Clinical Advances.
M. Filicori and C. Flamigni, editors.

Infertility and spontaneous abortion — the role of luteinizing hormone

Ariel Zosmer[1] and Seang-Lin Tan[2*]

[1]*Clinical Research Fellow/Clinical Lecturer, Department of Reproductive Endocrinology, The Middlesex Hospital, University College London and The London Women's Clinic, 113/115 Harley Street, London;*
[2]*Senior Lecturer/Consultant, Department of Obstetrics and Gynaecology, King's College School of Medicine and Dentistry and Medical Director, The London Women's Clinic, 113/115 Harley Street, London, UK*

Abstract. The efficiency of any infertility treatment has been traditionally evaluated in terms of pregnancy rates. However, for infertile patients, a favourable result is nothing less than a live and healthy baby. The obstetric outcome of pregnancies resulting from infertility treatment is therefore an extremely important issue. In recent years, attention has focused on the effect of luteinizing hormone (LH) hypersecretion on reproduction. In this paper we will review the evidence for an adverse effect of high LH levels on conception, miscarriage and live birth rates. Recent data which suggest that reduction of LH levels may improve reproductive outcome will also be discussed.

Introduction

While pregnancy is the stated aim of any infertility treatment [1], the most important outcome to patients is the probability of a live birth [2], so that the obstetric outcome of pregnancies resulting from infertility treatments is an important consideration [3]. This is especially important as many patients return for a series of treatment cycles having previously successfully achieved a pregnancy with a first course of treatment [4,5].

In vitro fertilization (IVF) is a successful treatment whose results in terms of pregnancy, miscarriage and live birth rates compare favourably with that of spontaneous pregnancy in the fertile population [1,6,7]. The results are even more impressive when luteinizing hormone-releasing hormone (LHRH) agonists are used [8].

In recent years, attention has been drawn to the association between luteinizing hormone (LH) hypersecretion and poor obstetric outcome. The evidence to support such an association, as well as recent data which suggest that reduction of LH levels may be beneficial, is discussed.

---

[*]*Address for correspondence:* Dr S.-L. Tan, The London Women's Clinic, 113/115 Harley Street, London W1N 1DG, UK.

Hypersecretion of LH and impairment of fertility

The evidence for the impairment of fertility by hypersecretion of LH is derived from numerous studies of spontaneous menstrual cycles, induction of ovulation and assisted reproduction.

In a recent field study, Regan and co-workers [9] prospectively followed up 193 women (mean age 30.7 years) with regular menstrual cycles who were planning to become pregnant. In all cases, a serum LH level was measured on day 8 of the cycle. 88% (130/147) of the patients with normal LH levels (<10 IU/l) conceived compared with 67% (31/46) of those with high LH levels (>10 IU/l) ($p < 0.015$).

A similar correlation has been demonstrated in women with polycystic ovaries [10]. In an analysis of 556 women with ultrasonically-diagnosed polycystic ovaries, it was found that the mean serum LH concentrations in women with proven fertility were significantly lower compared with those of women who complained of infertility (mean 6.7, range 5.1–8.8 IU/l vs. 11.3, range 10.2–12.6) [11]. Homburg et al. [12] studied 54 infertile women with clomiphene-resistant polycystic ovarian syndrome (PCOS) and related outcome of therapy to basal serum LH concentrations. Serum LH concentrations at the time of maximum follicular growth were significantly lower in women who ovulated (mean 9.4, range 2.9–35.4 IU/l) compared with those who remained anovulatory (mean 29.0, range 7.0–50.0 IU/l). Similarly, basal LH concentrations were significantly lower in those who conceived (mean 6.2, range 2.9–8.5 IU/l) compared with those who did not (mean 17.9, range 4.0–50.0 IU/l).

Stanger and Yovich [13] were the first to report the adverse consequences of high LH levels in the context of IVF. They demonstrated that oocytes obtained from women undergoing IVF who had a serum LH level greater than one standard deviation above the mean on the day of human chorionic gonadotrophin (hCG) administration had a significantly reduced rate of fertilisation and cleavage. Out of ten clinical pregnancies, none occurred in the patients with high LH levels. This relationship was confirmed in a series of 200 patients [14] in whom it was found that elevated urinary LH excretion in the 2 days prior to hCG administration was associated with poor oocyte quality and embryo viability, and with reduced pregnancy rates. Patients with an endogenous LH surge were excluded from the analysis. More recently, MacDougall and colleagues [15] compared the IVF outcome of 76 patients with ultrasonically diagnosed polycystic ovaries with that of 76 patients who had normal ovaries and who were matched for age, cause of infertility and ovarian stimulation regimen. They found that fertilisation rates in the patients with polycystic ovaries were significantly lower than in those with normal ovaries ($52.8 \pm 3.4\%$ vs. $66.1 \pm 3.4\%$, $p = 0.007$).

Hypersecretion of LH and miscarriage rates

In the context of spontaneous conception and anovulatory infertility, the association between hypersecretion of LH and miscarriage rates has been increasingly realised in the last few years. In the field study earlier described [9], the miscarriage rate in patients with normal serum LH levels (<10 IU/l) was 12% (15/147), compared to 65% (20/46) in patients with high LH levels (>10 IU/l) ($p < 10^{-8}$). Similarly, a study of women attending a recurrent miscarriage clinic demonstrated that 82% had polycystic ovaries detected by ultrasound [16] and associated abnormalities of follicular-phase LH secretion [17]. With regard to induction of ovulation for anovulatory infertility, Homburg et al. [12] reported, in a study of 54 patients with clomiphene-resistant PCOS treated with pulsatile luteinizing hormone-releasing hormone (LHRH), that the mean basal LH level in those who miscarried (17.9 IU/l) was significantly higher than in those who had ongoing pregnancies (9.6 IU/l) (p = 0.01).

In the context of assisted reproduction, Balen et al. [18] studied the risk factors associated with miscarriage rates in 1,060 IVF pregnancies. They found that the mean age of women with ongoing pregnancies was significantly lower compared with that of women who miscarried (32.18 ± 3.86 compared with 33.17 ± 4.09 years, p = 0.008). The miscarriage rate was 23.6% in women with normal ovaries compared with 35.8% in those with polycystic ovaries (p = 0.0038). There was a highly significant difference between the miscarriage rates in patients who received clomiphene citrate and gonadotropins, compared with those who had pituitary desensitisation with the LHRH agonist buserelin (Suprefact, Hoechst, Hounslow, UK) before ovarian stimulation with gonadotrophins (long protocol) [19], (31.1% compared with 19.1%) (p=0.001). There was, however, no significant difference in miscarriage rates between those who received the short [20] or ultrashort [21] protocols of buserelin compared with those who had clomiphene citrate and gonado-tropins, implying that the pituitary desensitisation with buserelin (rather than the omission of clomiphene) was responsible for the improved results. Interestingly, the beneficial effects of long buserelin seemed to be primarily in patients who had polycystic ovaries. There was no difference in the miscarriage rates in women with normal ovaries who received clomiphene citrate (20.3%) or long buserelin regimen (25.5%). There was, however, a highly significant difference in miscarriage rates in women with polycystic ovaries who received clomiphene citrate (47.2%) and those who received the long buserelin regimen (20.3%) (p = 0.0003).

All these data point very strongly towards an adverse effect of LH hypersecretion on reproductive performance. Exposure of the developing follicles to high levels of LH, as is the case in women with polycystic ovaries, is strongly associated with increased miscarriage rates. This is true for patients who are treated with clomiphene citrate and gonadotropins, as well as for those treated with the short or ultrashort LHRH agonist protocols. In the latter, follicular growth is initiated before pituitary desensitization occurs, thus allowing the developing follicles to be exposed to the high LH levels. In contrast, in the long LHRH agonist protocols suppression of pituitary LH secretion is achieved before follicular growth is initiated, which may explain the significantly lower miscarriage rates.

Mechanism by which elevated LH levels impair reproductive performance

Oocytes are maintained in the first meiotic division from their first appearance during intrauterine life until just before ovulation when oocyte maturation is completed. Since oocytes undergo spontaneous maturation when they are cultured in vitro, an intrafollicular oocyte maturation inhibitor (OMI), related to cyclic adenosine monophosphate (cAMP) [22], has been postulated to exist in vivo. OMI, which is suppressed by the midcycle surge of LH, maintains the meiotic arrest of the oocyte at the diplotene stage of prophase 1. Studies in pigs have demonstrated that if ovulation is induced prematurely with hCG, there is an increase in the rate of polyspermic fertilisation [23]. Similarly, it has been found that delaying the insemination of rats after ovulation increases the number of abnormal pregnancies [24]. These findings support the notion that there is a species-specific interval between ovulation and fertilisation and that if this interval is exceeded, the aged oocytes are at increased risk of reproductive failure. Sustained high levels of LH during the late follicular phase may be sufficient to decrease the levels of cAMP (OMI) in the oocyte, thus allowing premature meiotic resumption. Hypersecretion of LH may, therefore, profoundly affect the process of oocyte maturation such that the released oocyte is either unable to be fertilised, or if fertilised, miscarries [12].

Improvement of reproductive performance by lowering LH levels

Recently, there has been preliminary data which suggest that correction of LH hypersecretion may improve reproductive performance. Armar and co-workers [25] studied 21 patients with clomiphene-resistant PCOS. Laparoscopic ovarian diathermy was performed with four applications to each ovary. They found that there was a decline in the mean serum LH concentration from 19 ± 1.2 IU/l preoperatively to 10.4 ± 1.2 IU/l ($p < 0.001$) by the follicular phase of the next cycle. Seventeen of the 21 patients resumed regular spontaneous ovulation, three ovulated in response to clomiphene citrate and 11 became pregnant. The mean time to ovulation was 32 days.

Another promising line of treatment is the administration of LHRH agonist therapy. Johnson and Pearce [26] induced ovulation in 21 pairs of women with PCOS and recurrent spontaneous abortion and found that there was a significantly lower miscarriage rate (2/20 vs. 11/20) in those treated with buserelin and FSH compared with those treated with clomiphene citrate alone. Abdalla et al. [27] compared the outcome of 14 pregnancies following treatment with clomiphene and hMG, in an IVF/gamete intrafallopian transfer programme, with 33 pregnancies in which ovarian stimulation had been with buserelin and hMG. They found a significantly lower rate of early pregnancy loss, defined as loss of pregnancy within 6 weeks of oocyte retrieval, in the group that received, compared with the group that did not receive, buserelin (three out of 33 vs. five out of 14). There was, however, no significant difference in the rate of miscarriage that occurred after 6 weeks of gestation.

More recently, we used life table techniques to relate the results of IVF to the ovarian stimulation used [28]. The data consisted of information on almost 2,900 women who had one stimulation regimen exclusively throughout all treatment cycles, namely, human menopausal gonadotrophin (hMG) ± clomiphene citrate (CC), follicle-stimulating hormone (FSH) ± CC, and long, short and ultrashort protocols of buserelin plus FSH or hMG. There were no significant differences in cumulative conception and live birth rates between those who received short or ultrashort buserelin regimens and those who had FSH ± CC or hMG ± CC. However, the cumulative conception rate was significantly higher in those women treated exclusively with the long buserelin regimen (59% after three cycles) compared with that of women who only had hMG or FSH ± CC (39% after three cycles) ($p = 0.001$), and compared with that of women who only had short or ultrashort buserelin regimens (22% after two cycles) ($p = 0.0001$). The cumulative live birth rate was similarly significantly higher in the women treated exclusively with the long buserelin regimen (55% after three cycles) compared with that of those who only had hMG or FSH ± CC (29% after three cycles) ($p = 0.0001$) and compared with that of women who had short or ultrashort buserelin regimens (17% after two cycles) ($p = 0.005$). When the results were analysed using a multiple logistic regression model, it was found that after allowing for possible confounding factors such as age, cause of infertility, number of IVF attempts and year of treatment, women who were stimulated with the long buserelin regimen were more than 60% more likely to conceive and almost twice as likely to have a live birth, compared with women who received hMG or FSH ± CC. Pituitary desensitisation with buserelin produced the highest pregnancy and live birth rates in all age groups and for all causes of infertility. The superior pregnancy and live birth rates and reduced miscarriage rates provide additional reasons to favour the routine use of LHRH agonists besides the increased convenience and reduced monitoring this method of ovarian stimulation affords [29].

Conclusion

Although the precise role of LH in the pathogenesis of infertility and miscarriage is still being debated, and the mechanisms underlying the association between LH hypersecretion and adverse reproductive outcome are speculative, there is considerable data to support a cause-effect relationship between high serum LH levels and reduced pregnancy, increased miscarriage and reduced live birth rates in spontaneous cycles, as well as in the context of ovulation induction and assisted reproduction. Pituitary desensitisation, presumably by preventing exposure of the developing oocytes to hypersecretion of LH, significantly increases the probability of pregnancy and live birth following IVF treatments.

References

1. Tan S-L, Steer C, Royston P, Rizk P, Mason BA, Campbell S. Lancet 1990; 335:299.

2. Tan S-L, Royston P, Campbell S, Jacobs HS, Betts J, Mason BA, Edwards RG. Lancet 1992; 339:1390−1394.
3. Tan S-L, Doyle P, Campbell S, Beral V, Rizk P, Brinsden P, Mason BA, Edwards RG. Am J Obstet Gynecol 1992; 167:778−784.
4. Shenfield F, Doyle P, Valentine A, Steele SJ, Tan S-L. Hum Reprod 1993; 8:60−64.
5. Tan S-L, Doyle P, Maconochie N, Edwards RG, Balen A, Bekir J, Brinsden P, Campbell S. Pregnancy and birth rates of live infants after in vitro fertilization in women with and without previous in vitro fertilization pregnancies: A study of eight thousand cycles at one center. Am J Obstet Gynecol (in press).
6. Shoham Z, Zosmer A, Insler V. Fertil Steril 1991; 55:1−11.
7. Hull MGR, Eddowes HA, Fahy U, Abuzed MI, Mills MS, Cahill DJ, Fleming CF, Wardle PG, Ford WCL, McDermott AM. Br Med J 1992;304:1465−1469.
8. Tan S-L, Maconochie N, Doyle P, Campbell S, Balen A, Bekir J, Brinsden P, Edwards RG, Jacobs HS. Cummulative conception and live birth rates after in vitro fertilization with, and without, the use of the long, short, and ultrashort protocols of the luteinizing hormone releasing hormone agonist, buserelin. Am J Obstet Gynecol (in press).
9. Regan L, Owen EJ, Jacobs HS. Lancet 1990;336:1141−1144.
10. Adams J, Franks S, Polson DW, Mason HD, Abdulwahid N, Tucker M, Morris DV, Tucker M, Jacobs HS. Lancet 1985;ii:1375−1378.
11. Conway GS, Honour JW, Jacobs HS. Clin Endocrinol 1989;30:459−470.
12. Homburg R, Armar NA, Eshel A, Adams J, Jacobs HS. Br Med J 1988;297:1024−1026.
13. Stanger J, Yovich J. J Obstet Gynecol 1985;92:385−393.
14. Howles C, Macnamee MC, Edwards RG. Hum Reprod 1987;2:17−21.
15. MacDougall MJ, Tan S-L, Balen A, Jacobs HS. Hum Reprod 1993;8:233−237.
16. Sagle M, Kiddy D, Mason HD, Dobiransky D, Polson DW, Franks S. Br Med J 1988;297:1027−1028.
17. Watson H, Hamilton-Fairley D, Kiddy D, Bray C, Armstrong P, Beard R, Bonrey R, Franks S. J Endocrinol 1989;(suppl):abstract 25.
18. Balen A, Tan S-L, MacDougall J, Jacobs HS. Hum Reprod 1993;8:959−964.
19. Kingsland C, Tan S-L, Bickerton N, Mason BA, Campbell S. Fertil Steril 1992;57:804−809.
20. Tan S-L, Kingsland C, Campbell S, Mills C, Bradfield J, Alexander N, Yovich J, Jacobs HS. Fertil Steril 1992;57:810−814.
21. Macnamee MC, Howles CM, Edwards RG, Taylor PJ, Elder K. Fertil Steril 1989;52:264−269.
22. Downs SM. In: Bavister BD, Cummins, Roldan ERS (eds) Fertilisation in Mammals. Serono Symposia, Norwell, USA, 1990;5−16.
23. Hunter RHF, Cook B, Baker TG. Nature 1976;260:156−158.
24. Austin BR. In: Austin CR, Short RV (eds) Reproduction in Mammals. Part 1. Germ cells and Fertilisation. 2nd edn. Cambridge, UK: Cambridge University Press, 1982;46−62.
25. Armar NA, McGarrigle HHG, Honour JW, Howlownia P, Jacobs HS, Lachelin GCL. Fertil Steril 1990;53:45−49.
26. Johnson P, Pearce JM. Br Med J 1990;300:154−156.
27. Abdalla HI, Ahuja KK, Leonard T, Morris NN, Jacobs HS. Fertil Steril 1990;53:473−478.
28. Tan S-L, Balen A, Doyle P, Brinsden P. Gynecol Endocrinol 1993;7(suppl):50.
29. Tan S-L, Balen A, Hussein El, Mills C, Campbell S, Yovich J, Jacobs, HS. Fertil Steril 1992;57: 1259−1264.

Predictors of miscarriage in menotropin ovulation induction for anovulatory polycystic ovarian syndrome

M. Wingfield[1], S. Clarke[3], X. Li[1], P.I. McCloud[2], H.G. Burger[3], G. Kovacs[1], N. McClure[1] and D.L. Healy[1]*

[1]*Department of Obstetrics and Gynaecology, Monash University, Melbourne;* [2]*Department of Mathematical Statistics, Monash University, Melbourne;* [3]*Prince Henry's Institute of Medical Research, Melbourne, Australia*

Abstract. The objective of this study was to examine the relationship of baseline, preovulatory and postovulatory serum estradiol, progesterone and LH levels and age with pregnancy outcome in polycystic ovarian syndrome patients undergoing hMG ovulation induction. The setting was a tertiary referral ovulation induction clinic analysing all available data over 5 years. There were 108 pregnancies from a total of 519 cycles in 204 women. The main outcome measures were ovulation pregnancy ending in miscarriage before 20 weeks gestation or continuing after 20 weeks pregnancy. Of the endocrine parameters considered, none were significantly different in nonconception and conception ovulatory cycles. Miscarriage was associated with elevated postovulatory serum E_2 values. Patient age, basal serum E_2, LH and progesterone levels were not related to pregnancy outcome.

Introduction

Spontaneous miscarriage is tragic for any couple and particularly for those with a history of infertility. Increasing efforts are therefore being directed towards identifying those women who are at high risk of miscarriage. This will provide appropriate counselling and perhaps delay pregnancy until identified risk factors have been addressed.

Much excitement has been generated in recent years by the reporting of an association between raised serum LH (luteinising hormone) levels in the follicular phase and miscarriage in patients with spontaneous cycles or polycystic ovary syndrome (PCOS) [1–5]. These studies have provoked attempts to lower serum LH values prior to conception using either GnRH analogues [6,7] or ovarian electrocautery [6].

In a preliminary report of 44 subjects we found that age and follicular phase estradiol (E_2) were shown to be better predictors of pregnancy outcome than serum LH [8]. Because this data was novel, we have prospectively collected details of patients in our programme in the 3 years subsequent to those already reported. In this

---

Address for correspondence: Prof David L. Healy, Department of Obstetrics and Gynaecology, Monash Medical Centre, 246 Clayton Road, Clayton 3168, Victoria, Australia. Tel.: +61-3-550-5374. Fax: +61-3-550-5389.

total of 204 consecutive individuals, basal serum LH, E_2 or age were not predictive of miscarriage.

Patients and Methods

We have reviewed the histories of all women with PCOS attending our ovulation induction clinic between January 1989 and July 1993. There were 108 pregnancies from a total of 519 cycles in 204 women. Polycystic ovarian syndrome was diagnosed by ultrasound (≥10 peripheral ovarian cysts ≤8 mm in diameter and increased ovarian stroma) in the presence of clinical features (oligomenorrhoea/amenorrhoea and/or hirsutism) and/or endocrine abnormalities (elevated LH:FSH ratio, testosterone >3.5 nmol/L (1.01 ng/ml; and/or DHEAS >7.5 nmol/L (2.76 mg/ml). Other causes of infertility were excluded by two semen analyses and laparoscopy. All patients had failed to conceive after at least six cycles of clomiphene citrate.

Within 1–4 days of the start of menstruation or progestogen-induced withdrawal bleed, basal serum E_2, LH, and progesterone (P) levels were measured and human menopausal gonadotropin (hMG) therapy (Pergonal: Serono, Melbourne, Australia; or Humegon: Organon, Melbourne, Australia) begun. The standard initial dose was 75 IU (ultrasound range, 37.5 to 225 IU/day). After 5 to 7 days this was adjusted according to the serum E_2 and US determined ovarian follicular response. When the largest follicle had a mean diameter ≥16 mm (and provided no more than 3 follicles were >14 mm and serum E_2 was <4,000 pmol/l (1,090 pg/ml), human chorionic gonadotropin (hCG; Profasi: Serono) 3,000 IU i.m., was given. The typical peak serum E_2 was 1200 pmol/l prior to hCG. hCG luteal phase support (1,500 IU i.m.) was given on days 3, 6 and 9 after the ovulatory hCG injection if serum P was <50 nmol/l (15.7 ng/ml) and provided serum E_2 was <3,000 pmol/l (817 pg/ml).

Pregnancy was diagnosed if serum βhCG levels were >30 mIU/ml 16 days after the ovulating hCG injection. Ultrasound was performed approximately 2 weeks later to confirm that the pregnancy was viable and intrauterine. Biochemical pregnancies (n = 3) were excluded from the analyses. There were no ectopic pregnancies.

All serum hormone levels were measured by RIA. For E_2 a kit (Biomediq, Melbourne, Australia) was used, interassay and intra-assay coefficients of variation (Cvs) <4% and <5%, respectively. For P an Amerlex-M progesterone RIA kit (Amersham, Melbourne, Victoria, Australia) was used, interassay and intra-assay Cvs were <5% and <10%, respectively, within the ranges measured. For serum LH, the Baxter diagnostic kit (Pacific Diagnostics, Brisbane, Queensland, Australia) was used, interassay and intra-assay Cvs were ≤6.5% and ≤8.5%, respectively.

Pregnancy outcome was recorded as a miscarriage if ultrasound scanning of the uterus showed nonviability or if the pregnancy ended spontaneously before 20 weeks gestation [9]. Patients' age, previous fertility and obstetric history and hormone profiles during the current conception cycle were compared for pregnancies ending before and after 20 weeks gestation.

The Genstat and Glin statistical packages were used. Logistic regression analysis two-way analysis of variance and chi-squared analyses were used as appropriate.

Results

Patients' age and past history are illustrated in Table 1. By two-way analysis of variance, age, the years of infertility or a past history of miscarriage were not significantly different in those whose pregnancy ended spontaneously before 20 weeks compared to those whose pregnancies progressed for 20 weeks or more.

Table 2 illustrates mean values of basal (day 1–4) and preovulatory serum E_2, LH and P_4 concentrations. Also shown are levels of E_2 and P_4 on day 3 following the ovulating hCG injection and serum βhCG levels on day 16 following hCG injection.

Contrary to the preliminary work from this department [8], analysis of this follow-up study with a larger group of women, showed no significant difference in basal E_2 levels between women who had miscarried and those who continued their pregnancy. Patients who miscarried tended to be older and have lower basal serum E_2, but this did not reach statistical significance. The only significant difference was in serum E_2 levels 3 days following hCG injection where E_2 levels were higher in the miscarriage group.

Logistic regression analysis was also performed for the variables of basal E_2 and age. No significant difference was detected between those who miscarried and those whose pregnancies continued ≥20 weeks (χ^2 = 1.95 and 0.56, respectively).

Contingency tables were constructed dividing age around its median value of 31 and basal E_2 around its median value of 120 pmol/l. The odds ratios for miscarriage of age >31 or basal serum E_2 ≤ 120 were again not significant (1.07 and 1.69, respectively).

Analysis of the three-way dependence between duration of pregnancy, age and basal serum E_2, using the above median values as cutoff points, accepted the hypothesis of no three-way interaction between basal E_2, age and outcome (χ^2 = 0.08, df = 1, P = 0.5).

Table 1. Age and past history of women with pregnancy ending after <20 or ≥20 weeks gestation

	Pregnancy population	Delivery <20 weeks	Delivery ≥20 weeks	Probability[a]
Age (y)	30.21 (0.38)[b] n = 108	31.00 (0.66) n = 33	29.87 (0.46) n = 75	0.17
Infertility (y)	3.63 (0.36) n = 50	3.78 (0.63) n = 16	3.56 (0.45) n = 34	0.78
Previous miscarriage (no)	0.44 (0.08) n = 108	0.64 (0.17) n = 33	0.35 (0.09) n = 75	0.10

[a]Delivery <20 weeks vs. ≥20 weeks; [b]Mean (SEM).

Table 2. Hormone levels in stimulated cycles leading to pregnancies ending after <20 or ≥20 weeks gestation

	Pregnancy population	Delivery <20 weeks	Delivery ≥20 weeks	Probability[a]
Basal E_2	148.80 (6.39)[b] n = 108	141.82 (11.83) n = 33	151.87 (7.61) n = 75	0.47
Basal P_4	2.37 (0.28) n = 108	2.32 (0.23) n = 33	2.39 (0.39) n = 75	0.91
Basal LH	7.48 (0.62) n = 89	6.60 (1.30) n = 26	7.85 (0.70) n = 63	0.37
Pre-hCG E_2	1574.77 (104.41) n = 107	1831.21 (236.87) n = 33	1460.41 (106.49) n = 74	0.10
Pre-hCG P_3	3.44 (0.64) n = 99	2.57 (0.32) n = 28	3.78 (0.89) n = 71	0.40
Pre-hCG LH	7.89 (0.73) n = 92	6.88 (1.19) n = 27	8.30 (0.91) n = 65	0.38
Post-hCG P_4	27.26 (3.21) n = 59	30.30 (6.69) n = 21	25.57 (3.39) n = 38	0.49
Post-hCG E_2	1092.71 (234.41) n = 59	1761.90 (623.10) n = 21	722.89 (85.64) n = 38	0.03
Day 16 βhCG	4209.71 (2570.39) n = 59	840.53 (541.36) n = 19	5810.08 (3771.56) n = 40	0.37

[a]Delivery <20 weeks vs. ≥20 weeks; [b]Mean (SEM);
Pre-hCG: on day of ovulating hCG injection;
Post-hCG: Luteal phase, 3 days following hCG injection;
Post-hCG: Luteal phase, 3 days following hCG injection;
Day 16: 16 days following hCG injection;
E_2 values pmol/l, P_4 nmol/l, LH MIU/Ml, βhCG MIU/Ml.

Discussion

For as many as 50% of couples undergoing ovulation induction, the initial joy of a positive pregnancy test is soon replaced by the despair of spontaneous miscarriage [10]. While the cause of miscarriage is unknown in the majority of cases, several factors have been proposed to increase the risk of exposure to subsequent miscarriages. Identification of these risk factors aids doctors and counsellors in giving the couples reasonable expectations of pregnancy outcome.

Maternal age

The association of age and miscarriage is controversial. Preliminary studies from this department [8] demonstrated that, among 44 women with PCOS undergoing menotropin ovulation induction, patients aged >29.5 were more likely to have their pregnancy end <20 weeks compared with patients ≤29.5 years. However, this follow-up study of 204 consecutive women with PCOS failed to confirm this association.

Other recent studies also have failed to show a significant association between age and miscarriage. Tulppala et al. [11] studied 50 women with a history of recurrent spontaneous abortion and 20 healthy control women. The mean age was similar in both groups but this may have been biased by the greater number of women with PCOS in the miscarriage group. Those with PCOS were significantly younger than women with normal ovaries and may have factors other than age predisposing them to miscarriage. Similarly, Sagle and colleagues [12] found no relationship between age and miscarriage in patients and controls where, again, patients had a history of recurrent miscarriage and a higher incidence of PCOS.

Other studies of women with spontaneous [13] or IVF [14] pregnancies showed no age difference between those miscarrying and those having successful pregnancies. In a large series of 50 spontaneous abortions in 407 pregnancies [15] age was not related to miscarriage though the authors note that few patients were in the older age groups. This may be important as Querby and co-workers [16] have recently shown that increasing maternal age results in a progressive rise in miscarriage rate only until the age of 30, beyond which the effect of increasing age is minimal. Our own data would need further analysis of the younger patients to assess this point.

The most likely mechanism by which advancing age might increase miscarriage risk is by increasing the incidence of chromosome abnormalities. Recent developments in chorionic villus sampling procedures enable successful karyotyping in up to 99% of spontaneous abortion samples and reduce contamination by maternal cells [17]. The reported incidence of chromosomal aneuploidy in first trimester pregnancy losses ranged from 55 [18] to 100% [19]. When maternal age has been analysed in these studies, aneuploid fetuses were found more frequently in older women [17,18]. Multiple logistic regression analysis in the study of Cowchock and associates [18] showed maternal age to be an important predictor of chromosome abnormality, specifically trisomy.

With the introduction of human in vitro fertilisation (IVF) techniques it has become possible to karyotype preimplantation embryos and oocytes. The reported incidence of chromosomal abnormalities in human oocytes after superovulation for IVF range from 20 to ≥50% [20,21]. A recent study by our colleagues [22] has shown a similar incidence of aneuploidy (20%) in oocytes from nonstimulated or natural cycles in infertile women. This latter study showed no significant difference in the age of patients from whom karyotypically normal and aneuploid oocytes were retrieved. However, the age range of patients in the study was small and all women suffered from infertility.

In summary, we believe that the influence of age on risk of miscarriage is unproven. However, because of the presence of variables which are not controlled for in all studies, it is important that, at least for the present, age should be assessed as a possible confounding factor in future study of miscarriage risk.

History of previous miscarriages

It is generally accepted in clinical practice that women with one or two miscarriages suffer from sporadic abortion not requiring investigation compared to those with a history of three or more consecutive miscarriages. Regan and colleagues have studied this issue in a group of 407 women [15]. The risk of spontaneous abortion was greatly influenced by past reproductive history. Surprisingly, women with only one prior miscarriage had a significantly higher rate of subsequent miscarriage than primigravidas or women with a history of only successful pregnancy (20 vs. 4–5%). The outcome of the last pregnancy also influenced the outcome of the study pregnancy: if the previous pregnancy had been successful, only 5% aborted in the study pregnancy compared to 19% of women whose last pregnancy ended in abortion. The study did not address the impact of increasing numbers of previous miscarriages.

This, however, was examined by Quenby and co-workers [16] who found that, in women with a history of either two or three previous miscarriages, the risk of miscarriage in the subsequent pregnancy was similar (21 and 23%) but rose rapidly following four or more prior miscarriages. Both of these studies controlled for maternal age and found it to either not [15], or to a limited degree only [16], affect the risk of miscarriage. Past history was a much stronger predictor of outcome.

In our study, we failed to show a relationship between spontaneous abortion and a history of prior miscarriage (Table 1). However, we have not yet further analysed the prior miscarriage data according to whether or not the prior miscarriage occurred in the pregnancy immediately preceding the index pregnancy. Based on the studies described above [15,16], this variable requires more detailed analysis.

Fertility

It is being increasingly recognised that a major determinant of the success of infertility treatment is the duration of prior infertility [23]. Higher rates of spontaneous abortion have been described in women undergoing infertility treatment compared to controls [24–27]. The assumption has been that the increased rate of abortion is related to the drugs used to induce ovulation [27]. Other confounding features in this group of patients include older age and obesity [28], ovarian hyperstimulation syndrome [29] increased incidence of chromosomal abnormalities [30] and increased incidence of multiple pregnancy [27]. However, the influence of the duration of infertility or miscarriage risk has not been studied in these reports. In our study the duration of infertility was not significantly different in women who miscarried compared to those with successful pregnancies (Table 1).

Hormonal predictors of miscarriage

In our study described in this chapter we have attempted to assess E_2, P and LH levels throughout the entire cycle of ovulation induction in women with PCOS. Serum LH as a predictor miscarriage is discussed elsewhere in this book and therefore will not be reviewed here. Serum βhCG levels 16 days following ovulation have also been studied (see Table 2). Statistical analysis is not yet complete, but our initial results show no significant difference in basal endocrinological profiles between women who subsequently miscarry and those with successful pregnancies (≥20 weeks). We do find significantly elevated serum E_2 levels on day 3 following hCG injection in women who subsequently miscarry. This may induce endometrial changes which permit implantation but promote spontaneous abortion. If confirmed, such data might be used to predict pregnancy outcome [31].

References

1. Regan L, Owen EJ, Jacobs, HS. Lancet 1990;336:1141–1144.
2. Turner MJ, Lancet 1991;337:742.
3. Howles CM, MacNamee MC, Edwards RG, Goswamy R, Steptoe PC. Lancet 1986;2:521–522.
4. Homburg R, Armar NA, Eshel A, Adams J, Jacobs HS. Br Med J 1988;297:1024–1026.
5. Homburg R, Eshel A, Armar NA, Tucker M, Mason PW, Adams J. Br Med J 1989;298:809–812.
6. Gadir AA, Alnaser HMI, Mowafi RS, Shaw RW. Fertil Steril 1992;57:309–313.
7. Homburg R, Levy T, Berkovitz D, Farchi J, Feldberg D, Ashkenazi J, Ben-Rafael Z. Fertil Steril 1993;59:527–531.
8. McClure N, McDonald J, Kovacs GT, Healy DL, McCloud PI, McQuinn B, Burger HG. Fertil Steril 1993;59:729–733.
9. World Health Organization. Acta Obstet Gynaecol Scand 1977;56:247–253.
10. Yen SSC. Clin Endocrinol 1980;12:177.
11. Tulppala M, Stenman UK, Cacciatore B, Ylikorkala O. Br. J Obstet Gynaecol 1993;100:348–352.
12. Sagle M, Bishop K, Ridley N, Alexander FM, Michael M, Bonney RC, Beard RW, Franks S. BMJ 1988;297:1027.
13. Whittaker PG, Stewart MO, Taylor A, Lind T. Br J Obstet Gynaecol 1989;96:1207–1214.
14. Edelstein MC, Seltman HJ, Cox BJ, Robinson SM, Shaw RA, Muasher SJ. Fertil Steril 1990;54: 853–857.
15. Regan L, Braude PR, Trembath PL. BMJ 1989;299:541–545.
16. Quenby SM, Farquharson RG. Obstet Gynecol 1993;82:132–138.
17. Strom CM, Ginsberg N, Applebaum M, Bozorgi N, White M, Caffarelli M, Verlinsky Y. J Assist Reprod Genet 1992;9:458–461.
18. Cowchock FS, Gibas Z, Jackson LG. Fertil Steril 1993;59:1011–1014.
19. Sorokin Y, Johnson MP, Zador IE, Uhimann WR, Drusan A, Koppitch FC, Moody J, Evans MI. Am J Med Genet 1991;39(3):314–316.
20. Wramsby H, Liedholm P. Fertil Steril 1984;41:736–738.
21. Wramsby H, Fredga K, Liedholm P. N Eng J Med 1987;316:121–124.
22. Gras L, McBain J, Trounson A, Kola I. Hum Reprod 1992;7:1396–1401.
23. Jansen RP. Fertil Steril 1993;59;5:1041–1045.
24. Ben-Rafael Z, Fateh M, Flickinger GL, Tureck R, Blasco L, Mastroianni. Obstet Gynaecol 1988; 71:297–300.
25. Jansen RPS. Am J Obstet Gynecol 1982;143:451–473.
26. Shoham Z, Zosmer A, Insler V. Fertil Steril 1991;55:1–11.
27. Ransom MX, Bohrer M, Blotner MB, Kemmann, E. Fertil Steril 1993;59:567–570.
28. Bohrer M, Kemmann E. Fertil Steril 1987;48:571–575.
29. Ben-Rafael Z, Dor J, Mashiach S, Blankstein J, Lunenfeld B, Serr DM. Fertil Steril 1983;39:157–161.

30. Oelsner G, Serr DM, Mashiach S, Blankstein J, Snyder M, Lunenfeld B. Fertil Steril 1978;30:538–544.
31. Yamashita T, Okamoto S, Thomas A, MacLachlan V, Healy DL. Fertil Steril 1989;51:304–309.

Management and obstetrical outcome of multiple pregnancies

J. Salat-Baroux and J.M. Antoine

Departments of Obstetric Gynecology and Biology of Reproduction, Hôpital Tenon, 4 Rue de Chine, 75020 Paris, France

Abstract. The use of ovulation-inducing agents has increased the number of multiple pregnancies about 10-fold. The increased rate of maternal and fetal complications in this series of 82 twin and 10 triplet pregnancies managed and delivered in our unit led us to the following conclusions: embryo reduction is not necessary in the case of triplet pregnancies, but early diagnosis is essential to prevent prematurity; maternal rest is required, together with cesarian section and the presence of a well-trained pediatric team. These measures can reduce perinatal mortality from 30 to 6% and neonatal mortality to 4.2%. However, the most important approach to the problem of multiple pregnancies is prevention.

Introduction

While the spontaneous incidence of multiple pregnancies, according to Hellin's previsions (1985), is only one twin pregnancy out of 89 and one triplet pregnancy out of 7,921 [1], the incidence of pregnancies resulting from assisted medical technics has been multiplied by a factor of at least 10 [2]. Many publications [3–5] have underlined the frequency of maternal and, above all, fetal complications and the need for early specific management, particularly of triplet and quadruplet pregnancies. However, these studies are retrospective, do not always compare induced and spontaneous pregnancies, and rarely mention the number of patients lost to follow-up; finally, the results are not analyzed according to whether or not selective embryo reduction was used [6]. We took all these elements into account in this series at the Tenon Hospital, which focused on twin and triplet pregnancies. The findings are discussed in the light of a French multicenter study on triplet and higher-order pregnancies, in which we participated [7].

Twin pregnancies

Patients and Methods

We compared the outcome of all twin pregnancies managed in our hospital, whether they were the result of in vitro fertilization (IVF) or simple ovarian stimulation, or occurred spontaneously. Between April 1987 and March 1992, 3,913 oocyte recovery procedures were carried out in our IVF center, yielding 906 pregnancies (23.2%).

There were 187 spontaneous miscarriages (20.6%), 50 ectopic pregnancies (5.5%), seven therapeutic abortions (0.8%) and 662 ongoing pregnancies (73.1%). Of these latter, 521 (78.7%) were singleton, 128 (19.3%) twin and 13 (2%) triplet pregnancies. Only the 82 IVF twin pregnancies (64.1% of total) were taken into account, as all were managed and delivered in the unit. They were compared to 17 twin pregnancies resulting from simple ovarian stimulation and 121 spontaneous twin pregnancies. These 220 twin pregnancies were analyzed retrospectively for maternal, obstetrical and pediatric data.

It must be underlined that term was defined either in real weeks of amenorrhea (WA) (for spontaneous and stimulated pregnancies) or in corrected WA (for IVF: from the date of transfer plus 2 weeks). Ultrasonographic diagnoses, hypertension, labor and premature rupture of the membranes were defined according to Seoud et al. [3]. Intrauterine growth retardation was determined from the French curves [8], and prematurity was evaluated from 26 WA and not 24 WA as in many Anglo-Saxon series [4]. The IVF and ovarian stimulation groups were compared with the spontaneous pregnancy groups by means of the chi-squared and Student's tests, with the threshold of significance set at $p < 0.05$.

Results

Maternal age was significantly higher in the IVF group than in the spontaneous twin pregnancy group (33.5 ± 4.1 vs. 30 ± 5.1 years; $p < 0.0001$). The proportion of primiparas was also higher (68.3 vs. 48.8%; $p < 0.01$).

The first ultrasonography was done earlier in the IVF group (8.5 ± 3.2 vs. 12.9 ± 4.6 WA; $p < 0.001$), while the proportion of women who underwent cervical cerclage (36.6 vs. 8.3%; $p < 0.001$) and progesterone therapy (100 vs. 76.9%; $p < 0.001$) was higher.

The frequency of threatened premature delivery (TPD), arterial hypertension, intrauterine growth retardation (IUGR), hyperuricemia >360 µmol/ml, and thrombocytopenia <150,000 platelets/ml was similar in the three groups (Table 1). Hospital admissions during pregnancy were not more frequent, but they occurred earlier (22.8 ± 8.5 vs. 26.9 ± 6.9 WA; $p < 0.0003$), due to the higher proportion of cerclage in

Table 1. Complications during 220 twin pregnancies (Hôpital Tenon, France)

	IVF (n = 82)	Stimulation (n = 17)	Spontaneous (n = 121)
TPD	41 (50%) NS	9 (52.9%) NS	67 (55.4%)
Hypertension	12 (14.6%) NS	4 (23.5%) NS	19 (15.7%)
IUGR	13 (15.9%) NS	3 (17.6%) NS	14 (11.6%)
Uricemia > 360 µmol/ml	16 (19.5%) NS	2 (11.8%) NS	18 (14.9%)
Thrombocytopenia < 150.000	19 (23.2%) NS	0 (0%) NS	20 (16.5%)

TPD = threatened premature delivery; IUGR = intrauterine growth retardation.

Table 2. Term at delivery among 220 twin pregnancies (Hôpital Tenon, France)

	IVF (n = 82)	Stimulation (n = 17)	Spontaneous (n = 121)
< 28 weeks	3 (3.7%)	0	4 (3.3%)
28–29 weeks	2 (2.4%)	0	1 (1.0%)
30–31 weeks	2 (2.4%)	0	7 (5.8%)
32–33 weeks	7 (8.5%)	0	10 (8.3%)
34–35 weeks	13 (15.9%)	2 (11.8%)	12 (10.0%)
> 36 weeks	55 (67.1%)	15 (88.8%)	87 (71.9%)
Mean (SE)	35.6 ± 2.9	37.1 ± 2.5	35.8 ± 3.8

early pregnancy. Cesarian sections were more frequent (64.6 vs. 44.6%; $p < 0.01$), while the indications were comparably distributed (in particular, uterine scarring, breech presentation of the first twin, and acute fetal distress).

Finally, there was no difference with regard to the term at delivery (mean 35.6 ± 2.9 WA), intrauterine, perinatal and postpartum deaths, birth weight, length, sex ratio, or birth defects. The proportion of infants transferred to pediatric units was similar in the three groups (Tables 2 and 3).

Triplet and higher-order pregnancies

Material and Methods

It is difficult to analyze the only quintuplet pregnancy (3 sacs, one of which was monoamniotic and contained three embryos), which resulted in fetal loss at 17 WA after reduction at 14 WA, or the three quadruplet pregnancies, one of which led to a spontaneous miscarriage at 4 months, while a double embryo reduction was carried

Table 3. Pediatric prognosis in 220 twin pregnancies (Hôpital Tenon, France)

	IVF	Stimulation	Spontaneous
No of fetuses	164	34	242
Intrauterine deaths	2 (1.2%)	0	4 (1.7%)
Still births	1 (0.6%)	0	2 (0.8%)
Live births	161 (98.2%)	34 (100%)	236 (97.5%)
Body weight D1	2322 ± 494 g	2531 ± 323 g	2388 ± 560 g
Body weight D2	2193 ± 395 g	2476 ± 278 g	2325 ± 623 g
Birth defects	5 (3.1%)	0	6 (2.5%)
Transfers:			
Pediatric Unit	18	5	32
Intensive care	13	1	24
Total	31 (19.3%)	6 (17.6%)	56 (23.7%)
Postpartum deaths	3 (1.9%)	1 (2.9%)	3 (1.3%)
Overall deaths	6 (3.7%)	1 (2.9%)	9 (3.7%)

out in each of the other cases and led to a single ongoing pregnancy.

This study of triplet pregnancies extends over a 10-year period, from 1983 to 1993: out of 52 pregnancies diagnosed by ultrasonography between 6 and 7 WA, four (7.7%) resulted in miscarriage, while 18 twin pregnancies (34.6%) were viable, after spontaneous embryo disappearance of two of the three embryos in four cases, and one in 14 cases, before 10 WA. One embryo reduction was performed in four further cases (7.7%), leading to the loss of the entire pregnancy in two cases. The remaining 26 pregnancies (50%) continued as triplet pregnancies, but only 10 were monitored and delivered at the Hôpital Tenon; the other 16 were investigated on the basis of questionnaires and were included in the national multicenter cohort. We first give the data for the 10 pregnancies for which the complete files were available.

These 10 triplet pregnancies were obtained by IVF, after replacement of frozen embryos in six cases. Table 4 shows the yearly frequency of triplet IVF pregnancies diagnosed at the first ultrasonography.

Maternal age was lower than in the group of twin pregnancies (32.1 ± 10 years). The number of US scans was 4–7 (5.5 ± 1.0). The term at diagnosis was between 6 and 7 WA, and all the patients underwent cerclage between 11 and 18 WA (13.7 ± 2.1 WA).

Complications arose during pregnancy in eight of the 10 cases (threat of premature delivery in seven cases, between 25 and 32 WA, associated with anemia in five cases, pruritis, thrombocytopenia and metrorrhagia in the other two cases). The term at admission to hospital varied from 25–33 weeks (mean 30 ± 2.35); the hospital stay lasted 7–56 days (mean 29.6 ± 15.6 days) and all the women received betamimetic drugs. Cesarian section was carried out routinely, between 29 and 37 WA (34 ± 2.3 WA): at 29 WA in one case, between 32 and 33 WA in five cases, at 34 WA in one case, and between 36 and 37 WA in three cases.

Table 4. Outcome of triplet IVF pregnancies diagnosed at the first ultrasonography

Yearly distribution								
Year	n	FCS	Reduction to twins	Spontaneous reduction to single	FCS reduction	Ongoing twin pregnancy	Ongoing triplet pregnancy
1983	1	–	–	1	–	–	–
1984	2	–	–	–	–	–	2
1985	6	1	1	1	–	–	3
1986	1	–	–	1	–	–	–
1987	5	–	1	–	–	–	4
1988	6	–	4	–	–	–	2
1989	6	1	2	–	1	–	2
1990	8	–	2	–	–	1	5
1991	1	1	–	–	–	–	–
1992	5	–	–	1	1	1	2
1993 (Nov)	11	1	4	–	–	–	6
Total	52	4	14	4	2	2	26

All the living children (12 girls and 18 boys) were viable; the birth weights of the first-, second- and third-born were between 1,300 and 3,040 g (2054 ± 575 g), 1,300 and 2,780 g (1973 ± 377 g), and 1,230 and 2,560 (193 ± 353 g), respectively.

Although there was no perinatal or neonatal mortality, the majority (23/30, 76.7%) of the living children were transferred to the neonatal intensive care unit for 1—42 days (mean 12.5 ± 10.4) and there were numerous complications (respiratory distress, n = 10; low birth weight, n = 7; maternofetal infections, n = 5; and enterocolitis, n = 3).

Discussion

The increasing frequency of multiple pregnancies in assisted medical procreation centers working with obstetrical units (one triple pregnancy per 1,149 pregnancies, out of a total of 27,577 pregnancies reported over a 10-year period by Pons et al. [5]) calls for uniform expression of the results from one publication to the other, a complete analysis of obstetric and neonatal complications, and recommendations on the best way of minimizing such pregnancies. The problems in comparing data from retrospective international series [9—11] are due to the following factors:
1. Losses to follow-up: 49 (3%) out of 1,686 clinical pregnancies monitored between 1987 and 1989 in 14 French IVF centers were lost to follow-up [7]. Losses to follow-up reached 12% after birth;
2. Definition of term: in this study and in the French multicenter cohort study, 14 days were added to the date of oocyte harvest to determine the theoretical date of the woman's last period, while this is not the case in other series [9]; and
3. Prematurity is evaluated differently from one country to the next: in the USA and Australia [9,10], prematurity and low birth weight are measured for all births occurring after 20 WA, compared to 28 WA in France.

Although several recent studies [12—14] have shown a higher risk of prematurity and low birth weight in IVF than spontaneous multiple pregnancies, essentially related to the patients' medical background, no such difference was found in our series for twin pregnancies.

In contrast, our findings confirmed the high maternal and fetal risk in triple and higher-order pregnancies. With regard to the maternal risk [15], the threat of premature delivery predominates (nearly 90% of the cases), with hospitalization around the 30th WA for 7—56 days. All the published series report similar rates of complications: 100% in the series of Pons et al. [5], 32.3% in that of Seoud et al. [3], and 82.2% in that of Olivennes et al. [7]. Arterial hypertension was also very frequent (six cases out of 10), as was anemia (eight out of 10). Seoud et al. [3] reported values of only 38.6 and 23.1%, respectively, but their criteria were far stricter than ours. Other frequent complications were thrombocytopenia, bleeding in the 1st and 2nd trimesters and the HELLP syndrome, although premature rupture of the membranes was no more frequent than in the group of twin pregnancies (15.4 vs. 13.8%). We did not observe more cases of eclampsia or pre-eclampsia than in the twin pregnancies.

Fetal and neonatal complications were far more problematic than in the twin pregnancies.

The rate of prematurity before 36 WA was high (seven out of 10 cases, with a mean of 34 ± 2.3 WA). Pons et al. [5] reported a figure of 91.6%, with a mean of 34.8 ± 1.0 WA, while Olivennes et al. [7] reported 82.2% between 28 and 36 WA. If triplet and quadruplet pregnancies are combined, the figures are even more alarming: 31% in the series of Mellier et al. [16]. Among the 156 triplet births analyzed by Levene et al. in 1992 [4], the median gestational age at birth was 33 weeks.

Low birth weight

The triplets' birth weight ranged from 1,230 to 3,040 g, with a mean of 1,987 ± 400 g; there was no significant difference according to birth order, and the mean gestational age was 34 ± 2.35 WA. In our series, like in Olivennes' first series [7], the rate of low birth weight (<10th percentile on Lubchenko's curve (1963)) was 60%. It is interesting to note that among the 26 triplet and four quadruplet births studied by Seoud et al. [3], none of the neonates was below the 10th percentile for body weight. It thus appears that infertility is far more important in this respect than the multiple pregnancy itself: in the study by Williams et al. [17], the risk of having a low birth weight was 2.3 times higher in infertile patients (adjusted relative risk). However, the role of arterial hypertension should not be overlooked [12].

The mortality rate among the 10 sets of triplets managed in our center was zero, but it should be remembered that only 26 (50%) out of a total of 52 triplet pregnancies were viable. Perinatal mortality varied according to the mode of delivery (6% in a series of 24 patients managed by Pons et al. [5], and 15—30% in a series in which the vaginal approach was chosen, with a higher risk for the third fetus [18]. It is true that the vaginal route is usually adopted when labor has not been controlled medically and when the prematurity is extreme (<28 WA). Indeed, prematurity is the most important factor in mortality, along with low birth weight and arterial hypertension and the "transfuseur-transfusé syndrôme". The mortality rate climbs still further in the case of quadruplet and higher-order pregnancies (25—81.9% in some series such as Olivennes' multicenter study [7]. However, it should be pointed out that in the series of Seoud et al. [3] and Mellier et al. [16], this corrected neonatal mortality rate (after 28 WA), which was difficult to determine in our short series, was 36.8% in the French multicenter study, but fell sharply to 4.2% when delivery occurred after 28 WA. Neonatal complications, however, remain frequent: 76.7% of the neonates in our series were transferred to a pediatric unit and 14 of the 23 infants required neonatal intensive care, particularly for respiratory distress (50% of neonates). Comparable results have been obtained in other series, Seoud et al. [3] reporting 64% of admissions to a specialized pediatric unit and 36.9% to a neonatal intensive care unit, and Olivennes reporting 71.8% [7]. However, these complications and their outcome depend closely on the way in which the infants are managed at birth. Finally, the rate of birth defects was about 6.7% in all reported series [3], although it was only 2.9% in the French multicenter study [7].

Management of multiple pregnancies

These results call for a discussion of the way in which the pregnancy and delivery must be managed. The first question is that of selective embryo reduction: it is undeniably necessary in case of quadruple and higher-order pregnancies [19,20], but the indications are more problematic in the case of triplets, except in the presence of uterine scarring. Whatever the technique used (transcervical, transvaginal or transabdominal, depending on the term, between 10 and 16 WA) the risk of complications (infections, abortions in 15% of cases, and prematurity) remains high. Boulot et al. [21] consider that selective reduction prolongs the pregnancy by no more than 1 or 2 weeks, while Perrero et al. [6] showed in a comparative, unrandomized series that neither body weight (2,227 ± 478 vs. 2,239 ± 399 g), nor term (35.5 vs. 35.7 ± 2.5 WA) was improved by reduction.

Thus, while prevention remains the primary aim, several measures must be taken during pregnancy, the cornerstone of which is early diagnosis. Seoud et al. and ourselves diagnose IVF multiple pregnancies by means of ultrasonography between 6 and 7.5 WA. In the case of spontaneous triplet pregnancies, however, the diagnosis may take place much later, at about 17 WA according to Pons et al. [5]. Optimum management calls for monthly examinations and frequent US scans (5.5 ± 1). The patient must be advised to stop work and to rest from the 22nd to the 24th WA onward, while hospital admission is neither obligatory nor desirable in every case. Only rest is truly effective: in our series hospitalization did not significantly prolong the term, except in cases of patent maternal complications (arterial hypertension or HELLP syndrome). However, some teams continue to hospitalize systematically all patients from the 26th WA onwards [16].

All the patients in our series underwent cerclage, although other groups only use this measure in case of local indications, with no reduction in the rate of premature births [3–7].

We do not administer steroids, unlike many authors, including Keith et al. [22]. The only reported benefit was in a series of 12 patients with a mean term of 33.9 WA treated by Pons et al., in which there were no respiratory complications. Benedetti et al. [23] consider that the combination of betamimetic drugs and steroids is contraindicated. Spasmolytic drugs and progesterone are the main elements in the prevention of prematurity. Finally, the mode of delivery is no longer controversial: the mortality rate of 15–30% with the vaginal route (according to the type of presentation and the last-born) can be cut to 4% by elective cesarian section [16–18]. The main advantages are a reduction in trauma, obstetric procedures and neonatal infections, as well as the fact that each infant can be treated by a specialized team.

All international and multicenter studies tend towards the same conclusions: early diagnosis improves the management of multiple pregnancies, the cornerstone of which is rest in order to avoid extreme prematurity (less than 28–30 WA). The prognosis of spontaneous and IVF twin pregnancies is now similar, while that of triplet pregnancies can be improved by good obstetrical management and routine cesarian section; the prognosis of quadruplet and higher-order pregnancies remains grim and justifies selective embryo reduction.

References

1. Olofsson P. Eur J Obstet Gynecol Reprod Biol 1990;35:159—171.
2. Collins MS, Bleyl JA. Am J Obstet Gynecol 1990;162:1384—1392.
3. Seoud MAF, Toner JP, Kruithoff C, Muasher S. Fertil Steril 1992;57:825—834.
4. Levene M, Wild J. Br J Obstet Gynecol 1992;99:607—613.
5. Pons JC, Fernandez H, Diochin P, Mayenga JM, Plu G, Frydman R, Papiernick E. J Gynecol Obstet Biol Reprod 1989;18:72—78.
6. Perrero R, Burke S, Hendrix ML. Obstet Gynecol 1991;78:335—338.
7. Olivennes FJS. Les grossesses après procréations médicalement assistées. Paris, Thèse Université Paris XI, Faculté de Médecine Paris Sud, No 5076, 1992.
8. Leroy B, Lefort F. Rev Fr Gynecol 1971;66:381—396.
9. National perinatal statistics unit, Sydney. Fertil Soc Austr 1988;1030—4711.
10. Elster AD, Bleyl J, Crown TE. Obstet Gynecol 1991;77:387—393.
11. Sassoon DA, Castro LC, Davis JL, Hobel CJ. Obstet Gynecol 1990;75:817—820.
12. MRC Working Party on Children conceived by In Vitro Fertilization. Br Med J 1990;300:1229—1233.
13. Tan S-L, Doyle P, Campbel S, Beral V, Rizk B, Bridsen P, Mason B, Edwards RG. Am J Obstet Gynecol 1992;162:778—784.
14. Olivennes F, Rufat P, Andre B, Pourade A, Quiros MC, Frydmand R. Hum Reprod 1993;8:1297—1300.
15. Antoine JM, Gomes A, Uzan S, Alvarez S, Cornet D, Tibi Ch, Mandelbaum J, Plachot M, Salat-Baroux J. J Gynecol Obstet Biol Reprod 1990;19:901—907.
16. Mellier G, Claris D, Andra Ph, Chabert Ph. Fr Gynecol Obstet 1991;86:629—633.
17. Williams RL, Creasy RK, Cunningham GC, Hawes WE, Norris FD, Tashiro R. Obstet Gynecol 1982;59:624—629.
18. Michlewitz H, Kenedy R, Kawada C. J Reprod Med 1981;26:243—249.
19. Doumergues M, Nisand I, Mandelbrot L, Isfer E, Radunovic N, Dumez Y. Fertil Steril 1991:55:805—811.
20. Salat-Baroux J, Aknin J, Antoine JM, Alamovitch R. Hum Reprod 1988;3:399—405.
21. Boulot P, Hedon B, Pelliccia G, Deschamps F, Arnol F, Humeau C, Molinat F, Laffargue G, Mares P, Viala JL. J Gynecol Obstet Biol Reprod 1991;20:309—316.
22. Keith LG, Ameli S, Depp OR, Hobart J, Keith DN. The northwestern University triplet study II: 14 Triplets Pregnancies at 5th International Congress of the International Society for Twins studies. Amsterdam, The Netherlands. September 15—19, 1986.
23. Benedetti TJ. Am J Obstet Gynecol 1983;146:1—6.

General discussion

Ovulation induction regimens: is a consensus possible?

Marco Filicori and Carlo Flamigni
Reproductive Medicine Unit, University of Bologna, Bologna, Italy

This chapter reports the final general discussion held on January 22nd, 1994, at the completion of all the invited presentations of the Conference "Ovulation Induction: Basic Science and Clinical Advances", held on January 20–22, 1994, in Palm Beach, Florida. This discussion tried to draw some firm conclusions and indications for clinical management of ovulation induction procedures. Provocative questions were posed by the chairpersons of the session (Drs Filicori and Flamigni) and answers and comments were given by the audience. The discussion was minimally edited and the chapter is organized in such a manner as to maintain the sense of participation and interest that was present during the meeting.

Pulsatile GnRH vs. gonadotropins: which comes first?

M. Filicori (I): Our first provocative question regards the timing of pulsatile GnRH use in ovulatory disorders; should this therapeutic tool be used before or after exogenous gonadotropins?

S. Franks (UK): The policy we tend to adopt in our unit is to give the patient a chance to make the decision regarding low-dose gonadotropin therapy and pulsatile GnRH. We find that in our experience the chance of multiple pregnancy is similar; thus, it's a matter of whether the patients prefer to carry around a pump or to have daily injections.

H. Jacobs (UK): I think that even before you consider clomiphene or hormone levels one should weigh the patient, determine body mass index, and not treat people if they're subnormal weight. I think it might be helpful to measure prolactin concentration as well thyroxin.

D. Baird (UK): The important thing to do is first of all to make the diagnosis, and I'm assuming that we're talking about women with hypogonadotropic hypogonadism who are progesterone negative. In my view, I think you would have to have a very good reason for not trying pulsatile GnRH as a first line resort for somebody who had hypogonadotropic hypogonadism and who has a pituitary gland which responded to GnRH. Furthermore the reason is evident, in spite of what Steve Frank says, as it is almost impossible to avoid multiple pregnancy in an appreciable number even with careful gonadotropic therapy in women with hypogonadotropic hypogonadism. I'm sorry to say it, but there are some very able people who have tried it since Carl Gemzell in 1958. As he summed up, the problem still remains to avoid multiple pregnancy. There's no doubt in my mind, and I've been saying this for years, that you do somebody no service at all to either have twins or triplets. So unless they have an aversion to needles I think the first line treatment should be pulsatile GnRH and that message should get over loud and clear. I think it's almost bordering on the unethical to do a randomized trial between pulsatile GnRH and gonadotropins in this present day and age.

M. Filicori (I): We may begin to obtain some consensus; would anybody disagree with what David Baird just stated on the treatment of hypogonadotropic hypogonadism?

R. Jewelewicz (USA): I think we should do the most effective treatment in the shortest period of time and the least expensive. I don't understand why in the United States pulsatile GnRH did not become as widely used as it should.

N. Santoro (USA): In the USA we also have the doctrine of informed consent and usually after clomiphene does not work for patients, what we do is try to present them with the information, because that's really the appropriate clinical juncture, in my opinion, at which pulsatile GnRH should be considered vs. gonadotropin, and the best we can do for our patients is give them the information and have them make the decision as to which way they would like to proceed. Patients see gonadotropins as more efficient, which has been very difficult for me to believe, but I have to say that I've seen that in clinical practice and some patients are willing to brave those risks. I think another down side of pulsatile GnRH therapy that needs to be considered is that when you get away from the more ballistic approach of ovulation induction and you're growing a nice single follicle it can take longer. We tend to think of time in 6-month blocks when we're giving gonadotropin therapy and when we give pulsatile GnRH I think we need to extend that to almost 10—12 months before we consider the therapy a failure. That type of time delay can be a negative selling point for patients when they're considering this form of therapy.

M. Filicori (I): I have a very short comment on this. I think it depends on the gonadotropin regimen. If you're talking about low-dose gonadotropin I think that the data that were shown at this meeting indicate that the chances both of ovulation and conception are almost superimposable upon pulsatile GnRH. It's only when you use large traditional doses of gonadotropins that you significantly increase your chances of conception, but you do so because you make more eggs available and as you do that you also increase your chances of hyperstimulation and multiple pregnancy. So really it's not so much GnRH vs. gonadotropins, but rather which type of gonadotropin regimen you apply.

W.F. Crowley, Jr. (USA): Could I just ask for a show of hands: how many people use gonadotropins first in hypogonadotropic patients after clomiphene fails? How many people use pulsatile GnRH first? And then let me ask just the people from the United States to vote on the same question. The outcome of the vote is that the ratio is 3:1 in favor of pulsatile GnRH in Europe and the opposite ratio in the USA. We have done everything possible to convince people to use pulsatile GnRH in the USA, but we haven't been very successful. Actually, I'm really amazed that so many people are using pulsatile GnRH in the USA in spite of the difficulty in getting pumps and the peptide. I'm very pleased with the Europeans, and I think we must congratulate the Italian group for being much more effective proselytizers then we were. Having an industrial partnership is very important here; all academic advances can't be brought to patients without partnerships between industry and academics, and without an industrial partner, no matter how good an innovation is. Nevertheless, a prospective study comparing pulsatile GnRH and gonadotropins results and costs will be essential to convince people. To ensure penetration of pulsatile GnRH into practice, it's going to have to be shown in a contemporaneously done study that it has a lower cost.

L. O'Dea (USA): People who are most experienced in a particular of treatment mode will do best in that particular mode. I think it's something to bear in mind; it's a question of what do you do best for your patients. Furthermore, the practicality of the pump treatment needs to be considered; for some women who are working or need to travel this may not be an optimal regimen. The third problem in the United States is the fact that pulsatile GnRH is not yet registered for this application and this can be a problem for those of us who are trying to get insurance coverage for our patients. So I think there have been a number of reasons why people are more comfortable or continue to be more comfortable with gonadotropin therapy. But in general I would agree with the consensus that in this particular indication, pulsatile GnRH is the primary mode of therapy.

S.C. Pang (USA): Do you use heparin in the GnRH solution and how much?

M. Filicori (I): Well, if you use intravenous GnRH there's no question as to whether you should use heparin, because otherwise you end up with a lot of catheters clotted. If you use subcutaneous GnRH you should not use heparin, because then you end up with a lot of hematomas and this has been clearly established several years ago. In the intravenous solution we use about 100 units of heparin per ml.

H. Jacobs (UK): It's very important that we should not assume that the only way to give GnRH is through the intravenous route. Dr Filicori showed a compilation of data from his group where the intravenous therapy only was used and about 100 pregnancies in around 600 cycles of therapy were obtained. We used entirely subcutaneous therapy and we achieved around about 100 pregnancies in around 400 cycles. So people mustn't go away with the notion that subcutaneous route doesn't work and it isn't an option. It's the better option to maintain patient autonomy.

M. Filicori (I): So I think we can take this as the last comment on pulsatile GnRH and it's very well taken. I think there is no objection basically that the choice of route of administration is up to the individual physician and the patient and how comfortable each of us feels.

Gonadotropins: which preparation to use?

C. Flamigni (I): The next question is which gonadotropin preparation to use out of hMG, purified FSH, highly purified FSH, and recombinant FSH.

M. Filicori (I): As a first issue we would like to remind you what David Baird showed in his presentation, i.e., that basically there is no difference between using hMG or purified FSH, and so the provocative question is whether you agree or not.

D. Baird (UK): I think with the exception of the few cases with hypogonadotropic hypogonadism that don't have a pituitary where you should be giving them some LH along with the FSH of the current gonadotropin preparations which are available on the market, you should use the cheapest because I don't think there's any difference between them.

M. Filicori (I): Do we have a consensus on this?

Audience: Yes.

J. Schoemaker (NL): No, I don't think so. I think we should bear in mind that in general when we can do a job with one drug we should not use any combination drug. Moreover, when we have a real drug we should not use an extract. None of us will use the extract of digitalis anymore; any cardiologist will treat these patients with digitalis despite the fact that the extract of digitalis is probably much cheaper than the drug as such. New drugs such as recombinant FSH and LH are coming. I think that whenever it is possible to obtain results with a single drug we should do so, and not use two drugs.

S. Franks (UK): I just want to add my support to what David Baird said. As yet there has been no study which shows an increase in efficacy of one gonadotropin preparation over another. The point that Joop Schoemaker makes about using the purest preparation is fine, but not if that preparation costs 3 times as much. So it is up to the drug companies to bring the cost of the recombinant gonadotropin down to the cost of the currently available urinary gonadotropins; if they do so there will be no problem about using them.

C. Flamigni (I): Dr. Franks, in which cases would you consider it necessary to give LH.

S. Franks (UK): Well, I think in women with undetectable levels of LH (e.g., <2 U/L, immunoassay) and hypogonadotropic amenorrhea.

R. Homburg (IL): If the recombinant hormones do turn out to have the same price as urinary preparations, they do have one additional advantage and that is because of the purity and the low protein content they can be given subcutaneously, which means the patient can self-administer this medicine. And this can translate into a major advantage by eliminating a nurse or a doctor to inject them.

S. Franks (UK): Nevertheless, when urinary FSH is given by pulsatile subcutaneous infusion very few patients have anything more then a very minor local skin reaction.

M. Filicori (I): So what you're saying is that even the present preparations could be given subcutaneously rather than intramuscularly?

S. Franks (UK): I'm not recommending it, but it has yet to be shown that there are fewer local reactions with the highly purified preparations.

C. Howles (CH): I work for Serono. We now have on record 12 cases of patients who previously had extremely severe adverse reactions to urinary gonadotropin administration and who had no problems whatsoever when treated with the highly purified FSH preparation we recently launched in Europe. I think that shows quite clearly that there is a difference between these preparations.

Audience: It was suggested that if treatment is started with FSH followed by hMG the response may improve in the poor responders. What do you think?

M. Filicori (I): There may be actually some evidence suggesting that if your goal is to achieve mono-ovulation, hMG could be more effective. If you use a very purified FSH preparation it's more likely that you end up with several follicles. Thus, if the goal is to induce mono-ovulation some LH in your preparation may actually be advantageous.

C. Howles (CH): In the work of Dr Shoham with Howard Jacobs, where they treated hypogonadotropic patients with either FSH or hMG, no difference was found in the number of large follicles that grew. So I think there's no evidence to support your statement.

M. Filicori (I): This issue has never been addressed specifically. However, there is at least one paper in the literature which is a study by Venturoli from our unit who showed greater follicle development by using purified FSH preparations.

D. Baird (UK): I think there is plenty of scientific data to suggest that LH physiologically plays a role in helping select a single dominant follicle, but I'd have to say at the moment I don't know of a clinical regimen which would help achieve that by using LH. And that was why I said that I don't really think there's any difference between hMG or purified FSH for indications other than hypogonadotropic hypogonadism.

E. Loumaye (CH): I would like to attract the attention of the audience to the regulatory and the registration aspects of these drugs. hMG preparations were registered about 30 years ago and have demonstrated a good safety profile. However, they contain numerous bioactive proteins, growth factors, cytokines, immunoglobulins; whether or not these compounds are really toxic is very difficult to demonstrate, but if you have the opportunity to avoid them it would be preferable from a regulatory and a pharmaceutical standpoint. Without resorting to mass hysteria, I question if it is still acceptable after 20 years to extract medications from the urines of hundreds of thousands of donors and copurifying them with infectious agents, drugs or metabolites. I don't know if it is really relevant, but urine is probably the last human fluid from which we are still allowed to extract pharmaceutical preparations. So the question has to be raised and at least evaluated as fairly as possible. Some allergic reaction to hMG preparations could be related to contamination by antibiotics copurified in the process. With the tight controls of in vitro production it is possible to avoid this type of problems.

M. Filicori (I): I think we're all applauding the attempt of the pharmaceutical industry to devise synthetic ways of producing gonadotropins.

C. Flamigni (I): Any disagreement is about their price and not the efficacy and safety of these drugs.

D. Baird (UK): When I said we should use the cheapest preparation I meant of the preparations which are currently available. One would have to ask and try to make an evaluation, for example, of whether the reduction in allergic reaction that you get with highly purified FSH is worth paying twice the amount per ampoule, considering that the majority of people whom you inject with regular FSH or hMG have no problems. And indeed, in our experience they can self-inject either intramuscularly or subcutaneously, although maybe Scottish women are particularly sturdy.

H.J.T. Coelingh-Bennink (NL): I hate to get involved in some type of marketing discussions on the preparations because I think this is a scientific meeting where we should discuss scientific issues and look at randomized appropriate studies and not quote all types of things that people are saying. I think that we, as industry representatives, would make ourselves rather ridiculous if after 30 or 40 years showing that urinary gonadotropins are safe, we now suddenly come up with threatening stories suggesting that the same drugs are dangerous. I think we should look very carefully at our recombinant hormones, look very carefully at what they do, how effective they are, how potent they are, and we should present facts to you and you should decide for yourself what to do. As far as the content of the ampoules is concerned, our development will be with 50 units per ampoule.

D. Navot (USA): It should be remembered that the exact quantity of FSH in each hMG ampoule is probably less controlled than in the more purified FSH forms; this may change the individual response of each patient. In addition, hMG also appears to contain hCG to achieve an LH/FSH ratio of roughly 1:1. In a minority of patients, especially those on prolonged GnRH agonist protocols, this hCG may accumulate and may explain cases of premature luteinization and progesterone rise. Whether that will harm the egg or the endometrium, or probably to some degree both, is a fact that should be seriously considered.

N. Santoro (USA): As to low-dose gonadotropin regimens being able to achieve mono-ovulation, I believe that the agent that really does that the best far and away is pulsatile GnRH. When I see graphs of gonadotropin cycles showing LH, FSH, estradiol, and progesterone levels superimposable upon normal only then I'll believe that exogenous gonadotropins can do that.

R. Jewelewicz (USA): I would like to play the devil's advocate, speaking about mono and multiple ovulations. When people come to us for induction of ovulation there's only one aim and the aim is pregnancy. So we want to do the best we can to get a pregnancy in the least expensive, fastest, and safest way. I think that if you hyperstimulate to a certain extent your pregnancy rate is better; you have to take the risk of multiple pregnancy and hyperstimulation. Ideally, if we could switch from gonadotropins to GnRH using the pump you have a partial solution. As long as we don't have the pump in the United States I think everybody has to make up their own mind what they go after.

M. Filicori (I): Your point is very well taken; if you increase the dose of gonadotropins, you improve your chances of conception but you also increase your chances of complications.

H. Jacobs (UK): You certainly did a good job being the devil's advocate, but I'm not the devil's advocate. I don't think the objective of treatment is to get the patient pregnant, I think the objective of treatment is to get the patient pregnant with a singleton fetus. Actually, Dr Salat-Baroux gave a most beautiful presentation just earlier saying why we should go for singleton pregnancies. The complications of being a twin or a triplet or a quadruplet are very severe. There are complications that are met initially and are measured in monetary terms and Dr Crowley told us how much it costs. There are additional complications that last for the rest of the person's life and a French study showed psychiatric breakdown, marital breakdown, in relation to the domestic overload of people trying to bring up triplets and quads. And then of course as I keep saying, imagine being a quad competing for your mother's attention. It's a very tough situation and I can not understand why people want to go for a huge treatment dose to get the person pregnant quickly, when we all know that the maximum normal conception rates are about between 25 and 30% per cycle. All you have to do is keep the treatment going and you'll collect singletons at a normal rate, just as Dr Santoro says you do with GnRH. So I don't accept that and I think it's a very important principle that maybe needs to be debated, but it shocks me to think that it would seem to be as good a thing to do to get a bunch of twins and triplets rather than singletons.

D. Navot (USA): Certainly there are cultural and personal preferences in this. We are kidding ourselves to a large degree when we talk about obtaining monofollicular response with gonadotropins. Multiple pregnancies with gonadotropins are not preventable.

M. Filicori (I): Absolutely, I think we all agree with that.

D. Navot (USA): When we say that we are aiming at singleton I'm not sure that we are really close to achieving our aim. Mine is a single experience, but regards many thousands of hMG cycles. When you have two and sometimes three preovulatory follicles of 15 or 16 mm the chances of a conception are increased while the multiple pregnancy rate is between 10–20%.

R. Jewelewicz (USA): I have used gonadotropins for many years and I found it almost impossible to get a mono-ovulation. It doesn't matter how carefully you're going to monitor and how little gonadotropin you're going to give; that is because the difference between the minimal effective dose and the ineffective dose is very narrow and if you're going to get ovulation you're going to get multiple ovulations. However, if fetal reduction is employed we have a good opportunity to get a single pregnancy or at the most twins in the majority of cases.

M. Filicori (I): Let me briefly comment on this and remind you that fetal reduction may not be available in every country and that in certain countries it may be considered as highly controversial.

R. Homburg (IL): I don't think it's just a question of cultural background, as in spite of the same cultural background of Dr Jewelewicz I find myself in complete disagreement. While not being able to avoid multiple pregnancies completely with gonadotropins you can certainly go a long way towards it and it's all a question of the dose that you give. In our hands with the chronic low-dose therapy even in PCOs (who are renowned for having a high incidence of multiple pregnancies) we get exactly the same multiple pregnancy rate as with pulsatile GnRH. So you can reduce this complication.

W.F. Crowley, Jr. (USA): I would like to comment on fetal reduction. I think it should be left as a last resort for a number of reasons. Number one (and this comes from somebody who's pretty actively pro choice on a lot of other issues) we are talking about women who have been trying for months, if not years, to conceive; suddenly you have to turn their psychology around and consider fetal reduction. Certainly there will be an impact which is both immediate and long-term; that's hard to quantify but having seen people that have gone through it, it's something that we have to be sensitive to. I really believe there's a price to be paid. Secondly, the reproductive community has a very broad-based agenda with society. We have many things that we can offer and there are many important barriers that we're trying to push back with these new technologies. However, sometimes this leads to excess and if we don't self-correct on some of these issues, society and the legal system will be all too happy to intervene; this is an area where I think an active stance by the scientific community to limit its own technology would be most welcome.

D. Baird (UK): I think it's very important to clarify exactly what sort of group of people we're going to treat with gonadotropins. I totally agree with Dr Navot and Dr Jewelewicz and others that it is impossible or very difficult to achieve mono-ovulation in women with hypogonadotropic hypogonadism when you're giving gonadotropins. And that is because you've got to act like the hypothalamic pituitary unit in that system, because all the gonadotropins which are stimulating the ovary are exogenous. That's why I think pulsatile GnRH in those women is the preferred option. Now, paradoxically, it may actually be easier to achieve mono-ovulation in what I call normal gonadotropic amenorrhea where you still have a hypothalamic pituitary unit which is capable of responding by feedback and adjusting the endogenous level of gonadotropins. And I think that with the sort of chronic low-dose therapy which Steve Franks is using, the hypothalamic pituitary unit is probably adjusting to the dose of endogenous FSH during the emergence of the dominant follicle to reduce the concentration of endogenous FSH as selection takes place. We have always thought that it's very difficult to avoid hyperstimulation in people with PCO and people with endogenous gonadotropin. With the low-dose regimen you actually allow the feedback system to operate in the same way as you're trying to do with step-down regimens.

GnRH analogs: whether and when?

M. Filicori (I): I think that we really should move to the next issue on the agenda which is the use of GnRH analogs. The first provocative question is: should we use GnRH analogs at all in regular ovulation induction. Now we're not discussing assisted reproduction and we will only say a few things about assisted reproduction, as we have to. But let's first start with regular ovulation.

W. Braendle (D): I think we should use them, but we should not use them as a first line of treatment. We did once a comparative study and we saw that the combination was not better than hMG alone. However, in patients in whom we have a premature LH surge the combined therapy should be used.

J. Schoemaker (NL): I have the opposite position and I think that analogs should not be used in regular ovulation induction as the increase in FSH tends to be too large because of the changed pharmacodynamics, as I've shown in my paper. And, secondly, because you completely block the endogenous negative feedback which helps in monofollicular selection. So I would like to move that you should not use GnRH analogs in regular ovulation induction.

D. Baird (UK): I'd have to confess I don't know. Maybe in patients with raised basal LH this may reduce the incidence of early pregnancy loss. I haven't actually seen data in prospective randomized trials to convince me that the outcome in terms of take-home healthy babies and reduced pregnancy loss is improved by giving GnRH analogs. So in the Scottish term of law I think the case is not proven.

R. Homburg (IL): I think the one indication for using the analog in ovulation induction is with those cases of PCO who have high LH and I think that S.L. Tan pointed this out very clearly today. It's true that we haven't done a randomized trial, as we would need about 150 patients in each arm of the trial and that needs to be set up as a multicenter trial. However, we've already published at least two papers of comparative data, both in IVF and with ovulation induction in large numbers of PCO patients. If you can reduce by half the miscarriage rate by using the analog then I think this should be done. And if we talk about a cost/benefit index there's no point in getting these patients pregnant when about 35–38% are going to miscarry. That brings your cost/benefit index way up.

C. Flamigni (I): Dr. Homburg, in 1990 you published that in PCO the use of GnRH analogs was associated with a high rate of hyperstimulation.

R. Homburg (IL): Yes, in this comparison (gonadotropin cycles with and without analogs) we found a slightly higher rate of hyperstimulation associated with the use of GnRH analogs but we feel we can control this better now and the improvement in the miscarriage rates make it worthwhile.

C. Flamigni (I): However, there are other papers suggesting that analogs are not the best way to treat PCO.

R. Homburg (IL): Well, this is certainly not so in our experience; we get an increased pregnancy rate in PCOs with high LH for the very reasons that we heard earlier this afternoon.

C. Flamigni (I): In a paper by Stankompf (a randomized comparative trial) FSH was used alone and with leuprolide. After 200 cycles they found out that the pregnancy rate was 16% when leuprolide was not used and 4% when it was used. The protocol was changed by stopping leuprolide a little earlier and the pregnancy rate went up. So I'm not sure that there are no data in the literature not proving that giving analogs may be in some way dangerous for the results.

B. Fauser (NL): I think that you're referring to an abstract which was presented at the last American Fertility Society meeting. I think it should be taken into consideration that in this particular study there was no luteal support and this might very well explain the low pregnancy rate. Secondly, we performed a meta-analysis and published it 2 years ago in which we looked at the five prospective randomized trials then available which compared gonadotropins alone and gonadotropins plus agonists. It was surprising to us to find that the use of GnRH agonists was associated with a doubling in pregnancy rate.

M. Filicori (I): What about complications?

B. Fauser (NL): There was no difference in complications, such as hyperstimulation. The study was conducted in clomiphene-resistant anovulations, a majority of which is probably PCO.

S. Franks (UK): There is no prospective control study of sufficient size to be able to answer the question as yet about whether there's any difference in outcome of pregnancy with or without GnRH analogs. This type of study needs to be done.

M. Filicori (I): There's enough evidence, however, to say that one of the major advantages of using analogs in assisted reproduction, particularly if you use the long protocols, is that you get more follicles. Now if you get more follicles of course you have more chances of multiple conception and of ovarian hyperstimulation. If we use GnRH analogs we're going to end up with more follicles.

C. Howles (CH): Does anybody know what the minimum effective GnRH agonist dose is. What is the rationale for waiting 14 days prior to starting therapy? What about 10 days or 6 days? What is the cost of treatment? As far as I'm aware there are no studies to actually show the optimum treatment regimen and dose and I think that's something that one should look at.

M. Filicori (I): Again, we have to get back to assisted reproduction; two protocols are generally used, short and long and I think that the evidence points towards a higher number of follicles obtained with the long protocols. Why you get that is a subject of debate. As to the GnRH agonist dose, I always try to use enough GnRH analog to provide maximum suppression because that is the final goal of GnRH analog administration. You should remember that you cannot overdose with GnRH analogs.

M. Filicori (I): An additional add-on regimen that we discussed today is the addition of growth hormone. Let me state my point of view, which is basically that if you have a normal woman and you want to induce multiple ovulation, the addition of growth hormone would not improve the outcome of treatment. I believe that there is a general agreement on this statement. In other ovulatory disorders there's probably not enough evidence to identify which patient may benefit and whether or not it is really worthwhile.

R. Homburg (IL): I don't really think I've got more to add than what I gave in my talk. I think there is a very limited, small, select group who may benefit from the addition of growth hormone. I think those are the fairly rare cases of profound hypoestrogenism (WHO group I patient), e.g., hypophysectomized subjects. In addition, the use of GnRH analogs in IVF protocols may disturb growth hormone kinetics and pituitary reserve. Most of the evidence suggests that growth hormone can be beneficial for some patients, but we still haven't reached the stage (and I doubt whether we will do) where we can see in control trials a real improvement of the pregnancy rate which is really what we want.

How do we deal with the polycystic ovary syndrome?

M. Filicori (I): One of the major problems with PCO is the definition of this disorder; one of the difficulties of comparing studies coming from different groups in terms of results and outcome is that the definition of PCO changes so dramatically. Rather than discussing the definition of PCO which would require another 3-day conference, we should probably just debate hyperandrogenic anovulation.

E. Loumaye (CH): It seems that we consider as granted that clomiphene citrate is safe in terms of multiple pregnancy and abortion rate. We should also provide figures of these complications when we use clomiphene. I remember a very extensive study comparing clomiphene vs. gonadotropins, showing an increase of about 5% of miscarriage rate when you use clomiphene.

H. Jacobs (UK): I'd like to back up what Dr Loumaye is saying. You know clomiphene is one of the strangest drugs that we use. We've been worried about hMG being a mixture of a few hormones. What about clomiphene? A racemic mixture where the content of the isomers is incredibly lax, and that contains a mixture of an estrogen and an antiestrogen. Is like giving digitalis and quinidine to the same patient! It is a very strange compound and I've never really understood why the pharmaceutical industry hasn't responded by providing just an antiestrogen. In addition, as shown by Yen years ago, if you treat a PCO patient with high LH, clomiphene will push LH further up. And if you believe the LH story that this is bad for fertility, the use of clomiphene in a woman with PCO and high LH does not make sense.

C. Flamigni (I): Are you saying that you don't use clomiphene?

H. Jacobs (UK): We've never used clomiphene in people who have polycystic ovary syndrome and high LH. If their LH is normal we use it and then measure LH.

C. Flamigni (I): If you find the patient has high LH as you don't use clomiphene, what do you do?

H. Jacobs (UK): We move on to some other form of treatment.

D. Baird (UK): I'd just like to make a general point. The majority of normogonadotropic amenorrheas which include many PCO are treated initially with an antiestrogen and the other forms of therapy are reserved for people who haven't become pregnant following this treatment. And I think what we badly need are proper randomized control trials of, for example, primary treatment with low-dose gonadotropins vs. clomiphene.

W.F. Crowley, Jr. (USA): When you start to ask which therapy you're going to give in PCO, I'll bet that most groups are right and that each therapy is working in a discrete subset of PCO patients. So I would say before we start to treat PCOs and start to talk about its generic therapy, the proper focus should be on sorting them out into discrete subsets and applying specific therapies to those subsets.

S. Franks (UK): I can agree with Dr Crowley up to a point; there are subsets of women with polycystic ovary syndrome whom you need to treat before giving induction of ovulation and that relates particularly to obese subjects with polycystic ovary syndrome. We know that outcome of their treatment is much better if they can lose weight.

M. Dommergues (F): Diagnostic difficulties exist between some cases of hypothalamic anovulation and some women who are PCO. Some diagnostic markers can be misleading, such as the number of follicles on sonograms or sometimes LH levels.

Audience: I want to ask Dr Franks what the exact effect of diet is with obese patients with so-called PCO, both in term of ovarian morphology and of response to therapy.

S. Franks (UK): A weight loss of 5% or greater of the initial body weight can result in a resumption of ovulatory cycles in the majority of subjects, without the need for induction of ovulation. As yet, we don't have any direct information about whether dose requirements for gonadotropin therapy in those women who don't ovulate spontaneously falls when they lose weight, but I suspect it will. I hope I have those data to present soon. I can't say anything about ovarian hyperstimulation.

C. Flamigni (I): Does initial weight have any influence on the results of losing weight.

S. Franks (UK): Apparently not in that it seems that calorie restrictions are probably the most important factor, because the mean body weight of the patients that we treated in that diet study was around 90 kg.

Audience: Have you any experience in repeating clomiphene after weight loss?

S. Franks (UK): Anecdotally yes. Women who don't respond well to clomiphene when they're obese tend to ovulate in response to clomiphene after weight loss, but we don't have sufficient data to be able to put that into a formal statement yet. As to ultrasound morphology during weight reduction, it does not change, nor does the hyperandrogenism. Sex hormone binding globulin levels go up as Dr Nestler mentioned and therefore free androgens actually decrease.

M. Filicori (I): I would sort of draw some conclusion. I don't think anybody disagrees that if you have a fat PCO patient we should try to make her lose weight, I think there is a consensus on that, but there's also a consensus that it's not very easy. A different issue that was raised earlier and that wasn't presented at this meeting is the use of surgical approaches for the management of PCO.

J. Gerris (B): What I missed in this otherwise very interesting meeting is a talk on ovarian trauma in PCO, whether you call it wedge resection, diathermy, laser vaporization, or punch biopsy, as there is increasing evidence, albeit not in double-blind randomized studies but in open series, that these techniques provide a good ovulation rate followed by an acceptable pregnancy rate. However, there are a lot of questions concerning adhesion.

R. Jewelewicz (USA): About 22 years ago it was demonstrated that in properly selected cases the success rate of wedge resection was quite high as far as induction of ovulation and pregnancy is concerned. Maybe now with sophisticated 3-dimensional ultrasonography we will be able to select the proper cases which can respond to surgical treatment.

R. Fischer (D): We have a large group of PCO patients that we treated with cautery of ovary after they didn't response to standard treatment. This is a series of over 200 patients now; they resumed ovulation in about 90% of the cases and 70% of the patient treated became pregnant. Some had repeated pregnancies.

H. Jacobs (UK): I will give you an account of my colleagues' operations on these patients because I'm not a surgeon. We've seen a lot of patients who've had ovarian diathermy and there's an extensive literature on this. There's no doubt it's a good method for inducing ovulation, and there's no doubt it also reduces LH concentrations and in controlled studies we've noticed that after ovarian diathermy the miscarriage rate is 12%, not the 30% that can be expected in polycystic ovary syndrome. However, that's not very careful scientific work. I was at the American Fertility

Society meeting late last year and there was a big session on ovarian diathermy, and what astounded me as I sat listening to it was the huge variation in the damage done to the ovary. Some of the photographs on what is done to the ovary are really quite staggering. I could never imagine that was done in the name of medical therapy. So there is a very important plea from me to gynecologists to define the dose of diathermy before they start doing it. That's actually not very well known at present.

S. Franks (UK): A brief comment about the role of diathermy. There is in fact one controlled randomized study from Bob Shaw's unit, where they had 30 patients. Two groups received gonadotropins and one group received diathermy and there were no significant differences in the outcome. It was admittedly a fairly limited study, but it is the only controlled study that's been reported comparing diathermy with gonadotropin therapy.

R. Fischer (D): I think that only the patients who don't respond to gonadotropins should be candidates for ovarian cautery because this treatment results in quite a large percentage of adhesions and you may convert these patients to mechanical infertility. And we do know of two cases of patients who, because of massive ovarian cautery, went into hypergonadotropic amenorrhea; thus, you have to be very careful with this method.

H.J.T. Coelingh-Bennink (NL): Before the IVF era we had patients in whom we couldn't induce ovulation even with pulsatile GnRH. In 15 patients we removed just one polycystic ovary and we left the other one. In 14 cases patients started ovulating regularly and several became pregnant. This is an interesting result. I wouldn't advocate it today but the mechanism is interesting.

M. Filicori (I): Would anybody like to comment on the gonadotropin dose we should use: low, high, standard, step-up, step-down?

S. Franks (UK): I'd like to comment on the possibility of limiting the number of multiple pregnancies with a low-dose gonadotropin regimen. Now it's not just at our center where we've got 7% multiple pregnancy rates (all twins); now we're hearing from other centers that are using the low-dose protocols routinely that it is possible to limit the number of multiple gestations and I think that is a very important advance in our thinking about induction of ovulation. It is not acceptable to have a 25–30% multiple pregnancy rate when it is avoidable.

C. Flamigni (I): However, with low-dose gonadotropins treatment may have to be prolonged excessively and that may not be acceptable to several patients who come from far away.

S. Franks (UK): There are certainly some patients who need a longer period of induction of ovulation, but as I showed in my data yesterday the average length of treatment is 14 days; in the study that Ernest Loumaye presented yesterday the length of the follicular phase was very similar, around 16 days.

C. Flamigni (I): The average of duration of these regimens is 22 days in Bologna.

M. Filicori (I): So may I sort of suggest that one possible approach would be to get started with a low-dose gonadotropin regimen if it is acceptable for the patient, then for nonresponders step up to regular gonadotropin ovulation induction, and for those who again do not respond turn to surgical laparoscopic management. Would that be acceptable for the audience or do we have any disagreement with that?

C. Flamigni (I): What follicular diameter do you consider optimal for stopping gonadotropin treatment? The literature suggests 16–20 mm. I would like to hear some opinions on that.

D. Meldrum (USA): I thought it was striking in Steve Franks' publication that the LH level increased on the last day of treatment and I believe that the criterion for hCG was 18 mm. A number of other publications using the low-dose regimen suggested triggering ovulation at 16 mm; this resulted in a trend towards a higher pregnancy rate.

S. Franks (UK): We haven't done the comparison of follicle size when we give hCG. So you may be right but we don't have the evidence to support that. As I mentioned yesterday, we tend to use 18 mm as a guide for giving hCG. I think quite an interesting question is what happens if you don't give hCG. Not everybody in our study had a spontaneous LH surge so that by the time their follicle reached 20 mm we lost our nerve and gave hCG. But it may be that the majority of subjects will actually ovulate when their follicles are the right size so it would be quite nice to know whether we need to give it at all.

C. Flamigni (I): I have data on what happens if you don't give hCG because we treated 24 patient with FSH and in four cycles we didn't give hCG; three of the four patients did not ovulate.

E. Loumaye (CH): Serono is developing 37.5 Unit ampoules which would really allow the chronic low-dose approach with FSH.

Can we limit complications?

M. Filicori: The last topic of the day is: can we limit complications? All of us probably agree that you monitor gonadotropin ovulation induction with ultrasound. What about daily estrogen evaluations? The provocative question is: does everyone agree that estrogen monitoring is mandatory in gonadotropin ovulation induction?

R. Jewelewicz (USA): I disagree. The cost of a rapid estradiol assay in New York now is $45–$60. If estrogen assays were free of charge I would run them every day. Conversely, in my practice I use two assays in a cycle, one after day 7 and one as close to ovulation as possible (day 10 or 12). Occasionally I will get another estrogen determination but in most cycles I use only two determinations.

J.M. Talbot (AUS): We've been using urinary estrogen measurements to monitor ovulation induction at a very low cost.

D. Healy (AUS): I don't think I've actually heard the word ovarian cancer mentioned here in the last 3 days; it has been suggested recently that infertility drugs may actually increase the risk of ovarian cancer.

M. Filicori (I): Let me just briefly comment on the issue of ovarian cancer. Almost a year ago when we were working on the program we invited Dr Whitmore (the author of the report about the association between fertility treatment and ovarian cancer) to this conference because we really wanted to have her insight and she declined our invitation to attend. So we didn't avoid the topic on purpose, we just couldn't get the right person to speak about it.

E. Loumaye (CH): On the ovarian cancer issue I think one of the best comments on this topic I've heard is from Dr Whitmore herself. She said that we should really address the issue and confirm or disprove these observations. And anyway, the increased cancer risk should be balanced against the individual need for having a pregnancy. I think that it's a very fair comment because many times when you consider an infertility or contraceptive treatment you have a balance between risks and benefit; the question should be properly and not speculatively addressed.

Index of authors

Adams, J. 255
Adashi, E.Y. 85
Antoine, J.M. 361

Baird, D.T. 135
Beltrami, V. 227
Berga, S.L. 91
Bergh, P.A. 319
Blankstein, J. 331
Boime, I. 177
Bouchard, P. 219, 291
Burger, H.G. 353

Campbell, R.K. 185
Cara, J.F. 65
Caraty, A. 291
Cedars, M.I. 115
Charbonnel, B. 291
Clarke, S. 353
Coelingh Bennink, H.J.T. 219
Crowley Jr, W.F. 255

Dahl, K.D. 57
Dal Prato, L. 125
Dalkin, A.C. 11
de Ziegler, D. 167
de Leeuw, R. 209
Devroey, P. 209, 219
Dommergues, M. 339
Dubourdieu, S. 291
Dumez, Y. 339

Erickson, G.F. 73
Evans, M.I. 339

Fanchin, R. 167, 283
Fares, F. 177
Fauser, B.C.J.M. 153, 219
Filicori, M. 239, 371
Flamigni, C. 125, 371
Franks, S. 145
Fraser, H.M. 291

Frydman, R. 283, 291
Furuhashi, M. 177

Galazka, A. 227
Gelety, T.J. 25
Giroud, D. 227

Haisenleder, D.J. 11
Hall, J. 255
Hamilton-Fairley, D. 145
Han, Y. 191
Harlin, J. 219
Healy, D.L. 353
Hillier, S.G. 47
Homburg, R. 307
Howles, C.M. 135, 227
Hsueh, A.J.W. 177

Jacobs, H.S. 267

Kang, I.S. 297
Kerrigan, J.R. 11
Khodr, G.S. 297
Kirk, S.E. 11
Knobil, E. 3
Kovacs, G. 353
Kuehl, T.J. 297

LaPolt, P.D. 177
Le Cotonnec, J.-Y. 227
Leroy, I. 291
Li, X. 353
Loumaye, E. 227

Macdonald, G.J. 191
Magarelli, P.C. 25
Magoffin, D.A. 25
Mannaerts, B. 209
Marshall, J.C. 11
Martin, K.A. 255
Mather, J.P. 57
McCloud, P.I. 353

McClure, N. 353
Meldrum, D.R. 277
Molskness, T.A. 57
Moyle, W.R. 191
Myers, R.V. 191

Navot, D. 319
Nestler, J.E. 103
Nishimori, K. 177

O'Dea, L. 227
Olivennes, F. 291
Østergaard, H. 307

Palermo, R. 319
Piazzi, A. 227
Polson, D.W. 145
Porchet, H.C. 227
Porcu, E. 125

Rebar, R.W. 115
Richards, J.S. 21

Sagle, M. 145
Sairam, M.R. 199
Salat-Baroux, J. 361

Santoro, N. 245
Schoemaker, J. 163
Sebok, K. 199
Shikone, T. 177
Shoham, Z. 219
Siler-Khodr, T.M. 297
Stouffer, R.L. 57
Sugahara, T. 177

Tan, S.-L. 347

van der Meer, M. 163
van Weissenbruch, M.M. 163
Venturoli, S. 125

Wang, Y. 191
White, D.M. 145
Wilshire, G.B. 245
Wingfield, M. 353
Woodruff, T.K. 57

Yasin, M. 11

Zeleznik, A.J. 37
Zosmer, A. 347

Keyword index

α 11
absorption 248
Acanthosis nigricans 104
activin 50
activin A 57
adhesions 385
administration of GnRH analogs 303
α-adrenergic blockade 15
age 148
albumin 328, 336
aldosterone 331
analog of GnRH 129
anasarca 325
androgen 48, 52
    substrate 28, 39
angiogenesis 322
angiotensin I 323
angiotensin II 322
angiotensin-converting enzyme 323
anovulation 103
antigonadotropic 87
antral follicles 209
antral stage 215
apoptosis 59
aromatase 39
arterial hypertension 362, 365
ascites 325
assisted reproductive 297
atresia 27, 209
autoimmune process 116

binding sites 68
birth defects 366
blood estrogens 333
body composition 246
bone density 119
buserelin 213

C-terminal peptide 178
calcium 299
capillary permeability 323
cerclage 362

cesarian sections 363
chimera 178
chimeric muteins 186
Chinese hamster ovary 227
CHO cells 194
chromosome abnormalities 357
clearance 136, 229
clinical monitoring 250
clomiphene 129, 382
clomiphene citrate challenge test (CCCT) 285
COH 225
cohort follicles 28
complications 386
controlled ovarian hyperstimulation 167, 283, 319 (*see also* COH)
corpus luteal function 303
corpus luteum 257
cost 264
cryopreservation 278
CTP chimera 181
cumulative conception rate 272
cytokines 324

Decapeptyl® 213
delay of hCG administration, 335
determinant loop 187
diarrhea 325
diazoxide 105
differentially regulate 16
diurnal rhythm 8
dominant follicle 25
dosage of pulsatile GnRH 258

E_2 and P replacement 168
E_2 and P substitution 167
early pregnancy 303
eclampsia 365
ectopic pregnancies 302, 362
egg donation 168
electrical activity 5
electrophysiological approach 8
embryo damage 297

endogenous GnRH secretion 241
endometrial receptivity 167
endometrium 169
estradiol benzoate 292
estrogen 29, 53
    production 39
    receptors 27
estrous cycle 13
expression vector 179
extraction 125, 228

fetal loss 341
fetal reduction 379
flare protocols 284
flare-up GnRH 283
follicle development 33
follicle growth 221
follicular development 320
follicular growth 229
follicular phase 246
follicular phase LH 242
folliculogenesis 37, 199
follistatin 51, 57
follitropin 199
free α-subunit 91
frequency 14, 240, 257
FSH 25, 115
    β 11
    analogs 204
    β gene 206
    threshold 163
    window 155

gene expression 11
GH 75
GHRH 76
GHRH-like protein 74
glandular stromal dyssynchrony 170
glucocorticoids 117
GnRH 3, 239, 245
    agonist 310
    agonist suppression 277
    analogs 379
    antagonists 130, 291
    -deficient 13
    dose 240
    hypersecretion 94
    in pregnancy 298
    pulse amplitude 16
    pulse frequency 16
    pulses 14
    pump 247
gonadotrope 12
gonadotropin 262, 371
    agonist 177
    dose 385
    reserve 241
    subunit 11
gonadotropin-binding specificity 185
Gonal-F™, 227
granulosa cell 22, 25, 48, 307
    maturity 213
growth hormone 73, 188, 307, 382

half-life 136, 202
hCG 212
HELLP syndrome 365
hemoconcentration 325, 326
heparin 373
high specific activity 228
higher-order pregnancies 365
highly purified FSH 374
history of previous miscarriages 358
hMG 125, 135, 374
hormonal predictors 358
hormone binding 191
hormone concentration 246
3β-HSD 30
human chorionic gonadotropin 177
human FSH β subunit 177
human menstrual cycle 246
17-α-hydroxylase deficiency 223
hyperandrogenic 241
hypergonadotropic amenorrhea 115
hyperinsulinemia 103, 104
hyperinsulinism 67
hypersecretion of LH 270, 348
hyperstimulation 129, 140, 145, 381
hypertrophy 26
hypogonadotropic hypogonadism 255, 372
hypothalamic amenorrhea 245

IGF binding proteins 66
IGF-I 29, 65, 75, 107, 307
    receptor 66, 75
IGF-II 65
IGFBP-4 and -5 78
IGFBPs 76
IGFs 73
IL-1 system 86

imminent hyperstimulation 334
incipient ovarian failure 312
indomethacin 324
inhibin 29, 48, 50, 220
insulin 65, 103, 104
    and the IGFs 68
    receptor 66, 104
    resistance 67, 103
insulin-like growth factor 48, 65 (*see also* IGF)
insulin-like growth factor-I (*see* IGF-I)
interleukin-1 85, 325
interleukin-6 325
intrafollicular oocyte maturation inhibitor (OMI) 350
intranasal 246
intraovarian mechanisms 28
intraovarian peptides 29
intrauterine growth retardation 362
intravenous 246, 256
isoelectric points 202
IVF-ET 221

Kallmann syndrome 137, 220
karyotypic abnormalities 116

Lasix 328
leukocytosis 325
LH 25, 127
    α 234
    β 11, 234
    pulses 3
    receptors 25
    secretion 6, 108
    surge 4, 21
LHadi™, 227
LHRH agonist 350
local inflammation 247
low birth weight 365
low-dose
    gonadotropin 145
    gonadotropin regimen 385
    step-up 157
    step-up 154
Lupron test 285
luteal support 280
luteinizing hormone 177, 347 (*see also* LH)

management of multiple pregnancies 367
maternal age 356
maternal morbidity 341

MCR 206
meiotic maturation 27
Metrodin 202
Metrodin HP® 232
mild hyperstimulation 332
miscarriage 138, 353
monkeys 7
monofollicular growth 165
mRNA 11
MUA 5
multicystic ovaries 109, 267
multifollicular ovaries (MFO) 109, 241
multiple
    births 137
    gestations 263
    pregnancies 361
    pregnancy 145, 239
mutagenesis 186

Nal-Glu 291
nausea 325
neonatal morbidity 341
neurotransmitters 299
neutrophilia 326
nocturnal slowing 7

obese women 246
obesity 99, 103, 148
oocyte
    donation 120
    quality 278
    retrieval 280
ovarian
    biopsies 117
    cancer 387
    enlargement 325
    hyperandrogenism 67
    hyperstimulation 239

P450 30
paracentesis 328
paracrine 47
    differentiation factors 30
    mechanism 32
pathophysiology 319
pathophysiology of OHSS 322
patient selection 250
PCO 279, 380
PCOD 227
PCOS 91, 127

pelvic ultrasounds 261
periovulatory period 291
pharmacodynamics 137
pharmacodynamics of FSH 165
pharmacokinetic parameters 202
pituitary 135
    desensitization 222
    escape 286
    FSH 200, 201
    neoplasm 119
PKC 26
placenta 298, 302
plasma expanders 328
pleural effusion 326
polycystic ovarian disease 163
    (see also PCO, PCOD, PCOS)
polycystic ovarian syndrome 91, 103, 138, 382
    (see also PCO, PCOD, PCOS)
polycystic ovary 267
    (see also PCO, PCOD, PCOS)
poor responders 277, 286, 312
pre-eclampsia 365
preantral follicle 38
preantral ovarian follicles 31
predict OHSS 333
pregnancy reduction 339
premature LH surge 293
premature ovarian failure 115
prematurity 365
preovulatory surge 34
price 376
primordial follicles 38
progesterone 23, 54
progesterone receptor (PR) 23
prorenin 323
prostaglandin 22
puberty 109
pulsatile GnRH 239, 246, 371
    dosage of 258
pulsatile gonadotropin-releasing hormone 255
pulse frequencies 93, 249
pulse generator 4
pulse shape 246
Puregon® 209
purified FSH 125, 126, 135, 141, 374

radioligand receptor assay 179
receptor binding 191
recombinant
    DNA technology 234

    FSH 199, 374
    hCG 191
    human FSH 209
    human LH 227
recruitment 320
reduce the dose of hCG 336
regimens of GnRH administration 240
regimens of pulsatile gonadotropin-releasing
    hormone 245
renin 323
routes 246

severe hyperstimulation 332
sex hormone binding globulin 70
    (see also SHBG)
sex steroids 47
SHBG 107
short regimens 283
singleton 378
slow frequency pulses 13
spontaneous abortion 242, 347
spontaneous miscarriages 362
step-down 153
step-up 154
steroid receptor 51
subcutaneous 246
α subunit 181, 200
β subunit 11, 187, 188, 200
superovulation 229
Suprecur® 213

TGF-β 29
theca interna 25
theca-interstitial cells 69, 87
thecal cell 48
threatened premature delivery 362
threshold 40
    concept 145
    level 234
    theory 37
thromboembolic phenomena 326
transabdominal needling 340
transcervical aspiration 340
transcription 13
transdermal 246
    systems 169
transforming growth factor 48
transvaginal needling 340
triplet 363
triptorelin 213

two-cell two-gonadotropin model 37

ultralong GnRH 281
ultrashort regimens 283
ultrasonographic monitoring 333
ultrasound guidance 340
urinary extracts 136
urinary FSH 126, 201
urine collection 228

volume expansion 328
vomiting 325

wedge resection 384
weight loss 383
wild type FSH 180
withholding hCG 334